Edited by
Howard Davies and
Beatrice Bressan

A History of International Research Networking

Related Titles

Sinnreich, H., Johnston, A. B.

Internet Communications Using SIP
Delivering VoIP and Multimedia Services with Session Initiation Protocol

2006

ISBN: 978-0-471-77657-4

Chlamtac, I., Gumaste, A., Szabo, C. (eds.)

Broadband Services
Business Models and Technologies for Community Networks

2005

ISBN: 978-0-470-02248-1

Matthews, J.

Computer Networking
Internet Protocols in Action

2005

ISBN: 978-0-471-66186-3

Edited by
Howard Davies and Beatrice Bressan

A History of International Research Networking

The People who Made it Happen

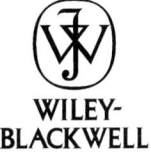
WILEY-BLACKWELL

WILEY-VCH Verlag GmbH & Co. KGaA

The Editors

Dr. Howard Davies
howard.davies@abington.plus.com

Dr. Beatrice Bressan
bb@beatricebressan.org

All books published by Wiley-VCH are carefully produced. Nevertheless, authors, editors, and publisher do not warrant the information contained in these books, including this book, to be free of errors. Readers are advised to keep in mind that statements, data, illustrations, procedural details or other items may inadvertently be inaccurate.

Library of Congress Card No.: applied for

British Library Cataloguing-in-Publication Data
A catalogue record for this book is available from the British Library.

Bibliographic information published by the Deutsche Nationalbibliothek
The Deutsche Nationalbibliothek lists this publication in the Deutsche Nationalbibliografie; detailed bibliographic data are available on the Internet at http://dnb.d-nb.de.

© 2010 WILEY-VCH Verlag GmbH & Co. KGaA, Weinheim

All rights reserved (including those of translation into other languages). No part of this book may be reproduced in any form – by photoprinting, microfilm, or any other means – nor transmitted or translated into a machine language without written permission from the publishers. Registered names, trademarks, etc. used in this book, even when not specifically marked as such, are not to be considered unprotected by law.

Cover Design   Adam-Design, Weinheim
Typesetting   Thomson Digital, Noida, India
Printing and Binding   T.J. International Ltd., Padstow

Printed in Great Britain
Printed on acid-free paper

ISBN: 978-3-527-32710-2

Foreword

The 20th anniversary of the Trans European Research and Education Networking Association, TERENA, took place in the summer of 2006. At this event, the idea arose that it would be interesting to write a "History Book" about how Europe got its act together and managed to create the globally most advanced facilities for research networking in the world – in spite of, originally, being far behind the United States.

The time also seemed to be ripe, since many of the original players in the field although now retiring were still around, so that the editors of such a "History Book" could still get input and feedback from many of the people who had been involved in this exciting development.

So it was decided to try to collect contributions from a fairly large number of people in the European research networking community, and have these contributions edited and put together by an editorial team consisting of Howard Davies – himself one of the original "networkers" in Europe – and Beatrice Bressan, a science writer from CERN (Conseil Européen pour la Recherche Nucléaire) with long experience in science dissemination.

As TERENA's President I was asked to provide the liaison with the editors, together with the Secretary General, Karel Vietsch, and we added a small editorial committee consisting of two networking pioneers, Lajos Bálint from Hungary and Claudio Allocchio from Italy.

So this is an attempt at writing a history of how the work of many brilliant people joined together and in the end produced a remarkable result – really put the European research area on the map as the first and foremost in high speed networking.

It is also a story about how complicated it can be to reach agreement on technical and organisational issues between so many different countries – how much work goes into getting the act together, when you are many different nations, each with experts and opinions; and a story about what it meant to Europe that liberalization came to the telecommunications market.

But apart from the telecommunications liberalization, it is not really a story about politics but, above all, a story about how engineers and scientists all over Europe joined forces to collaborate on the promotion of science and education, both in their home universities or research centers and in the remotest parts of the world.

A History of International Research Networking. Edited by Howard Davies and Beatrice Bressan
Copyright © 2010 WILEY-VCH Verlag GmbH & Co. KGaA, Weinheim
ISBN: 978-3-527-32710-2

The book is not the work of one person, and the styles of different parts bear witness to that, however, I believe the editors also got their act together and joined these different contributions into a very interesting whole. There is no attempt at completeness – a selection of topics had to be made, and also not all of the prospective contributors were able to provide contributions to the text – however, most main events are described here, and most invited contributors did agree to deliver.

One clear omission is that the intimate interplay in this development between high performance computing and high performance networking is not truly elucidated. Over the past decades, there is no doubt that this interplay has, at certain periods of time, been very strong and has played a crucial role in the development of the project. I personally saw how much it meant at the European level in the early 90s that the Director General of CERN, Carlo Rubbia, when chairing a high-level Advisory Committee for the EC (European Commission), made it an important issue to link high performance computing with high speed networking. I know that, at the national level, this has been decisive in many countries at certain periods of time.

On behalf of the TERENA Executive Committee I am happy to express our heartfelt thanks to all the people who took time out to write some pages of this history and I also think it appropriate to thank all the people involved in this process over the years – the heads of National Research and Education Networking Organisations, and their dedicated staff members. Without the "backbone" of all the research networks, the European connections would not be of any real value to anyone, and without the joint effort of the national organisations, there would not be a European association.

So this is not the story of a single individual who made an astonishing step forward – albeit there is also in the sequence of events at least one such story, the invention of the Web by Tim Berners-Lee – but it is the story of many individuals, all over Europe, making a collaborative effort that really has meant a big leap forward.

Dorte Olesen

President of TERENA and Director General of UNI•C,
the Danish IT Centre for Education and Research

Contents

Foreword *V*
Preface *XI*
List of Contributors *XIII*
Color Plates *XV*

1	**Early Days** *1*	
1.1	The Starting Point *1*	
1.1.1	The Data Communications Scene *1*	
1.2	Protocols and Standards *2*	
1.2.1	Interim Standards *3*	
1.2.2	Open Systems Interconnection *3*	
1.2.3	The Internet Protocols *4*	
1.3	European Coordination *5*	
1.3.1	Identifying the Need *5*	
1.3.2	Preliminary Steps *5*	
1.3.3	The First European Networkshop *6*	
1.4	RARE: From Proposal to Reality *11*	
1.4.1	Laying the Foundations *11*	
1.4.2	The First Step for COSINE *12*	
1.4.3	The Second European Networkshop *13*	
1.4.4	The Birth of RARE *13*	
1.4.5	The End of the Beginning *14*	
1.5	EARN, the First International Service in Europe *15*	
1.5.1	Preparation and Constitution of EARN *17*	
1.6	IXI *21*	
2	**The Role of Funding Bodies** *27*	
2.1	EUREKA and COSINE *27*	
2.2	EC and National Governments *31*	
2.2.1	Impact on the Internal COSINE Debates *33*	

A History of International Research Networking. Edited by Howard Davies and Beatrice Bressan
Copyright © 2010 WILEY-VCH Verlag GmbH & Co. KGaA, Weinheim
ISBN: 978-3-527-32710-2

3	**Organized Cooperation** *39*	
3.1	The Activities of RARE *39*	
3.2	The Gestation of DANTE *41*	
3.2.1	The Process and the Structure *43*	
3.2.2	Relationships with Other Bodies *45*	
3.2.3	Management and Staff *50*	
3.3	RARE and EARN: the Merger *52*	
3.4	RARE, EARN and TERENA *56*	
3.5	DANTE and TERENA *60*	
3.6	The Future of TERENA *62*	
3.7	The Value of COSINE *64*	
3.7.1	The Importance of the Achievements *65*	
3.7.2	COSINE Epilogue *67*	
3.8	RIPE and the RIPE NCC *68*	
4	**Different Approaches** *73*	
4.1	HEPnet *73*	
4.2	DECnet *77*	
4.3	EUnet *78*	
4.3.1	Precursors *79*	
4.3.2	The Network Grows Quickly *83*	
4.3.3	Cooperation with Emerging European Research and Academic Networks *84*	
4.4	Ebone *86*	
4.5	EMPB, European Multi-Protocol Backbone *93*	
4.6	EuropaNET *102*	
5	**The Interviews** *111*	
5.1	Dai Davies *111*	
5.2	Kees Neggers and Boudewijn Nederkoorn *118*	
5.3	Klaus Ullmann *126*	
6	**The Bandwidth Breakthrough** *135*	
6.1	TEN-34 *135*	
6.2	TEN-155 and QUANTUM *142*	
6.2.1	TEN-155 Takes Shape *144*	
6.2.2	Intercontinental and External Connectivity *150*	
6.2.3	The QUANTUM Test Program *151*	
6.3	Relations with Telecom Operators *152*	
6.4	Relations with Equipment Suppliers *154*	
6.4.1	Research and Education Networks as a Market *154*	
6.4.2	The Research and Education Community as a Technology Incubator *155*	
6.4.3	Research and Education Networks Need for Interoperability *158*	

7	**Support for Applications** *163*
7.1	Security and CERTs *163*
7.1.1	Establishing a Regional Identity *165*
7.1.2	Today's Activities *168*
7.1.3	The Trusted Introducer Service *169*
7.2	COSINE Sub-Projects *170*
7.3	Grids *175*
8	**Regional Perspectives** *179*
8.1	NORDUnet *179*
8.1.1	EARN, First Steps in European Collaboration *180*
8.1.2	RARE, Harmonizing European Development *181*
8.1.3	Ebone, the First Pan-European IP Backbone *182*
8.1.4	NSF, the American Connection *183*
8.1.5	DANTE, Coordinating European Networking *184*
8.1.6	Internet2, towards New Applications *185*
8.1.7	The 6NET Project, Testing IPv6 *186*
8.1.8	GLIF and Lambda Networking, the New Light *187*
8.2	CEEC *189*
8.2.1	External Support *189*
8.2.2	The EC's PHARE Program *190*
8.2.3	National Infrastructures *191*
8.2.4	Pan-European Connectivity of the CEEC *192*
8.2.5	European Projects *193*
8.2.6	The Significance of GÉANT *194*
8.3	Asia and Pacific *194*
8.3.1	Leased Line Connections *195*
8.3.2	Trans-Eurasia Information Network *196*
8.3.3	Trans-Siberia Link in the 2000s *197*
8.3.4	Network Development *197*
8.4	South East Europe and the Mediterranean *199*
8.4.1	GRNET/Greece and SEEREN *199*
8.4.2	ILAN/Israel *201*
8.4.3	EUMEDCONNECT *203*
8.5	Latin America *204*
8.5.1	A Very Brief History of Academic Networking in Latin America *206*
8.5.2	The ALICE Project and the RedCLARA Network *207*
8.5.3	New and Greatly Improved Research Networks in Latin America *211*
8.5.4	Collaborative Networked Applications in Latin America *213*
8.5.5	The Future of the Latin American Regional Network *214*
8.6	Russia *215*
8.6.1	The Origins of the Main Russian Research Networks *215*

9	**Transatlantic Connections** *221*
9.1	The "Welcome Guest" Period *221*
9.2	The Partnership Period *228*
9.2.1	Euro-Link *228*
9.2.2	GLIF - Global Lambda Integrated Facility *229*
9.2.3	TransLight/StarLight *230*
9.2.4	GLIF, Grids and the Future *231*
10	**A European Achievement** *235*
10.1	GÉANT *235*
10.2	GÉANT2, Creation of the First International Hybrid Network *242*
10.2.1	The Gestation Period *242*
10.2.2	Complex Procurement *243*
10.2.3	Roll-Out and Migration *245*
10.2.4	Switched Point-to-Point (p2p) Connections *245*
10.2.5	Cost Sharing *247*
10.2.6	Cross Border Initiatives *248*
10.2.7	Global Connectivity *249*
10.2.8	Conclusion *249*
10.3	The Impact of Research Networking *250*
10.3.1	The Impact on Individuals *250*
10.3.2	The Impact on Commerce *251*
10.3.3	The Impact on Entertainment *251*
10.3.4	The Impact on the Telecommunications Industry *252*
10.3.5	The Impact on Education and Research *253*
10.3.6	The Impact on the Environment *254*
10.3.7	The Political Impact *254*
10.3.8	The Impact on Standard Development Method *255*
10.3.9	Conclusion *257*

Further Reading *259*
Appendix A: The People who Made it Happen *261*
Appendix B: List of NREN Managers *273*
Appendix C: List of Network Names *279*
Appendix D: List of Acronyms *283*
Appendix E: List of Terms *293*
Appendix F: List of Units *303*
Index of Names *305*
Subject Index *307*
Picture Credits *317*

Preface

How do you get representatives of over 30 countries to manage the specification and implementation of a service which is then made available to all of them? How do you get several hundred highly qualified and independent-minded engineers to work together to find solutions to the numerous technical problems that arise while the service is being designed? How do you persuade funding bodies – which are often large and complex bureaucracies – that your proposals are more deserving of support than other demands on their resources? How do you persuade monopoly suppliers who believe that they know better than you what your requirements are to take your demands seriously? How do you – over a period of 25 to 30 years – increase the capacity of your service by six orders of magnitude, i.e. by a factor of a million while keeping the cost constant or even reducing it?

A facile answer common to all these questions might be "with difficulty". Yet there is a group of people, those who have been involved in the development of several generations of computer networks supporting scientific research, who can provide real answers to these questions.

This book records the main elements of the history of European research networking, including some of the mistakes and dead ends as well as the successes that were encountered along the way. It describes the principal steps which those involved in European research networking have taken, in collaboration with (and sometimes in competition with) their counterparts in North America and other world regions, in the development of the underlying telecommunications infrastructure which today supports the operation of the global Internet.

This is a story about people as well as technology; people as individuals and people acting through organisations, often their employer but also committees, working parties, task forces and so on. The developments described here have been to a very large extent collective activities. A large number of people (counted in hundreds if not thousands) have played some part and it would be impossible to name them all. It is also difficult to define a boundary between those whose influence on events has been so great that it would be invidious not to give them personal credit for their contribution and the larger mass of engineers, managers and administrators whose contribution has been significant but more routine. In general, the naming of individuals has been limited to the most senior person within any organisation or group and to cases where not naming someone would be counter-productive.

Some 30 people who have been deeply involved in some aspect of European research networking during the last 30 years were invited to contribute a part of the story. A few senior members of the community were interviewed. As might be expected, the contributions differed widely in style, length, and level of technical detail. They, and the interview transcripts, have been edited in order to remove overlapping descriptions of the same events, to get a reasonable balance in the treatment of different topics, and in some cases to re-order parts of different contributions in order to achieve a more logical flow. A consequence of the re-ordering is that there is not a one-to-one correspondence between the sub-chapters of the book and the list of contributors. A few of the contributions have been included with only small changes to the contributor's original text, many more have been changed significantly.

Cambridge and Pays de Gex
November 2009

Howard Davies
Beatrice Bressan

Acknowledgment

The Editors wish to acknowledge the support of TERENA (Trans-European Research and Education Networking Association) without which the production of this book would not have been possible. As well as providing the impetus for the book's development, TERENA and its Officers have been the driving force from conception to final print. TERENA's support has been paramount and is greatly appreciated.

List of Contributors

Claudio Allocchio
GARR
Rome
Italy

Lajos Bálint
NIIF
Budapest
Hungary

Vincent Berkhout
COLT
London
United Kingdom

Josephine Bersee
Hong Kong

Beatrice Bressan
Pays de Gex
France

Maxine Brown
University of Illinois at Chicago
Chicago
US

Brian E. Carpenter
University of Auckland
Auckland
New Zealand

Tryfon Chiotis
GRNET
Athens
Greece

Dai Davies
DANTE
Cambridge
United Kingdom

Howard Davies
Cambridge
United Kingdom

Thomas A. DeFanti
University of Illinois at Chicago
Chicago
US

François Fluckiger
CERN
Geneva
Switzerland

David Foster
CERN
Geneva
Switzerland

Fabrizio Gagliardi
Microsoft
Geneva
Switzerland

A History of International Research Networking. Edited by Howard Davies and Beatrice Bressan
Copyright © 2010 WILEY-VCH Verlag GmbH & Co. KGaA, Weinheim
ISBN: 978-3-527-32710-2

List of Contributors

Jan Gruntorád
CESnet
Prague
Czech Republic

David Hartley
Abingdon
United Kingdom

James Hutton
Abingdon
United Kingdom

Yuri Izhvanov
Moscow
Russia

Klaus-Peter Kossakowski
DFN-CERT
Hamburg
Germany

Glenn Kowack
US

Peter Linington
University of Kent
Canterbury
United Kingdom

Vassilis Maglaris
National Technical University of Athens
Athens
Greece

Boudewijn Nederkoorn
Utrecht
Netherlands

Kees Neggers
SURFnet
Utrecht
Netherlands

Michael Nowlan
Dublin
Ireland

Dorte Olesen
Uni-Copenhagen
Copenhagen
Denmark

Roberto Sabatino
DANTE
Cambridge
United Kingdom

Michael Stanton

Cathrin Stöver
DANTE
Madrid
Spain

Peter Tindemans
Netherlands

Stefano Trumpy
CNR-IIT
Pisa
Italy

Klaus Ullmann
DFN
Berlin
Germany

Jean-Marc Uzé
Juniper Networks EURL
Paris
France

Karel Vietsch
TERENA
Amsterdam
Netherlands

David West
DANTE
Cambridge
United Kingdom

Color Plates*

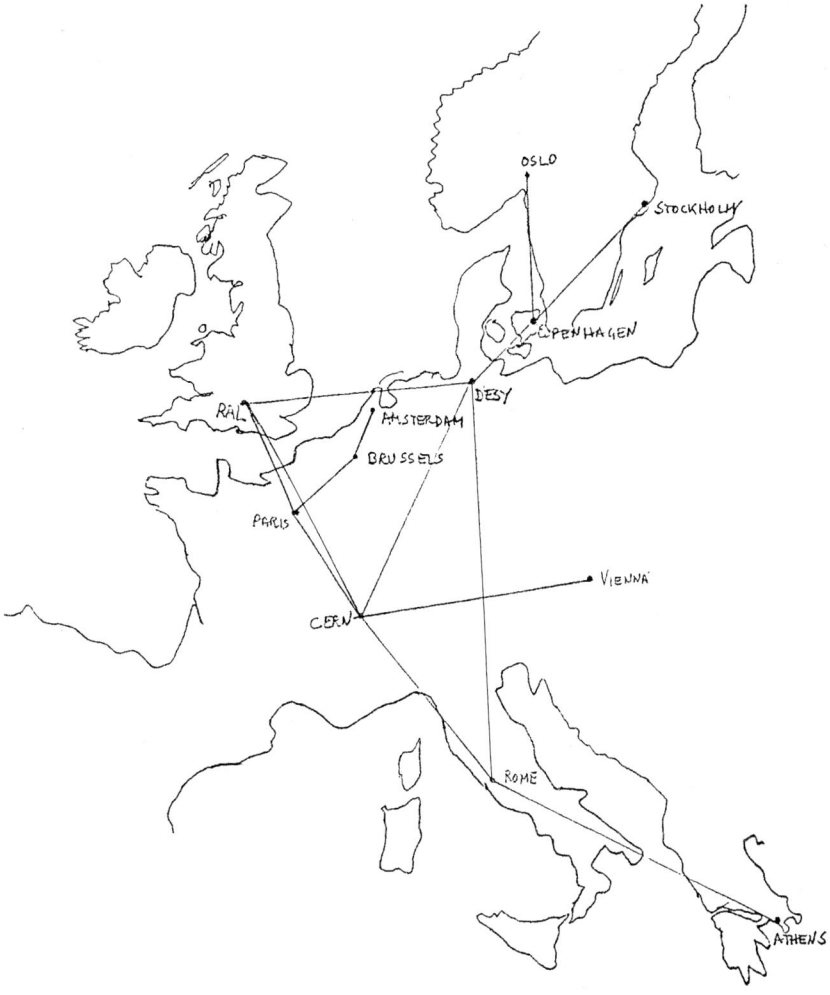

Figure 4.1 HEPnet planned configuration. (This figure also appears on page 75.)

*Note to the reader: The first figures in the color plates only exist in black and white. They have nonetheless been included because together with the color figures they help to illustrate the evolution of the network.

A History of International Research Networking. Edited by Howard Davies and Beatrice Bressan
Copyright © 2010 WILEY-VCH Verlag GmbH & Co. KGaA, Weinheim
ISBN: 978-3-527-32710-2

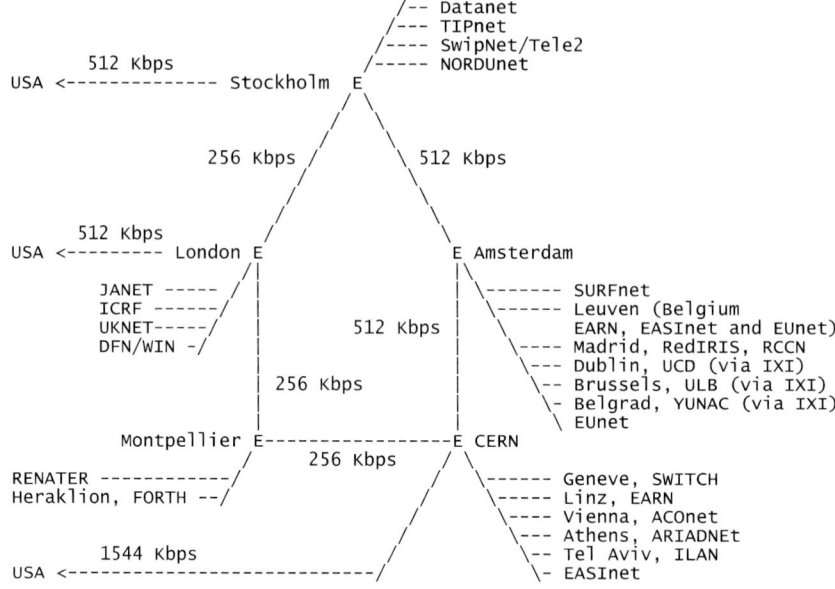

Figure 4.3 Initial Ebone 92 configuration. (This figure also appears on page 89.)

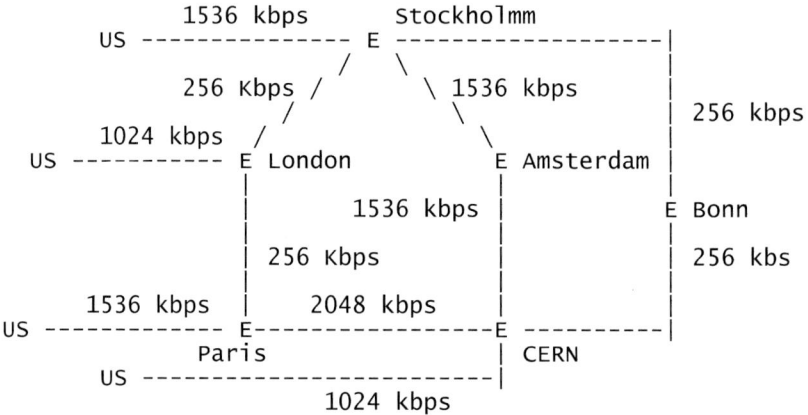

Figure 4.4 Ebone 93 configuration. (This figure also appears on page 91.)

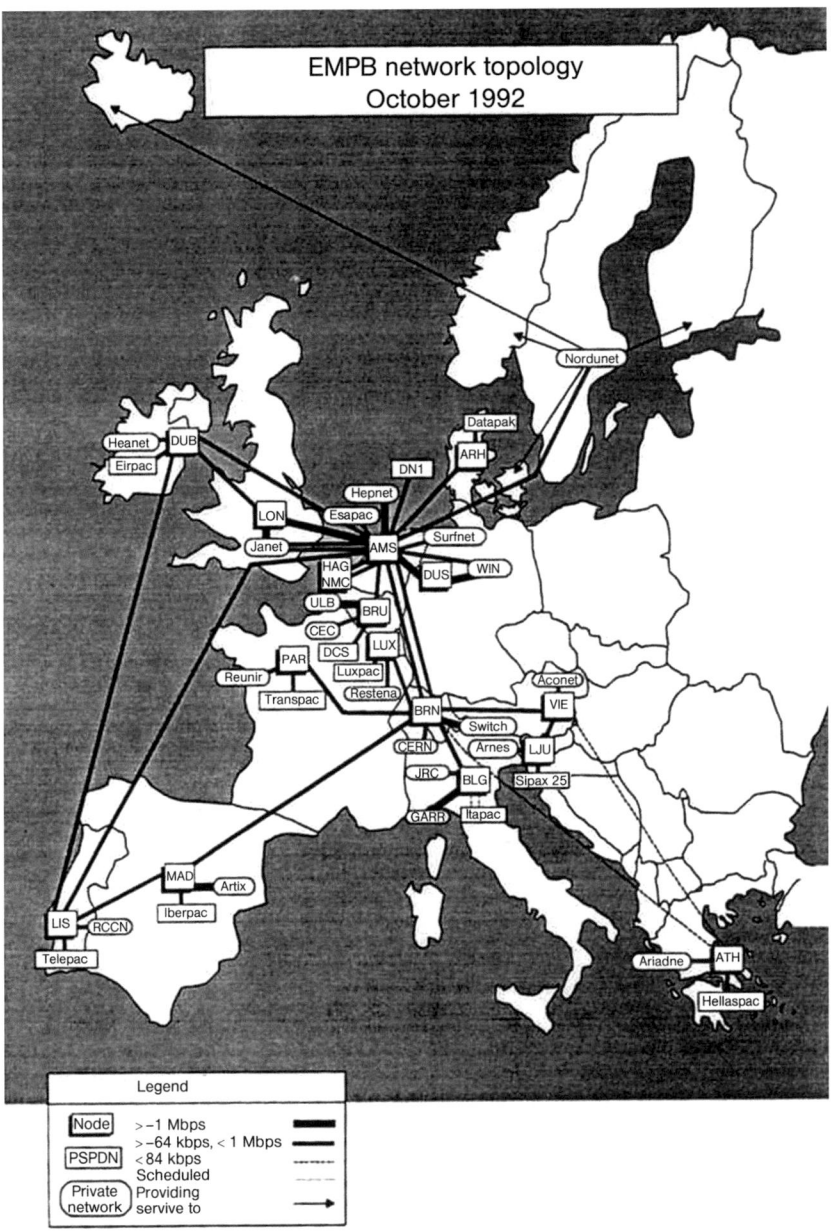

Figure 4.6 EMPB topology, October 1992. (This figure also appears on page 97.)

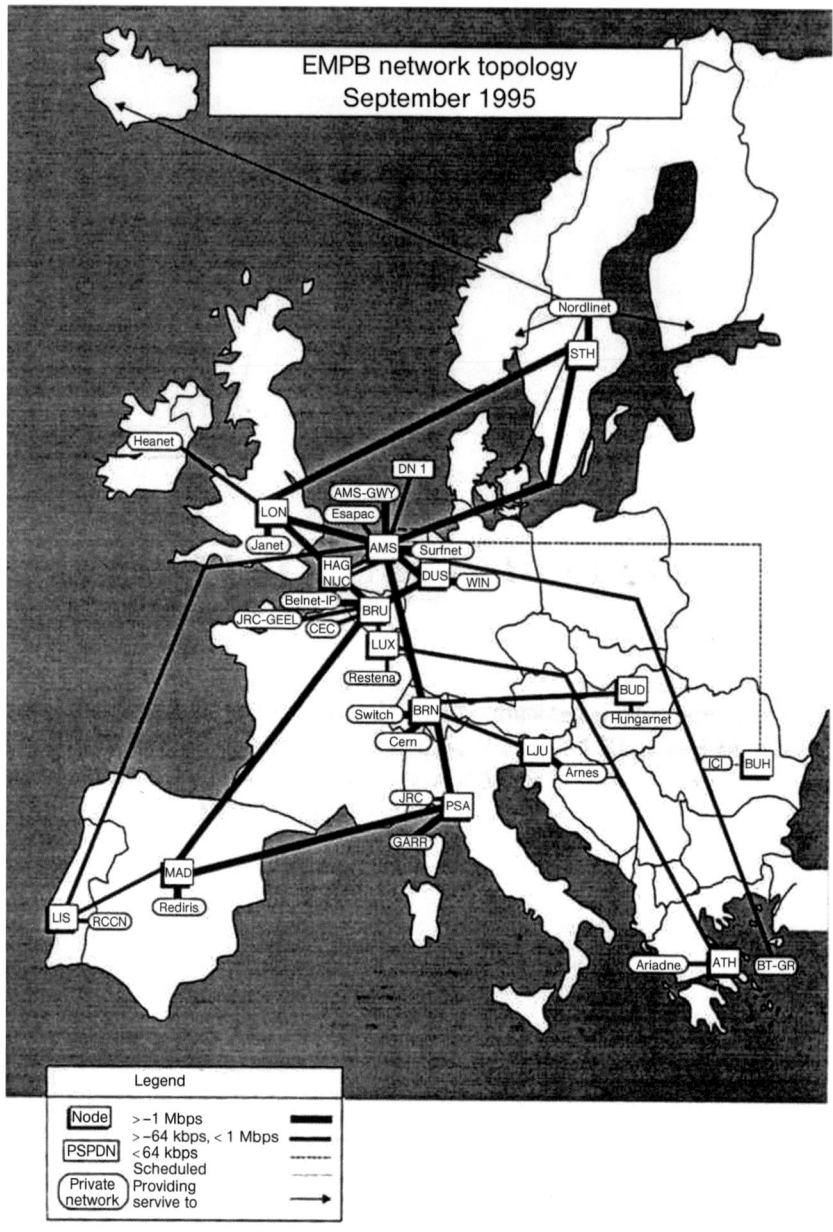

Figure 4.7   EMPB topology, September 1995. (This figure also appears on page 98.)

Color Plates | XIX

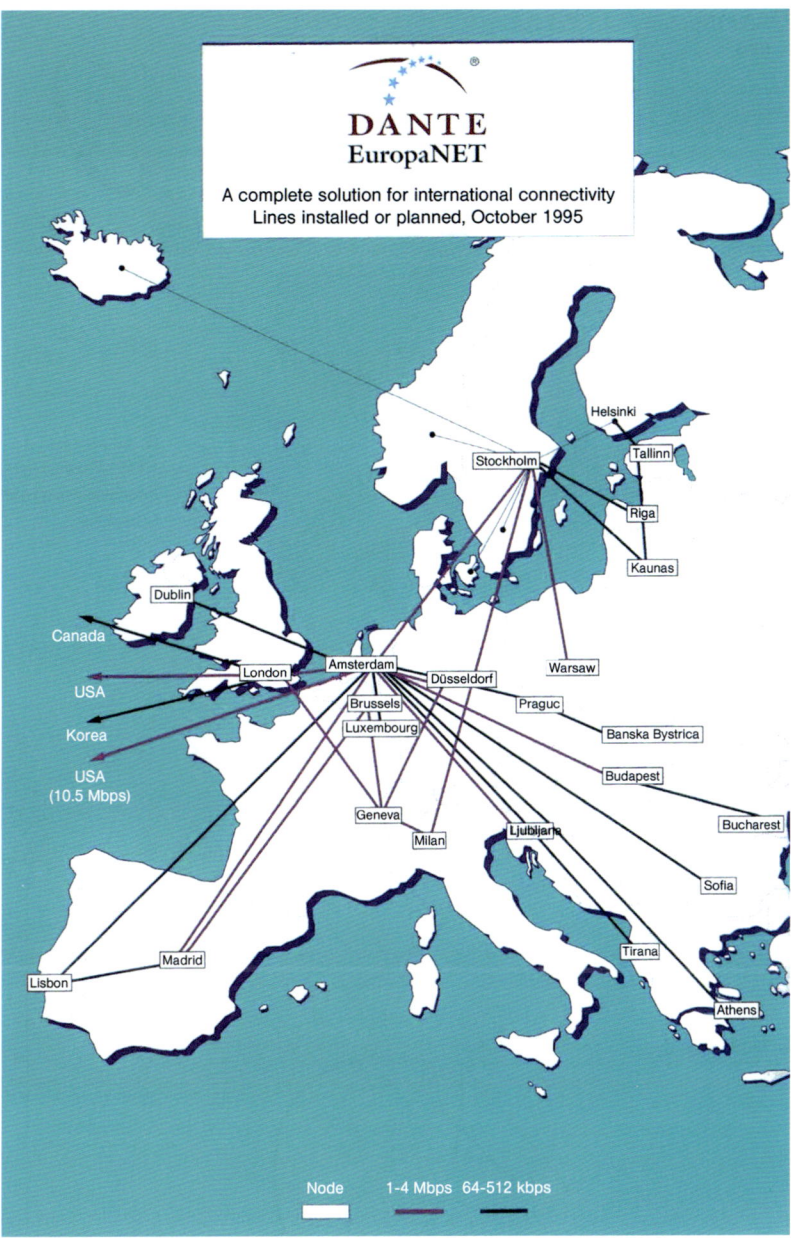

Figure 4.8 EuropaNET configuration. (This figure also appears on page 105.)

xx | Color Plates

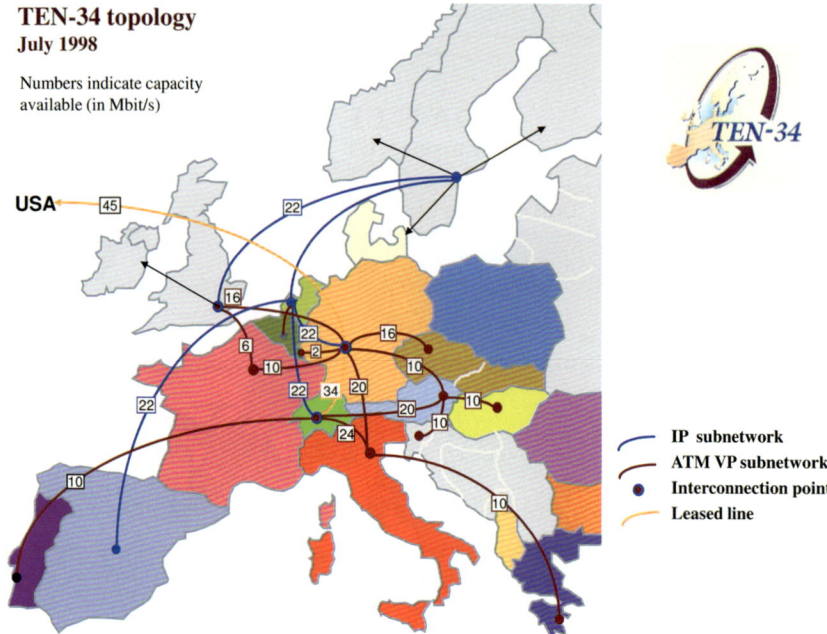

Figure 6.2 TEN-34 topology, June 1998. (This figure also appears on page 142.)

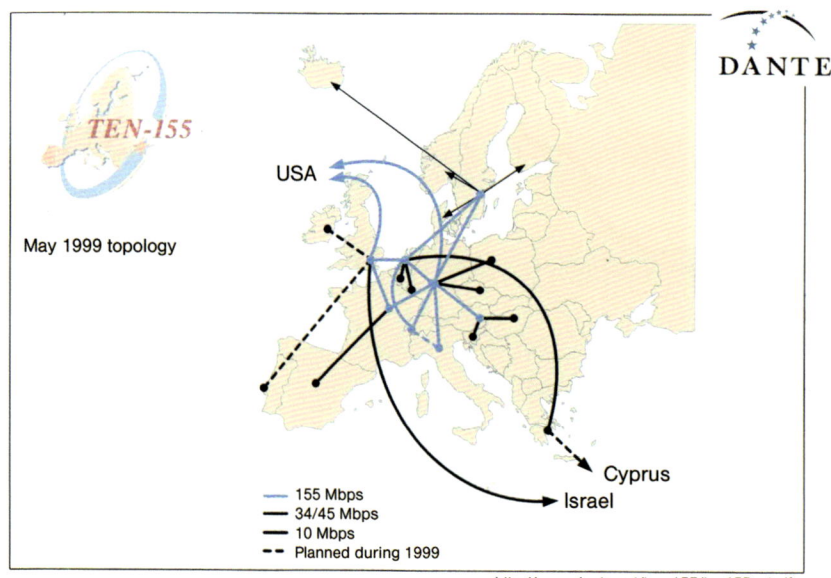

Figure 6.3 TEN-155 configuration, May 1999. (This figure also appears on page 145.)

Color Plates | XXI

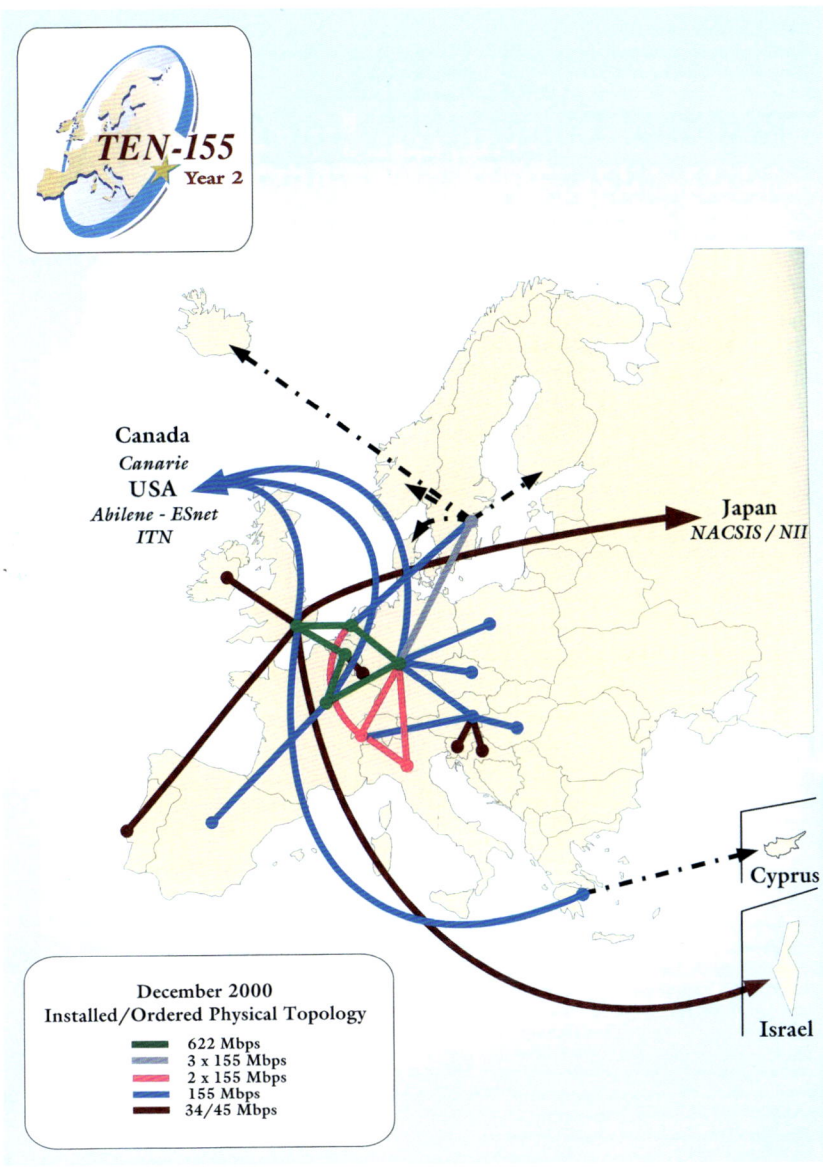

Figure 6.4 TEN-155 December 2000. (This figure also appears on page 148.)

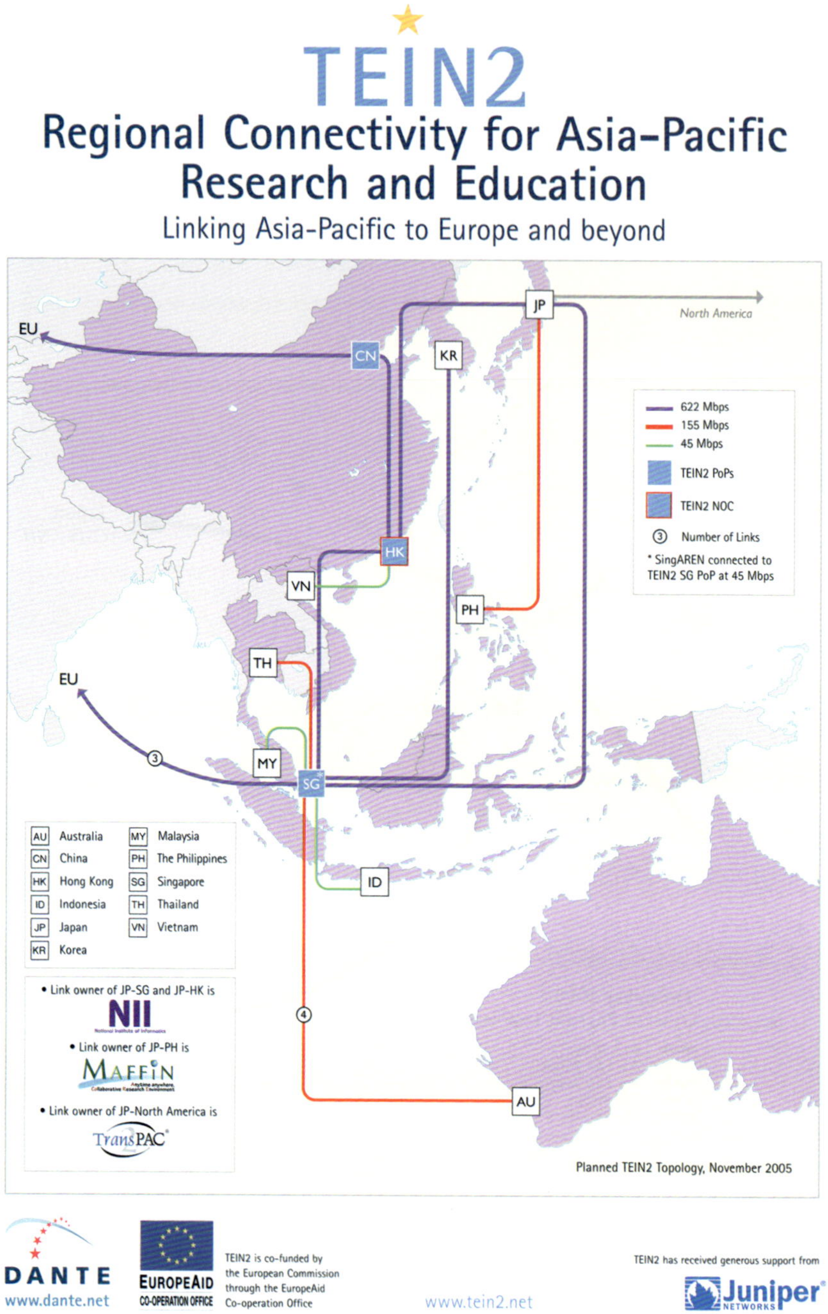

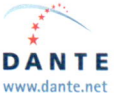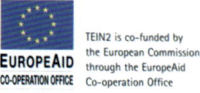

Figure 8.1 TEIN2 configuration. (This figure also appears on page 198.)

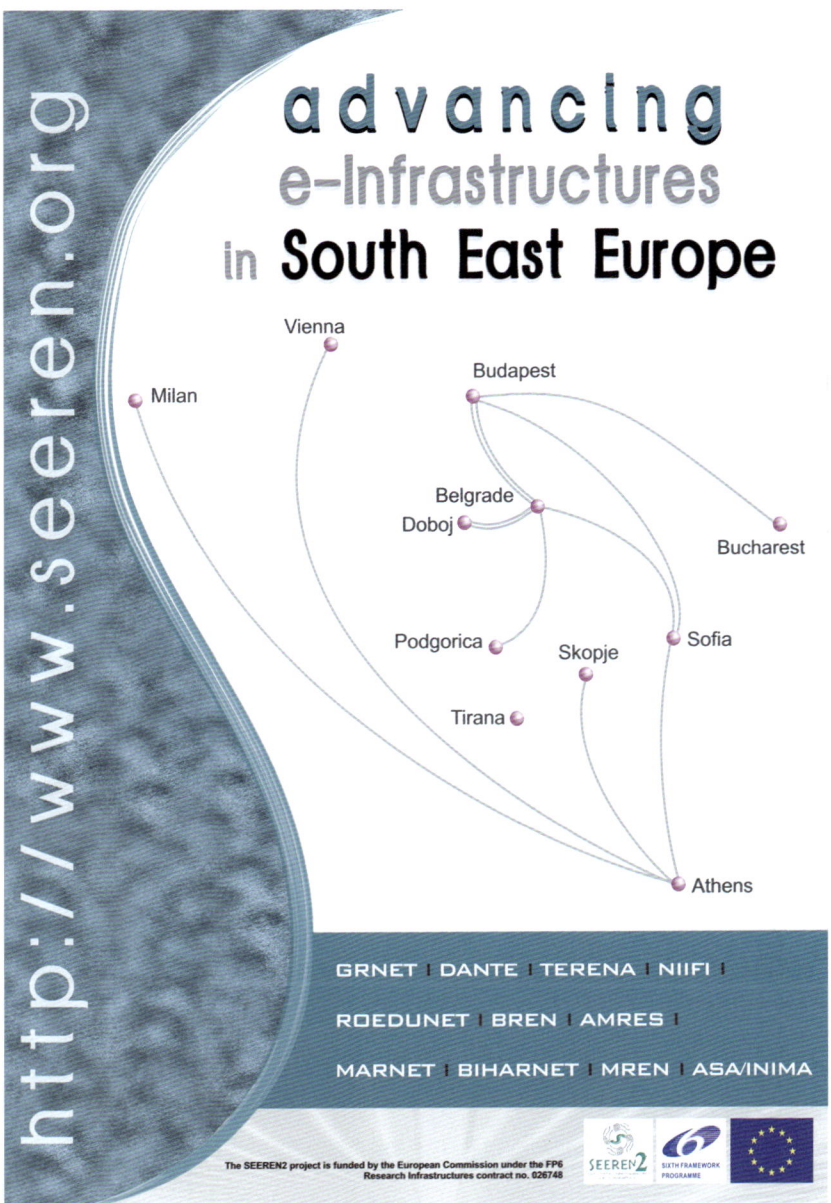

Figure 8.2 SEEREN configuration. (This figure also appears on page 201.)

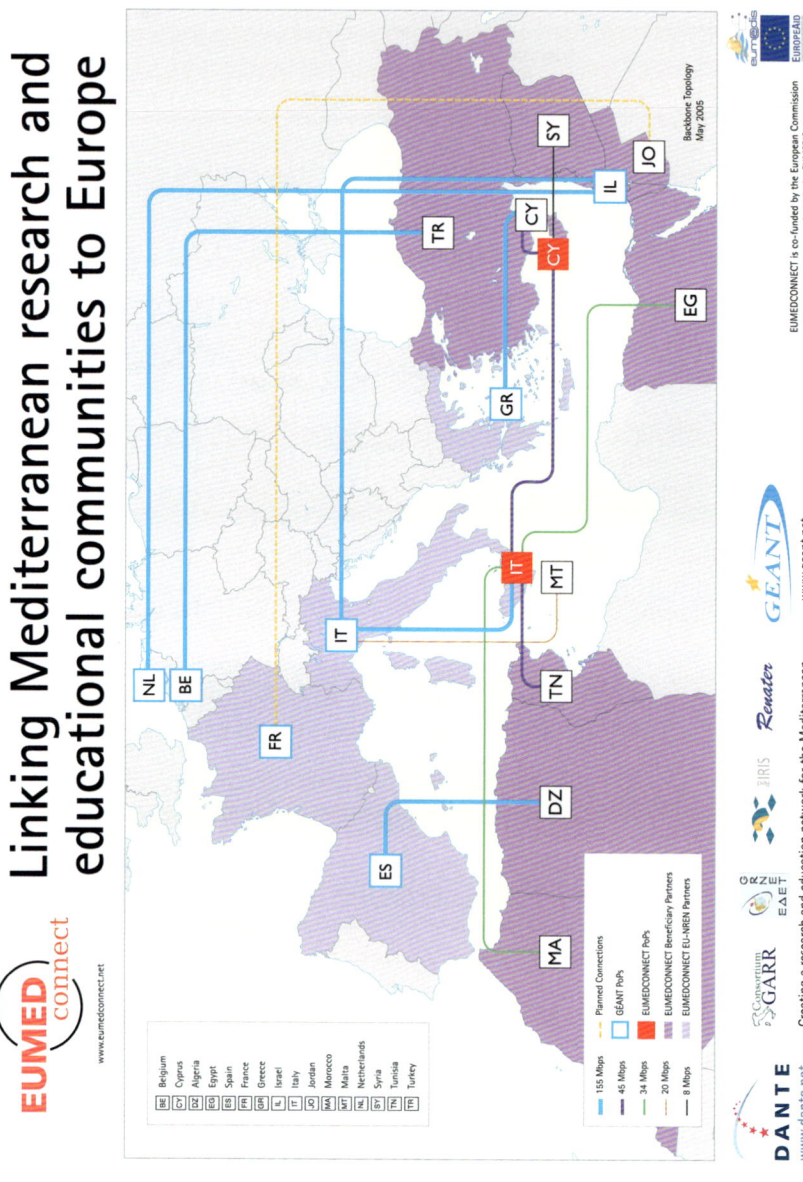

Figure 8.3 EUMEDCONNECT configuration. (This figure also appears on page 206.)

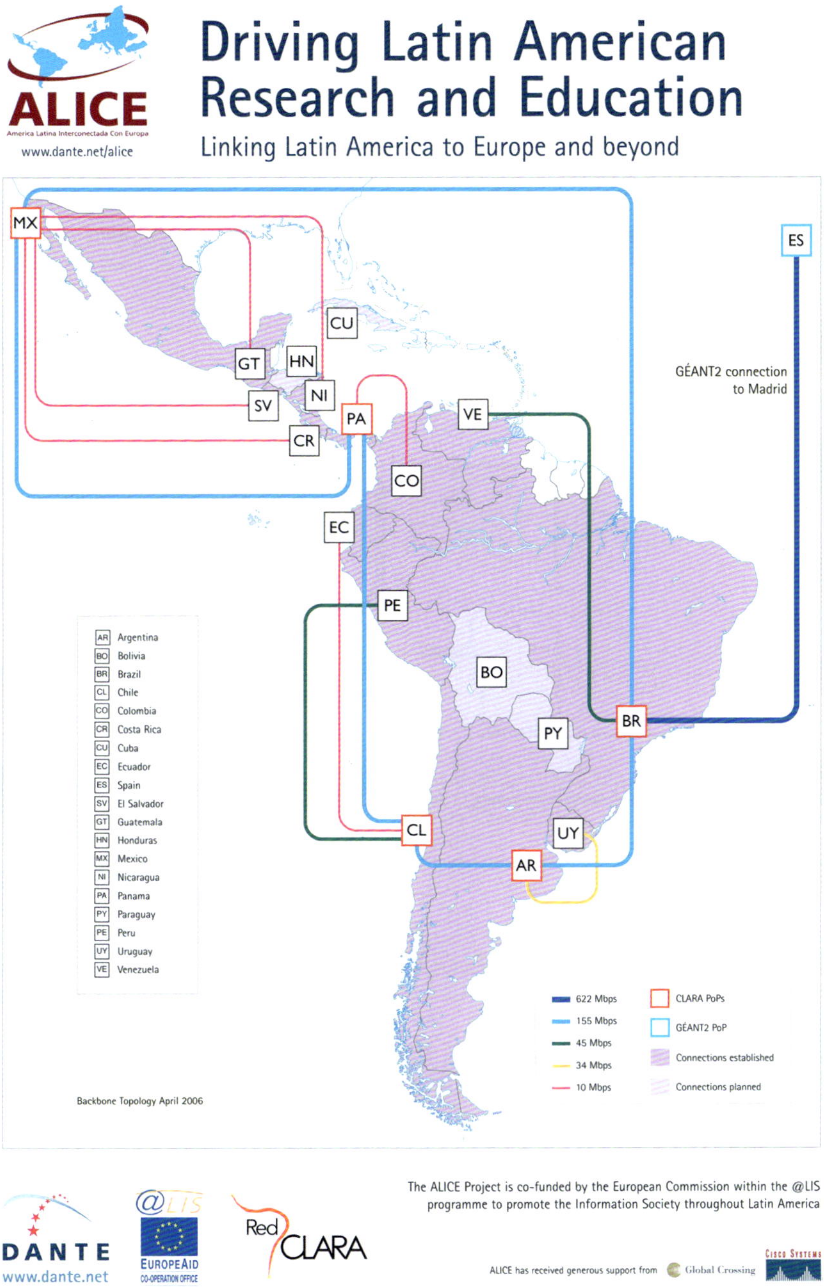

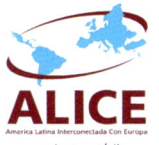

Figure 8.4 RedCLARA topology map, July 2007. (This figure also appears on page 210.)

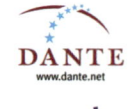

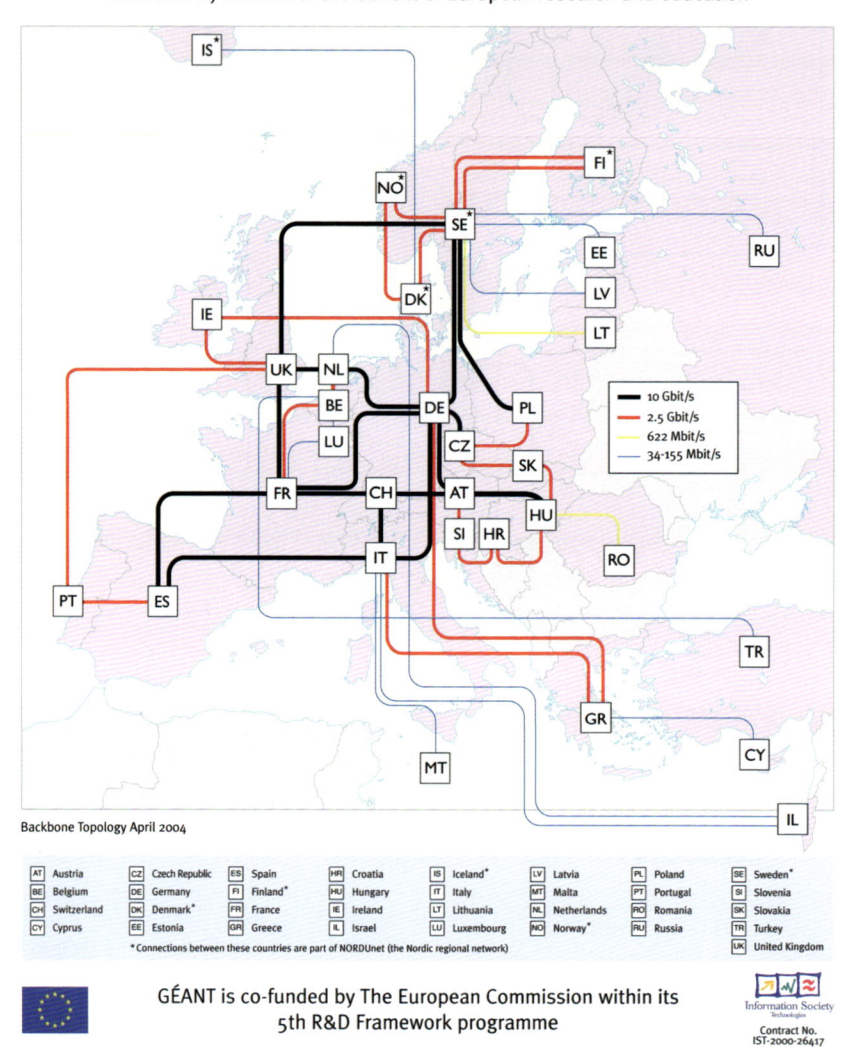

Figure 10.1 GÉANT configuration, April 2004. (This figure also appears on page 241.)

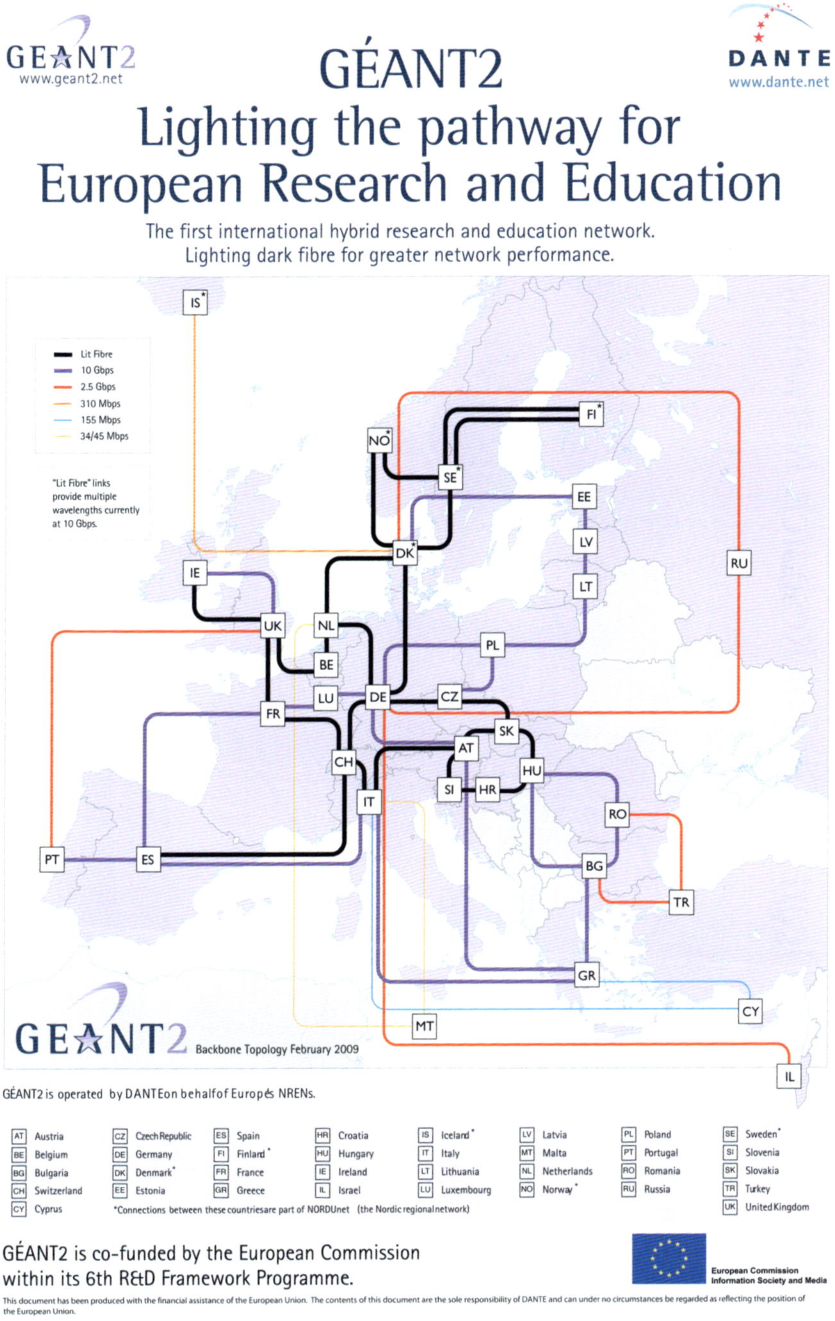

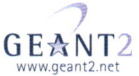 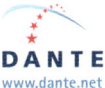

Figure 10.2 GÉANT2 configuration. (This figure also appears on page 246.)

XXVIII | Color Plates

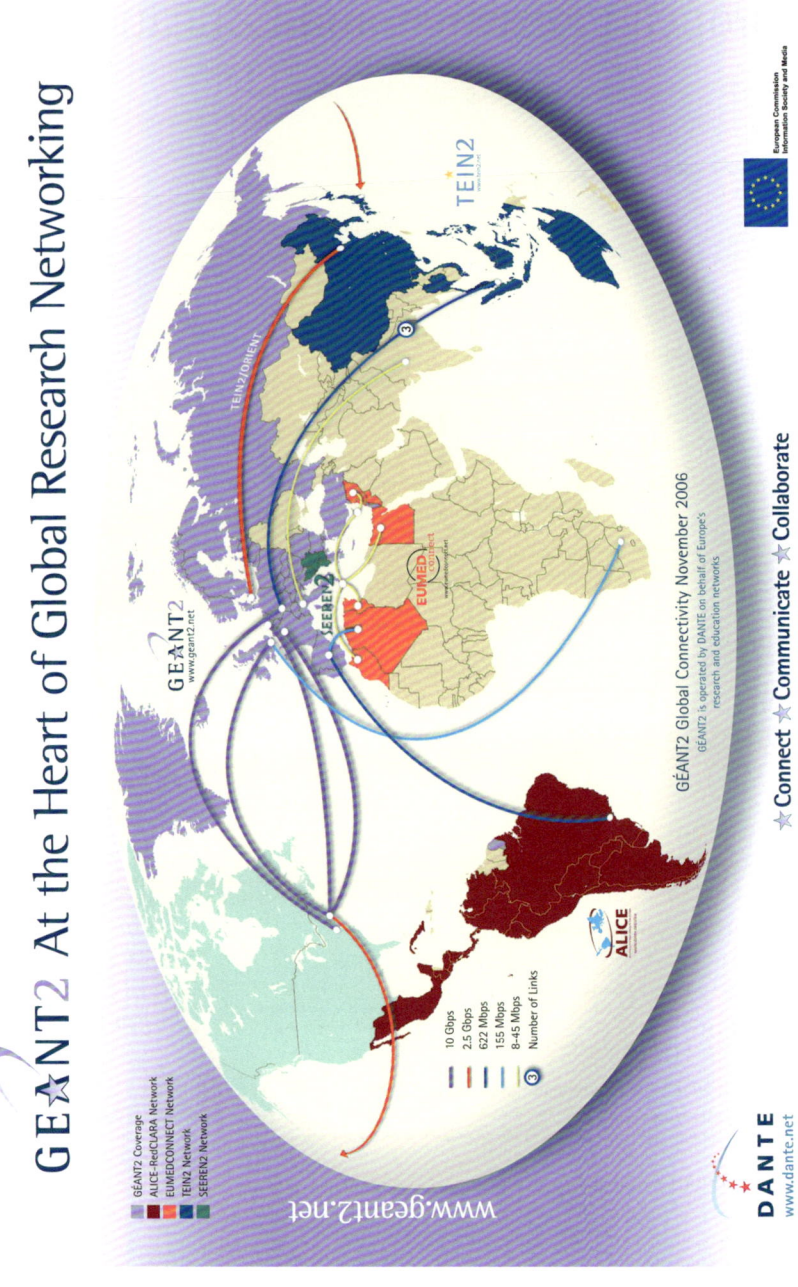

Figure 10.3 Global connectivity. (This figure also appears on page 256.)

1
Early Days

The national research and education networks which are interconnected to provide a seamless service across Europe are taken for granted these days. They have in fact followed different routes to reach this point. Using first-hand experience from some of those involved in their development, this chapter explains the steps that were taken, by whom, and the obstacles which had to be overcome. In addition to these individuals, entire organisations sometimes had to be cajoled to step into line from their differing positions. Different standards and protocols, changing requirements and attitudes, and different national positions all had to be taken into account in achieving the goals. The chapter focuses mainly on the years from the mid-1970s to the mid-1980s.

1.1
The Starting Point

In the early 1980s, almost all the countries in Europe were planning new networks. The technology existed, and the academic and research communities wanted to be able to use it. However, there was no coordination at a European level, just rapid national growth rates.

By the end of 1984, Scandinavia had a coordinated regional network, covering Denmark, Finland, Norway and Sweden. Austria and the United Kingdom each had operational networks, and Germany was in the middle of a major implementation programme leading to the full DFN (Deutsches Forschungsnetz) network. Ireland and Italy were also involved in implementation, and France, the Netherlands, Spain and Switzerland had plans they were about to implement.

Before describing the way all these were brought together on a European scale, we need to review the technologies that were available and the activities that form the backdrop to our story.

1.1.1
The Data Communications Scene

The early 1980s were the height of the age of large-scale multi-user mainframes, and the earliest remote access arrangements were stars of access links converging on

A History of International Research Networking. Edited by Howard Davies and Beatrice Bressan
Copyright © 2010 WILEY-VCH Verlag GmbH & Co. KGaA, Weinheim
ISBN: 978-3-527-32710-2

individual computer centers. These network links had their roots in the use of analogue leased lines connecting first generation modems at speeds starting at 300 bps but rising progressively to a few kbps. From the early 1970s to the early 1980s, most PTTs (post, telephone, and telegraph operating entities) introduced digital leased line services, although still primarily at speeds of 9.6 kbps or less. A few rather expensive 64 kbps services were introduced and the first megabit services were on offer in France and the United Kingdom, but not yet used in the emerging research networks.

The potential for merging the various star networks had already been shown; it had been demonstrated by the first phase of the ARPAnet (Advanced Research Projects Agency network) in the early 1970s and by the first ubiquitous campus network at the National Physical Laboratory in London at the same time. These were the first practical, general-purpose packet networks, separating the switching and routing from the hosts accessed, and setting the direction for the modern generation of data networks.

The first public packet switched network in the world, EPSS (experimental packet switching system), was opened by the United Kingdom Post Office in 1977; the British academic community played a leading part in its user community, particularly in the definition in 1975 of a set of so-called high level protocols to allow applications to communicate over the new network. In 1976, the CCITT (Comité Consultatif International Téléphonique et Télégraphique), the PTT standards body within the ITU (International Telecommunication Union) defined the first version of its X.25 packet switching recommendation, and all the European PTTs rapidly established plans for national packet switched services and for interworking between them. The first technically stable version of the X.25 recommendation was ratified in 1980. In the same year, the United Kingdom EPSS network was replaced by the X.25-based PSS (packet switch stream), and the German PTT introduced its DATEX-P (data exchange -packetized) X.25 network.

The transit arrangements between the national PTTs then gradually became operational, offering communication on a European scale. By the middle of 1985, a United Kingdom PSS customer, for example, could communicate with data customers in any of the COST (European cooperation in the field of scientific and technical research) countries except Turkey and Yugoslavia (although for Portugal, the call had to be initiated from there).

One thing this shows is that the prevailing view of networking at that time was one in which the PTTs played a large part. In their plans reported to the first European Networkshop in 1985, representatives of the research communities in all countries assumed that their infrastructure would be X.25 based, and all but Sweden and the United Kingdom planned either immediate or phased adoption of publicly operated networks as the basis of their networking activities.

1.2
Protocols and Standards

A crucial factor for any network to be successful is the choice of protocols (i.e. the rules that the computers in the network must follow in order to exchange signals and data) that it uses. Standardization is also an important consideration. For two computers to intercommunicate effectively, they must both be following exactly the same rules and procedures.

1.2.1
Interim Standards

The first implementers of networks had to invent their own protocols but only a few of these took root outside the domain for which they had been invented.

One set of protocols which did get more widely used was the set of so-called "Colored Books". This was a family of standards defined in the United Kingdom in the late 1970s and early 1980s, based on the experience gained from EPSS activities. Each book defined a protocol for one function or application, and each had a distinctive colored cover, giving it the obvious popular name. The main ones were:

- The Yellow Book – a network independent transport service
- The Green Book – character terminal protocols on PSS
- The Blue Book – a network independent file transfer protocol
- The Red Book – a network independent job transfer and manipulation protocol
- The Grey Book – the JNT mail protocol
- The Orange Book – Cambridge ring 82 protocol specifications
- The White Book – transition to OSI standards

The White Book was the final book in the series; it mapped out the intended transition from these interim standards. Published in 1987, the White Book was a plan worked out in response to a public declaration by the United Kingdom network funding body in January 1985 that it was committed to adopt the emerging OSI (open systems interconnection) standards; thus this decision had been taken before the main activities described here had even started.

However, the Colored Books were the basis of a thriving networking community over a period of more than ten years, and were the primary infrastructure in the United Kingdom for most of that period. They were also used in a number of other countries around the world but the real competition for acceptance as global standards turned out to be between the OSI and Internet protocol suites.

1.2.2
Open Systems Interconnection

It was widely accepted that ubiquitous networking would only happen if it was supported by a comprehensive set of open standards so that users could communicate no matter what equipment they used. Although the aim was agreed, the standards were not yet available and each pioneering networking group had to create some working set of protocols to get things going. Each equipment vendor also offered its own private solutions.

Some convergence process was urgently needed; to support this, in 1977, the ISO (International Standards Organisation) launched a comprehensive standardization program to provide OSI, a flexible architecture and a complete family of standards for the main functions that users were then demanding. This programme was carried forward by ISO during the next ten years, in close collaboration with, and later by joining forces with, the CCITT (later reorganized as the current ITU-T, the ITU telecommunication standardization sector) who were responsible for the standardization in the telecoms industry.

The technical merits and organization of the OSI standards process is a separate story in its own right, but its influence on the planning of academic networking was profound. Policy makers embraced the concept of open standards as an essential component of open markets; researchers welcomed the promise of vendor independence and open interchange of information; funding bodies welcomed the opportunity for efficient resource sharing. Open systems came to be seen politically as one of the essential elements for providing integration of the European infrastructure.

1.2.3
The Internet Protocols

Since the launch of the ARPAnet, its distinctive family of protocols had been evolving. Their development reached a plateau with the production of a re-worked and consolidated design by Jon Postel, leading to the publication of IPv4 (Internet Protocol version 4) in September 1981. IPv4 was trialled and then the transition away from the older NCP (network control programme) made in a final cutover in January 1983. At the same time the main focus for the network moved from the ARPA (Advanced Research Projects Agency) to the NSF (National Science Foundation), with the introduction of first CSNET (Computer Science NETwork) and then NSFnet (National Science Foundation network), with significant upgrades from 56 kbps to 1.5 Mbps circuits in 1984.

Although there is now a perception that the United States networking scene did not engage with the formal standards process, this was not in fact the case. There were many United States experts working within ISO, and there was a strong commitment to the idea of open standards. The responsibility for standards within the United States Government fell to the National Institute of Science and Technology (NIST), which formulated a Government OSI Profile (US-GOSIP, FIPS 146 - Federal Information Processing Standard 146 – not to be confused with the earlier UK-GOSIP) and eventually published it in 1988. This committed the United States Government to the concept of OSI and established an adoption timescale requiring transition to OSI for procurement purposes by 1990. The DoD (Department of Defense) signed up to this aim in principle. As we know, these plans did not mature, largely because of changes in economic factors such as the effect of bundling the TCP/IP (transmission control protocol/Internet protocol) family as a free component of the UNIX (Originally UNICS, uniplexed information and computing system) operating system. However, the environment in the mid 1980s was one in which a commitment to OSI was being promised by the United States and encouraged by European officials. More will be said later about how things actually evolved.

1.3
European Coordination

All these technologies created the basis for much broader European networking and the user experience from the early national pilots created a small but enthusiastic core of network supporters. People had seen what the networks could do and wanted to exploit them on a much larger scale.

From the earliest days, there was strong interest in following developments in the US but because of the practical difficulties of forming and operating intercontinental collaborations – the Atlantic Ocean was a bigger geographic obstacle than it is nowadays – a European approach to deal with specific European issues was the natural way forward.

1.3.1
Identifying the Need

Because of its commitment to open markets, the EC (European Commission), via the ESPRIT (European strategic programme for research in information technology) program, threw its considerable weight behind open networking developments in Europe. The EC was also the target of significant lobbying from national groups. The greatest impact was achieved between 1982 and 1984 by Professor Zander, who was in many ways the father of DFN, the German research network, and who spent a great deal of time and effort lobbying the EC and encouraging its political commitment to the process. He can justly be credited with stimulating action by the European institutions, particularly in the framework of the ESPRIT research programme. Collaborative academic and industrial research was increasing in importance in many European countries, and EC officials began a process of encouraging the separate networks to join together.

In the United Kingdom, the period from 1981 to 1984 had been one of unification of regional and discipline-specific networks to form the general purpose JANET (joint academic network); this was officially launched to mark the completion of this process in April 1984. This rationalization, under which all the existing regional networks serving universities and the central research support networks were brought into one organization with a single funding source, convinced those concerned of the benefits of harmonization. At the same time, the user groups now benefiting from the more effective communication with colleagues nationally became increasingly vocal about the need for similar connectivity across Europe. This message came particularly strongly from the large international experimental collaborations in astronomy and high energy physics (HEP).

1.3.2
Preliminary Steps

During the autumn of 1984, the JANET network managers and their colleagues from other networking interests, who were then all based at the Rutherford Appleton

Laboratory (RAL), were visited by Dr Nick Newman from the EC, who was contacting national groups and raising awareness of the European situation. He was also promoting the idea of cooperation on a European level.

Following this visit, Paul Bryant of the SERC (Science and Engineering Research Council) engineering support network, James Hutton (HEP), and Peter Linington, Head of the UK's Joint Network Team (JNT) and Network Executive (the JANET operations team), met in the JNT offices on 12 November 1984 to discuss how the kind of integration achieved in the United Kingdom might be encouraged throughout Europe. They decided that some kind of European technical networking summit was needed and, agreeing to pool their resources, set about contacting their colleagues to seek support.

There was an enthusiastic response, and it was clear that many groups were thinking along similar lines. Just before Christmas 1984, the United Kingdom group hosted a face-to-face meeting of the European prime movers at RAL where it was agreed that a larger workshop of all the appropriate representatives should be held. The EC agreed to host the event in Luxembourg and funding for participation was obtained from ECFA, the European Committee for Future Accelerators, ESF, the European Science Foundation, and COST-11. An organizing group was formed that expanded the circle of contacts and gathered background information about the situation in all the participating countries ready for the workshop.

1.3.3
The First European Networkshop

The first European Networkshop was held on May 14th and 15th 1985 in Luxembourg. It took place in meeting rooms made available by Barry Mahon of the EC's DG III (Directorate General III). About 60 people attended, and most of the agenda on the first day was taken up by presentations of the current activities and plans of the participants.

The resulting summary of national activities gives a good idea of both the diversity of practice and maturity, and the significant common themes across all the contributions.

The following thumbnail sketches are derived directly from the presentations used during the Networkshop:

Austria: Networking in Austria had reached the stage of a pilot linking Vienna, Graz and Linz, using the DATEX-P public X.25 service as a base. The pilot, ACOnet (Akademisches Computer Netz), was adopting an architecture in which local subnetworks and hosts were linked to the public network by gateways, operating at either the network or application level. Operations were supported by new gateway management tools, supporting down-line loading of code over X.25 and remote programme development.

Denmark: The core of the Danish activity was a long-established private X.25 network called Centernet, which linked NEUCC (Northern Europe University Computing Centre), RECAU (det Regionale Edb-center ved Århus Universitet), and RECKU (det Regionale Edb-center ved Københavns Universitet). It used the EUROnet (European network) transport protocol and supported a gateway to the public X.25 network. There were detailed plans for migration to the public X.25 service using standard off-the-shelf components. It had been decided that the protocols used in Denmark would be aligned with those used by DFN. Application plans included the early establishment of an electronic mail server.

Finland: FUNET (Finnish university network) had been launched in 1984, initially to provide terminal access to twelve university hosts via the public X.25 network. There were also closed sub-networks carrying manufacturer-specific protocols over X.25. The remaining university hosts were expected to be connected shortly. Early application use had focused on the popular KOM, a bulletin board system, and the PortaCOM conferencing system (originated by Jacob Palme in Stockholm), but electronic mail was seen as an important requirement. There were plans for a file transfer service, probably based on the UNINETT FTP (file transfer protocol). The University of Helsinki was using the GILT (get interconnection between local text system), teletext-based protocols.

France: A project had been launched at the start of 1984 to study the needs of the French research community. It involved all major research organizations and French industry. Its report, issued in February 1985, defined a network project that was under active consideration by the funding bodies. The hope was that implementation would start in late 1985. The plan placed emphasis on international standards, particularly for electronic mail (X.400) and international interworking. One distinctive requirement identified in France was for the support of high-speed file transfer using a broadcast satellite carrier.

Germany: DFN, Germany's flagship networking project, had been initiated in 1982. It was using the new OSI protocols, and was based on the public X.25 network (DATEX-P). The project was in response to a wide range of user requirements. Networking within the universities was well established, and therefore the need for WAN-LAN (wide area network–local area network) interworking was stressed. The user requirements were for interactive terminal access, file transfer, remote job entry and electronic mail. One distinctive requirement was the particular need to support graphics based on GKS (graphics kernel system) – a powerful (for its time) graphics software package – in both interactive and bulk transfer modes. The network would have no central accounting or logging mechanisms.

Ireland: There had been a university network in Ireland since 1979, based on EUROnet activity. This was currently in the form of a private X.25 network. A transition was in progress in which the initial network was being subsumed into a Higher Education Authority network (HEAnet), giving more complete coverage of the country. It would be based on the public X.25 service and was expected to be in operation during 1985–86. At the application level, the network used the United Kingdom Colored Book protocols; it also provided the COM (component object model) conferencing system for ESPRIT at UCD (University College Dublin).

Italy: There were two main networking activities in Italy. The longest-established was the network set up by INFN (Istituto Nazionale di Fisica Nucleare) for use by the HEP community and based on DECnet (network protocol design by DEC – Digital Equipment Corporation), and implemented on the VAX™ family of computers that it manufactured). More recently, a new initiative called OSIRIDE had been set up to create a pilot OSI network. Initially, this was to concentrate on file transfer, but with later targets of supporting electronic mail, conferencing, document transfer and, eventually, video conferencing.

Netherlands: There was no report on the Netherlands in the workshop summary, but the SURFnet proposal published the following autumn showed that detailed planning had been in progress since ministers had approved an initial proposal in December 1984. Requirements had been identified for file, job and image transfer, electronic mail and access to international facilities. There was already significant use of EARN (European academic and research network), and the plan called for connection of all institutions to the Dutch PTT's DATAnet 1 public network by 1987.

The SURFnet plan not only covered the provision of national connectivity, but made it part of a comprehensive strategy: each institution was required to produce a LAN plan by September 1986, together with a commitment for the Netherlands to play an active part in European coordination. The report committed to using OSI standards, while recognising the need for some pragmatic short-term upgrades to improve coverage.

Norway: UNINETT was based on research and development (R&D) starting in 1976 and had been in service since 1983. It supported interactive terminals, file transfer and conferencing. It was based on the use of public X.25 and on the ISO OSI reference model.

Spain: There were existing terminal access services and access networks to the major computing centers. However, strong user requirements based on Microelectronics (CAD, computer-aided design), HEP, AI (artificial intelligence), SoftEng (software engineering), computing center and supercomputer access were being articulated. This had led to Ministry support for a new project called the Interconexión de los Recursos InformáticoS (IRIS). IRIS was to report by June 1985, and a pilot was expected to start by the fall of 1985. The plans placed emphasis on international standards, European harmonization and the relationship to the public X.25 network (IBERPAC, servicio IBERico de conmutacion por PACkets).

Sweden: SUNET (Swedish university network), the existing solution in Sweden, was based on regional private X.25 networks and the use of the public X.25 services to connect them. It had been in operation since 1983. The network supported interactive terminal traffic, file transfer, electronic mail and conferencing.

Switzerland: A detailed study of user requirements and justification for a networking activity had been performed and the study report had proposed further technical work (jointly with the Swiss PTT) to establish a technical and organizational plan. The intended timescale called for a detailed plan to be produced in 1985–87, and for a network to be in service as of 1988.

United Kingdom: JANET in the United Kingdom had been based on a process of rationalization of existing networks, some of which had been in operation since the late 1970s. The unified network had been transferred to a single strategic and management organization early in 1984. At its formal launch, JANET was a private X.25 network with 10 transit switches connecting some 200 terminations, more than 50 of which were local networks. It connected a total of approximately 500 host computers, and 10 000 terminal access (PAD, packet assembler-disassembler) ports. It used the Colored Book protocols for terminal access (X.29), file transfer, job transfer and electronic mail. The JANET community was actively planning a transition to OSI, with the move to X.400 mail as a first step.

It was clear from these reports that there was a lot of activity and that support for X.25 and X.29 was already widespread. They indicated that in this environment, interworking of at least terminal services would be possible within Europe. However, other applications would need harmonization. Of the identified requirements, X.400 electronic mail seemed to be the most pressing. It was also clear that a lot more information needed to be collected and correlated. For example, there was no data about coverage and availability at a local level. There was also little information about how costs would fall on end users.

Informal discussions on the evening of May 14 led to the conclusion that a separate body was needed to act as a European focus and an outline of its mission and initial objectives was put to the final workshop session the following day. What was proposed was a networking association to promote peer-to-peer interworking and harmonization between the national academic and research networks, not the creation of a core international data network, since this was seen as best provided by the PTTs.

The rough outlines of the organization were proposed. The scope was to be Western Europe, which was then taken to mean the EEC (European Economic Community) and COST countries. In addition to the national members, the major European research laboratories such as CERN (Conseil Européen pour la Recherche Nucléaire) would also be eligible to join in their own right. A role was also seen for European industrial research laboratories and for significant user organisations, but not as primary members. ESPRIT was recognized as having a special status, as it represented an important group of infrastructure users within the scope of the association, but the EC would not be a member in its own right.

The stated aims were to provide a high-quality networking infrastructure for the support of research and academic endeavor on a European basis, by taking any necessary actions to ensure that this infrastructure adopted and exploited the most advanced technology available. This was understood to imply the creation of an international OSI network, involving as intermediate steps the short-term interconnection of existing non-OSI networks and the transition of existing networks to open standards.

Once these principles had been debated and agreed, a short summary resolution was put to the workshop and accepted without any objections. The wording proposed on that day is shown in Figure 1.1.

> **Recommendation A.200**
>
> *Considering*
>
> **that national academic networks exist or are planned in a large number of European Countries;**
>
> **that it is feasible, by coordination and harmonization of these national activities, to provide facilities on a European basis;**
>
> **that collaborative industrial research requires similar facilities;**
>
> *the meeting unanimously declares the view that an association should be established to promote the creation of a European research and academic networking infrastructure.*

Figure 1.1 The networkshop resolution.

The format and the bogus recommendation number in the text above were an irreverent, high-spirited, parody of the CCITT procedures in use at the time. Once it had decided to go ahead, the workshop did two more things. First, it asked all the representatives if their organizations were likely to participate actively, which they were, and then asked them to take this commitment back to their organizations for more formal ratification. Secondly, it drew up a list of priority items to be carried out in order to set the association up and start its work and attached to each item the name of a member prepared to take the lead in developing it.

The priority items covered both technical and organizational issues. On the technical side, there were:

- Coordination of message handling systems, primarily for X.400, including the EAN (electronic access network) software package (CERN)
- X.25 (84) harmonization of operational requirements (France)
- File transfer protocols and services (CERN)
- Full screen terminal working (United Kingdom)
- Collection (manual) of directory information, covering services, people and help contracts (EC)
- Exchange of operational information (Ireland)

And for the organizational items:

- Organization and support of the association (United Kingdom)
- Scope and mechanisms for liaison with CEPT (Conference of European Postal and Telecommunication Administration).
- Organization of the next European Networkshop, provisionally scheduled for mid-1986 (initially unallocated – Denmark subsequently volunteered).

The workshop ended on a very positive note. The technical and organizational tasks were to be started straight away. The association would be set up with a formal constitution so that it could hold funds and become self-supporting. It would seek financial support to help during the launch period but the members would not wait for these things to happen. Rather, they would move forward immediately in whatever way was open to them. This willingness to take risks and to make things happen without waiting for the formal niceties typified the spirit of optimism that pervaded the workshop, and indeed all the early stages of RARE's (Réseaux Associés pour la Recherche Européenne) history.

1.4
RARE: From Proposal to Reality

Despite the impatience to get things moving on the part of many of the people involved, it was necessary to go through a number of administrative steps to put a robust, stable and adequately funded organizational structure in place.

1.4.1
Laying the Foundations

After the Luxembourg workshop, the delegates went home and consulted their organisations. The Netherlands came back rapidly with an extremely positive response, backed by the charismatic and far-sighted Hans Rosenberg. He obtained support from SURF, the organization responsible for the Netherlands research network, to provide funding for the embryonic organization to pay for an interim secretariat. This secretariat was operated by James Martin Associates (JMA) in Amsterdam who got to work immediately and helped in the drafting of Articles of Association. This involved agreeing procedures and legal responsibilities, which were derived from a Dutch legal template. It was also necessary to agree a business plan, providing analysis of various proposed funding models to ensure that the association would indeed be self-sustaining in the longer term. The main burden of carrying this through fell on Rob Brinkhuijsen and Frank van Iersel of JMA.

One of the tasks that proved unexpectedly difficult was the choice of a name for the new entity. Many immediately intuitive names were already taken by existing organizations or led to acronyms that were already well established in members' home countries. The name "European Networking Association", although initially supported by many, would have been abbreviated to ENA, meaning Ecole Nationale d'Administration to any Frenchman. Other names proposed all seemed to be taken, confusing or even obscene in one country or another. Finally, the French name Réseaux Associés pour la Recherche Européenne, or RARE for short, was accepted despite some misgivings concerning future jokes about RARE implying half-baked ideas and from August 1985 that name was fixed.

Gradually the rest of the constitution came together, with a proposed structure in which a fully-representative Council of Administration delegated short term decisions to a smaller rotating Executive Committee. The Association was to have a President to chair both these bodies, a Vice-President, a Treasurer and eventually a Secretary-General as a full-time officer to oversee day-to-day business and run the permanent administration.

In parallel with the organizational work, this was a time of widespread lobbying for support. Members explained the objectives of the new body to their national organizations, to many European research groups, to international contacts such as the NSF in America, and to many parts of the EC. Finally, in December 1985, the officers of RARE met Michel Carpentier, the Director General of DG XIII (IST, Information Society Technologies) and his officials, and explained RARE's plans and goals to him. This led to a commitment from the EU (European Union) to fund the secretariat until regular support on a subscription basis could be put in place, thus providing bridging from the Dutch support.

Two important relationships with existing organizations were established during this preparatory period. First, the responsibility for liaison with the CEPT that Switzerland had undertaken to organize was progressed by Albert Kündig of ETH (Eidgenössische Technische Hochschule) Zurich. Kündig had moved to academia from the Swiss PTT and had a wide network of contacts. He laid the foundations for RARE's credibility with the PTTs, so that they began to see the organization in a positive light, and not as a potential threat.

The second key liaison was with EARN which, at the time, was also a relatively young organization and which was providing services based on the use of IBM equipment and protocols (see later for details). EARN was in many ways a natural competitor to RARE but there were several people who were involved in both organizations and there were clear advantages to cooperation. A series of meetings was held between Dennis Jennings, the President of EARN and Peter Linington, the President of RARE, in which common objectives were set out. This led later, after EARN had adopted a statement of intent on the transition to open standards, to EARN becoming an international member of RARE.

1.4.2
The First Step for COSINE

Although they were primarily academics, many of the members of the new association had strong links with their national industry or research ministries. These contacts were very supportive, and the discussion with industry ministries, particularly the BMFT (Bundesministerium für Forschung und Technologie) in Germany, the Ministry of Education and Science in the Netherlands and the Department of Industry in the United Kingdom, resulted in these bodies seeing RARE as a flagship for standards policy and, more generally, for open networking.

During the second ministerial conference in Hanover on November 5–6 1985, Andreas Vogel, an official from the BMFT, was lobbying other countries to get support for putting a project called COSINE, cooperation for open systems interconnection networking in Europe, on the first list of EUREKA (European Research Coordination Agency) projects that ministers would announce. A subsequent full meeting of COSINE participants in Bonn on February 19 1986 asked RARE to prepare the technical specification for the project by midsummer. (The required draft was delivered on time although the workshop set up to discuss it was not held until November 1986 because of the need for negotiations between EUREKA officials).

RARE was now in the position of being a contractor to the EUREKA programme before having its own legal existence! This put a very real pressure on the preparations for RARE's formal foundation.

1.4.3
The Second European Networkshop

The Second European Networkshop was held in Copenhagen on 26–28 May 1986. The whole of the July/August edition of the Computer Compacts Journal was dedicated to a report on the event, including an overview of RARE's mission and a feature interview with its President-elect. This edition also carried a full-page advertisement for the post of Secretary General of RARE!

The second Networkshop was a much more orchestrated and better planned event than the first; it was already more of a conference than an informal workshop. There was a series of activity reports covering the priority tasks set out by the conclusions of the first workshop, followed by technical sessions dealing with current technical challenges, new standards and longer-term opportunities such as broadband. There were also sessions looking at a number of EU industrial research projects and at plans from the PTTs for new services.

As well as being a forum for the interchange of information, the workshop also provided a sounding board for testing the level of support in the community and confirming that, after a year of largely organizational activity, the creation of the association was still welcomed at a working level within the research networks.

Associated with the main workshop, most of the technical working groups that RARE was setting up also met; these groups had started as task groups in response to the priority items identified in Luxembourg, but were already running smoothly with stable membership and with enthusiastic chairs able to take responsibility for their organization and for the delivery of results. There had been some changes in responsibilities of the Working Groups (WGs) during the year, and the line-up reporting in Copenhagen was (Figure 1.2):

- WG1: Message handling systems (Alf Hansen)
- WG2: File transfer, access and management (François Fluckiger)
- WG3: Information services exchange of operation information (Barry Mahon)
- WG4: Network operations and X.25 (Piet Bovenga)
- WG5: Full screen services (Brian Gilmore)
- WG6: Medium- and high-speed communications (Jacques Prévost)
- Task 7 – Liaison with CEPT performed *ad hominen* by Albert Kündig in direct collaboration with the secretariat, and so no separate working group was needed.
- WG8: Management of network application services (Mats Brunell).

1.4.4
The Birth of RARE

The formal establishment of RARE was activated by the signing of the constitution by the new officers in Amsterdam on 13 June 1986. Present at the ceremony were the key officers of the new organization, namely Peter Linington as the first President, Klaus Ullmann as Vice-President and Kees Neggers as Treasurer, plus long-term supporter and benefactor Hans Rosenberg and the Notary who witnessed the signatures (Figure 1.3). After some 22 international meetings to agree the details of the

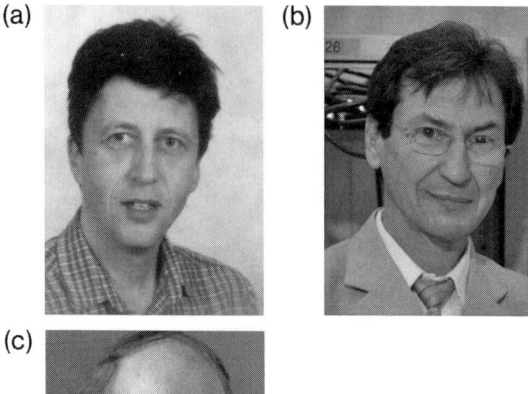

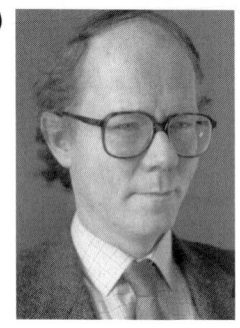

Figure 1.2 RARE working group leaders, 1986: (a) Alf Hansen, (b) François Fluckiger, Barry Mahon (no photo), Piet Bovenga (no photo), (c) Brian Gilmore, Jacques Prévost (no photo), Mats Brunell (no photo).

organization, the final signing was over in an hour, and was followed by a pleasant social lunch. RARE was now in existence; the initial RARE Executive Committee consisted of the three officers present at the signing, plus Birgitta Carlson, who brought a wealth of experience from the running of NORDUnet (Nordic university network). Francisco Ros was later co-opted as organizer of the third networkshop in Valencia.

The constitution allowed only one member per country, and limited eligibility for full membership to: Austria, Belgium, Denmark, Finland, France, Germany (Federal Republic), Greece, Iceland, Ireland, Italy, Luxembourg, the Netherlands, Norway, Portugal, Spain, Sweden, Switzerland, Turkey, the United Kingdom of Great Britain and Northern Ireland, and Yugoslavia. The document signed that day in Amsterdam was in Dutch and ran to 11 pages. However, the flavor of what was being agreed is given by the key clause shown in Figure 1.4, taken from the certified English translation provided at the time.

1.4.5
The End of the Beginning

Just over 18 months after its first international planning meeting, RARE was now an established organization with a constitution, a permanent secretariat and enough

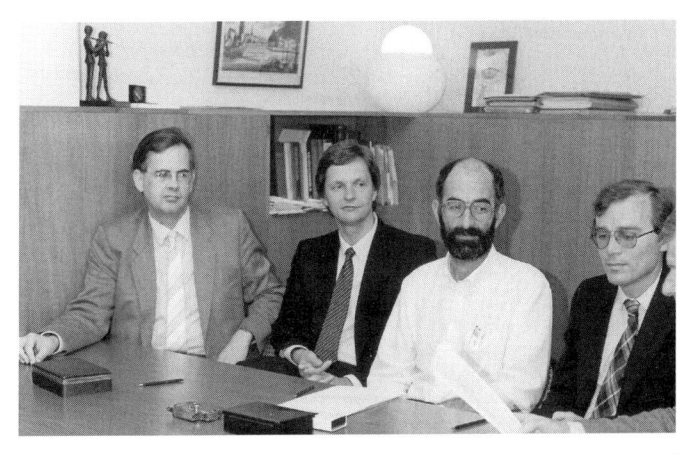

Figure 1.3 Adoption of the RARE constitution. Left to right: Peter Linington, Klaus Ullmann, Hans Rosenberg, and Kees Neggers.

resources to support its activity. Within this time frame, its influence had grown to the point where it was a recognized player in shaping European policy and it was a credible prime contractor for a major activity like the EUREKA COSINE project. It also had a thriving technical program supported by its working groups and, after two Networkshops, it was well on the way to establishing its long-running and well-respected conference series. RARE had arrived and the beginning was, so to speak, over.

1.5
EARN, the First International Service in Europe

The networks for the research and academic environments appeared as test-beds in different stages of evolution in various countries in the 1970s. Towards the end of the decade, some of these test-beds began to involve foreign partners and began to offer international services. To assert that EARN (European academic and research network) developed the first international network service in Europe is too strong. Yet, one can say that EARN was the first network in Europe offering an international service in a structured way. The diffusion of the research network services in the United States in the early 1980s was based mainly on networks such as ARPAnet, BITNET and CSNET. EARN constituted the European extension of the BITNET network. BITNET was a "store and forward" type network developed at the City University of New York by Ira Fuchs in 1981, initially baptized as "Because It's There Net" and later "Because It's Time Net".

The system was originally based on IBM's VNET (virtual networking) email system and used RSCS (remote spooling communications subsystem) and NJE (network job

> **RARE Constitution: Objectives - Article 4**
>
> 1. The objectives of RARE are to promote and participate in the creation of a high-quality European computer-communications infrastructure for the support of research endevour. It will take whatever steps are required to ensure that this infrastructure adopts the most advanced technology available, according to the principles of Open Systems Interconnection as defined by the International Standards Organisation (ISO), in order to ensure open international interconnection. It will wherever possible use the data carrier services of the European Postal, Telephone and Telegraph services.
>
> 2. In order to attain the above objectives, RARE shall, inter alia:
>
>   - remove technical and organisational barriers between national networks, by harmonizing their technical facilities;
>   - provide for the exchange of operational, directory and technical information;
>   - protect and serve the interests of RARE with respect to other organizations, in particular governmental, standardization, PTT and industrial bodies;
>   - where appropriate, set up and run common services and technical facilities;
>   - establish working groups to perform technical activities in line with the objectives of RARE;
>   - assist identified international user groups in the definition and provision of computer communications facilities;
>   - support and organize conferences.
>
> 3. RARE may negotiate and secure rights in the name of its members but has no authority to undertake obligations or liabilities in their name, unless so instructed by an express authorization from the members concerned.
>
> 4. Generating profits for the purpose of distributing the same among the members shall not be permitted.
>
> 5. RARE shall take an independent attitude towards political groups, whether national or international.
>
> 6. The language of communication within RARE shall be the English language, entirely without prejudice however to Article 22, paragraph 4, last sentence.

Figure 1.4 Extract from the RARE constitution.

entry) application protocols on IBM's VM (virtual machine) mainframe operating system. Later, RSCS was emulated on other popular operating systems such as DEC VMS (virtual memory system) and UNIX. The network was designed to be inexpensive but efficient, so it was built as a tree structure with only a single path from one computer to another. By the end of 1982 the network included 20 institutions in the United States. At this point IBM extended BITNET into Europe. Basically, BITNET began as a network for IBM computer users but was soon opened up to other manufacturers. This increased its appeal to the research and academic environments.

1.5.1
Preparation and Constitution of EARN

In 1982 the management of IBM research centers across Europe launched the idea of building a network dedicated to the research community. In 1983 the first dedicated lines were installed on a national basis. In the following year a set of international lines was deployed, including an intercontinental connection from Rome to the coordination centre of BITNET in New York.

The international lines were installed via an IBM-funded project to support the network over a four-year period. After the establishment of the first international links and the activation of the software, the European partners started to organize the network. An international network like EARN needed a good management structure to handle this organizational activity, distribute information, and address subsequent international issues.

It was a challenge to merge the operational experience gained in North America by BITNET with the requirements of the European research and academic community. The idea had been to define the role of an EARN coordinator for each country and create a Board of Directors. The first meeting of a group which would eventually become this Board was held in Geneva in February 1983; at another meeting later in the year, the participants agreed that Dennis Jennings would be their Chairman and President of the embryonic organization (Figure 1.5 and 1.6). During 1983 and 1984, there were four Board meetings to reach an agreement for the incorporation of the EARN Association in Paris on February 12.

The Articles of Association of EARN, registered in France, specified that EARN is a computer network open to any non-commercial academic and research institution located in Europe, the Middle East or Africa, aiming at information and data exchange to improve scientific collaboration. Looking through the statutes, the following items are notable:

- The geographical coverage includes the Middle East and Africa. This is connected to the fact that the sponsor of the initiative was IBM EMEA (Europe, Middle East and Africa) and that the international lines provided included these areas.

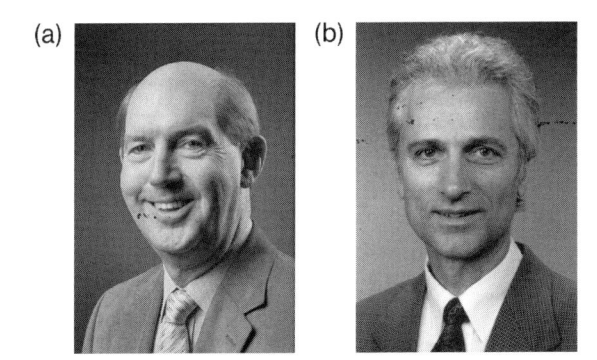

Figure 1.5 EARN Presidents: David Lord (no photo), (a) Dennis Jennings, (b) Frode Greisen.

- The non-commercial nature of the network: this referred not only to the potential partners but also to the utilization of the network.
- The importance and focus on information made available for public consultation.
- The national representation formed by the members of the Board of Directors: Stefano Trumpy was the acting director of EARN, Italy from the preparatory phase until 1990.
- The national contributions to ensure the annual budget for the association.
- The establishment of the following officers: President, Vice-President, Secretary General and Treasurer.

During the meeting of the Board of Directors in December 1984, David Lord was elected President, Dennis Jennings Vice-President, Stefano Trumpy Secretary-General and Jean Claude Ippolito Treasurer. During the October 1986 meeting, Dennis Jennings was elected President, David Lord Vice President and M. Hebgen Secretary-General. The Treasurer remained unchanged. Stefano Trumpy moved to the position of CEPT liaison. At the end of 1987 IBM considered that the network had reached maturity and withdrew its financial support.

In the beginning, IBM's assistance in creating EARN encountered some hostility due to the following doubts:

- Was it IBM's intention to boycott OSI protocols?
- Did IBM want to be the only acceptable manufacturer in universities and research institutions?
- Did IBM intend to dominate the market for networks?
- Telecom operators did not wish to support EARN's ideas.

The problem of the relationship between EARN and the CEPT was first raised during the EARN Board meeting of May 1984. EARN wanted to get support for the network from CEPT but the position of CEPT at that time was as follows:

- EARN, like all data networks, should use OSI protocols as much as possible.
- EARN should use the public X.25 network for its international links.
- Some CEPT members wanted to apply a form of volume charging for their leased lines.

CEPT then specified that these positions had to be considered as recommendations for the national PTTs. At the time, CEPT had a very conservative approach, later contradicted by history. For at least a couple of years, discussions had been very heated. The EARN Board closely monitored the relationships with the local PTTs. The EARN Board position, since the beginning, had been: "to agree to progress towards the adoption of X.25 and OSI but to ask for no volume-dependent component in tariffs for leased lines". In the beginning, British Telecom, the major telecommunications operator in the United Kingdom, wanted to impose one of the highest volume charges. Other PTTs across Europe proposed milder tariffs but the idea of a volume-related charge on top of the leased line cost was retained for some time.

An extract from a communication on the subject from Dennis Jennings to the Board, dated November 1985, reads as follows: "The connection of the United Kingdom on the basis of the imposition of this volume charge (one of the first and the highest), and EARN's implicit acceptance of this volume charge, sets a precedent for the imposition of a similar volume charge by every country PTT in Europe. EARN should never accept the imposition of such a volume charge." It could be said that Dennis Jennings was a good prophet as volume-related tariffs were later abandoned.

The reason for the CEPT position was the fear the PTTs had of losing their very rewarding income from telephone traffic to the networks. The introduction of the volume charges would compensate for this loss of telephone traffic. This situation was severely penalising to researchers in Europe when compared to the cost structure for leased lines in the United States.

The recent evolution of the Internet where VoIP (voice over Internet protocol) has gained momentum shows how conservative that position was. The imposition of using the public X.25 network for international connections was also a conservative position, one that might have been accepted as a compromise.

In 1985 the EARN Board discussed requests to join from institutions in Eastern European countries. At the time, a serious problem was the existence of COCOM (coordinating committee for multilateral export controls) export regulations that prohibited the export of sensitive technology (which covered almost all networking equipment) to communist countries. It was also not clear how the United States Department of Commerce would have reacted to the extension of EARN into Hungary and Poland, the countries which had asked to join EARN. These arguments seem quite amusing today but are linked to the political climate prevalent at the time. The conclusion of the Board was to move carefully and to investigate the position of the United States in this regard. During a Board meeting in October 1986 there was a vote concerning the request from South Africa to join EARN. The request was rejected with ten votes against and only one in favor – at the time, South Africa still implemented an apartheid regime.

There is no doubt that EARN helped spread usage of networks in European academic and research environments. In addition, EARN helped to weaken the domination of the telecommunications monopolies in Europe. EARN can take credit for setting up an international organization capable of designing and managing the network, as well as ensuring the financing of that infrastructure after the financial support of IBM ended in December 1987. At the beginning of 1987, EARN and BITNET were able to connect some 3000 scientific institutions (two thirds of them connected through gateways) with an estimated audience of 150 000 correspondents. Today these numbers do not seem so impressive, but until the early 1990s EARN provided the main instrument for cooperation in Europe amongst research and academic institutions.

The first gateways were activated by BITNET. The most relevant was the gateway to the IBM VM operating system. There was also a gateway to ARPAnet and one to CSNET. Columbia University developed the gateway to DECnet. A gateway was then

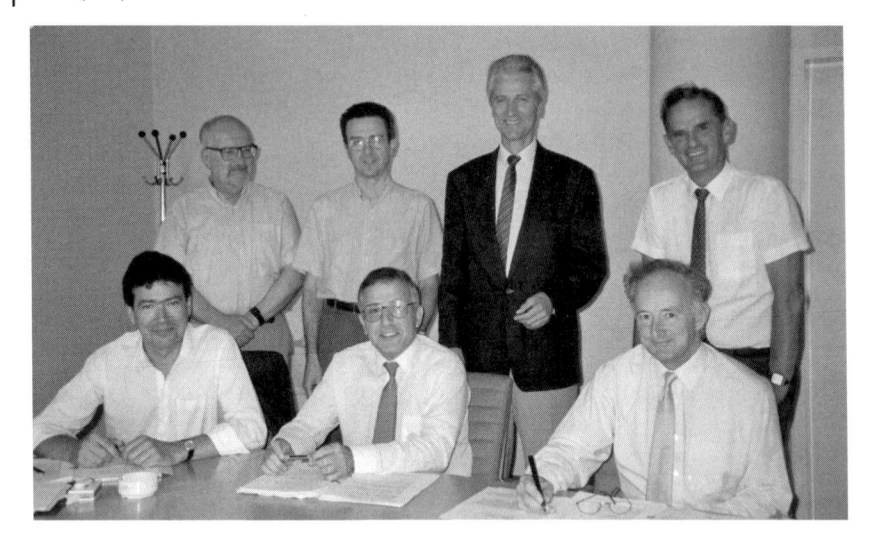

Figure 1.6 The EARN Board of Directors (about 1991). Back row, left to right: Hans Deckers (EARN Manager, not a member of the Board), Marco Sommani (Treasurer), Frode Greisen (President), László Csaba. Front row, left to right: Jean-Loïc Delhaye, Avi Cohen, Paul Bryant (Secretary).

developed for UNIX systems. These gateways were initially developed as test-beds. They were not easy to use and were subject to code errors but gradually became more reliable. Later the number of protocol emulators[1] would reach 32. In this way BITNET and EARN gained the reputation of a heterogeneous network.

The main services provided by EARN were:

- e-mail
- file transfer
- instant messaging
- resource sharing between computers in the network
- access to libraries and databases
- LISTSERV (mailing list server), a system based on a distribution list that supports interaction amongst groups of users with common interests.

The naming system adopted in the first years used the form "hosts.txt", a non-standard convention. ARPAnet adopted the DNS (domain name system) in 1984 and EARN adopted it in the late 1980s. In 1988, DEC began supporting EARN with funds. In 1991, EARN started to use the Internet for data transport and the justification for keeping an independent international structure alive progressively vanished.

By early 1993, RARE – through the COSINE project – had set up the IXI (international X.25 infrastructure) network and its plans for establishing an operational unit were well on the way to fruition. In April 1993, Marco Sommani

---

1) A protocol emulator is a device inserted on a line connecting two computers which use incompatible protocols. It manipulates signals and data passing between the two computers in such a way that it appears to each of them as though it was a compatible machine.

(Trumpy's successor as EARN's Italian Director) and Stefano Trumpy (who was also a member of the COSINE Policy Group, CPG) reported on the possible future of EARN and provided an evaluation of COSINE as follows:

- The COSINE project pulled together the wish for a pan-European network services organization based on the existence of well-organized national research networks while using a federated approach.
- COSINE helped link the research networks with the relevant financing bodies of the research and academic sector.
- COSINE ensured that RARE was involved with the organizational aspects of a pan-European network. The EARN Board tried to promote a role for EARN as one of the major service providers of the academic and research environment, but this failed due to the misconception that EARN was still linked with IBM.

COSINE failed to create user services for the broader community. But on a positive note COSINE created a managed multi-protocol backbone (EuropaNET, European multi-protocol backbone network) and a central structure OU (operational unit) that offered European-scale network services to the research networks. This OU still lacked structure but RARE had a fundamental role in defining that unit. A merger of EARN with RARE could be an excellent opportunity although it had recently been rejected, not through lack of initiative on EARN's part. If the proposal cannot be reformulated, an alternative partner should be found to make the best use of EARN's networking expertise gained over the last decade.

The relationship between EARN and RARE had been discussed for the first time as long ago as 1986 and there had subsequently been an exchange of representation on the two bodies; the EARN President had been nominated as the EARN representative on the RARE Council of Administration and RARE had become an EARN international member.

Despite these elements of cooperation, a merger with RARE was not generally favored within the EARN community and another year would pass before the topic was taken up again.

1.6
IXI

On completion of the COSINE specification phase as a result of the work undertaken by RARE during 1987/8, it was decided that the first step in the COSINE implementation phase (CIP) would be to establish a pan-European network for the academic and research community, which became known as IXI (International X.25 infrastructure).

The European PTTs were still mostly state monopolies. The concept that they should provide their customers with a "one-stop shop" for an international service was a novel one. They were contemplating setting up a joint MDNS (managed data network service) venture through the CEPT and at first it was thought that this service might be used to meet the research networks' requirement. In practice, the MDNS never materialized but an offer was received in October 1988 from the Netherlands PTT Telecom with several other telecom operators in Europe as sub-contractors.

Preliminary discussion within and between the organizations involved started in autumn 1988. Because of the urgency of setting up a service, it was decided that the technical planning and implementation of IXI would be carried out by staff from the research networks in parallel with continued negotiation of the COSINE implementation phase execution contract (CIPEC) with RARE. Since the CIPEC was not yet ready to be signed, RARE was not in a position to take responsibility for managing the funds required for IXI and the EC took on this role.

RARE established the IXI co-ordinating committee with one representative per participating organization to provide overall direction of the project and the IXI project team to provide day-to-day technical management. A contract between PTT Telecom (now KPN, Koninklijke PTT Nederland) and the EC acting on behalf of the CPG was signed in October 1989 and the pilot service started a few months later. The full IXI service was officially inaugurated on June 8 1990 in The Hague.

For the first few months, service availability and reliability were poor, due to software problems with the X.25 switches. These problems were mainly in the software modules that had been implemented to meet IXI's specific requirements. IXI was meant to be a one-year pilot service, but it continued until October 1992 when it was replaced by the European multi-protocol backbone (EMPB) network. By this time, the 64 kbps bandwidth was a major limitation. In addition, many of the connecting research networks were moving towards the use of IP (Internet protocol) rather than X.25.

The IXI project was started because it was clear that the international interconnections provided by the public X.25 networks were inadequate to support the European research community and match the bandwidth available nationally. Subject-specific networks, such as HEPnet (high-energy physics network), were starting to be established but it was clearly necessary to establish an interconnection for the national research networks for their general traffic. Although the initial target was for access at 64 kbps, it was a stated requirement that access at 2 Mbps should be available in due course because the requirements of this user community would obviously grow. In the research network environment, traffic was typically doubling every year.

There were many issues that had to be addressed in the IXI planning phase, technical, organizational and political. Many research networks had been created to support universities and government research laboratories and because of national connection policies (sometimes determined as a result of in-fighting between different ministries) could not widen their range of client organizations; others were already moving towards support for the whole education sector. "Acceptable use" rules also varied and while it was easy to get agreement that the transport of "commercial" traffic should be forbidden, there was no agreed definition of which traffic was "commercial".

Despite the PTTs' earlier exploration of the MDNS (or perhaps as a result of it) PTT Telecom in its lead role in IXI found itself in conflict with some of the other PTTs, particularly when it had to locate a network switch on another PTT's premises. Sometimes it was even difficult to get good quality service specified in the contract. Perhaps fortunately, the EC agreed to be the contracting party on behalf of the CPG, rather than RARE having to accept the risks involved. PTT Telecom was concerned, however, that the EC would try to use the contract to get the European PTTs to drop their restrictive practices. The EC was concerned that RARE should not be too flexible in the negotiations with PTT Telecom, to ensure that the EC's policy aims were met. It was issues like these that resulted in long drawn-out contract negotiations.

While the CIP execution contract was still being negotiated, RARE did manage to create the necessary working groups and project team by using experts from the national research networks, consultants and its own staff. All those involved found the project interesting, if challenging. The organizations accessing IXI also had to take responsibility for supporting their IXI connections, not only to support their own users but also to ensure that users from other networks could access them. RARE developed software to test both the initial delivery of network connections and the ongoing performance of the network as a whole. The initial acceptance tests ensured that a newly connecting network was able to reach all the other connected networks over IXI. There was concern from PTT Telecom that RARE's ongoing performance-monitoring would itself load the network unduly. Yet this extensive testing helped identify problems before they had an impact visible to the user networks; it also provided early availability and reliability reporting before it was available from PTT Telecom.

It was not straightforward to get digital connections (64 kbps) for all the COSINE countries for IXI and this issue was one that had to be pressed on PTT Telecom. The Nordic countries shared a single 64 kbps connection and JANET, the United Kingdom national research network, upgraded its connection to 128 kbps in July 1991. The other network connections remained at 64 kbps as the upgraded service, EuropaNET, was being tendered. In the case of Greece, 64 kbps was not provided until EuropaNET was rolled out. Slovenia connected in June 1991, as it happens at the same time as it separated from the Federation of Yugoslavia. Other countries in Central and Eastern Europe had connections to IXI, and later to EuropaNET, funded by the EU under the PHARE (Poland and Hungary: Assistance for restructuring their economies) program.

It was intended that IXI should provide connections for the national research networks, a limited number of international research centers and the public X.25 networks. The public X.25 connections enabled industrial and other researchers to use the IXI service without having to connect to their national research network. In Table 1.1 of IXI connections, the connections are categorized as NREN (National

Table 1.1 Numbers of IXI connections.

IXI connections	NREN	PSPDN	Sites	Total
April 1990	10	3	3	16
At end of 1990	12	4	7	23
April 1992	13	10	6	29

research and education network) including NORDUnet and PSPDN (packet-switched public data network), public X.25 networks sites) international research centers, such as CERN as well as the EC in Brussels.

IXI was the first pan-European network serving the whole research community. The experience gained from this was fed into the successor networks managed by DANTE (delivery of advanced network technology to Europe).

Leased Circuits

At the time when this story starts, telecommunication services almost everywhere in Europe were provided by the same government body that was responsible for the postal and telegraph services, commonly known as the PTT. The main exception was the United Kingdom where competition was first introduced by the grant of a licence to Mercury Communications in 1982, following the establishment of British Telecom as a state-owned company the previous year. When a PTT was split up, the branch which then offered telephone services joined the set of Public Telecoms Operators (PTO), later known as Public Network Operator (PNO). The national PNOs continued to hold a monopoly on the provision of telephone and data transmission services within their country. In some countries, the PNO was owned by the government; in the others, the PNO was controlled by the government.

Digital circuits had only recently been brought into use with 64 kbps adopted as the basic transmission speed, sufficient to handle a single phone call including the signaling needed for call set-up and other management functions. Digital technology was intended by the PNOs to improve the way in which voice telephone services were provided. However, the PNOs did not recognize the scale of the revolution that computers and digital technology would eventually provoke and they appeared to be primarily concerned with making improvements to their telephone services. Circuits could be leased from the PNOs but their use was subject to restrictions. In particular, the re-sale of the circuit capacity was forbidden and switching traffic between third parties was also not allowed.

International leased circuits were normally provided in the form of two "half circuits" one half circuit being provided by the PNO at each end. The tariff for each half circuit was specified in the standard price list of each PNO. If the circuit had to pass through a third country or countries, the additional cost would be reflected in the half circuit tariffs at each end; payment to the PNOs of the intermediate countries for the transit service they provided was handled by the PNOs at each end. The price of circuits bore very little relation to the cost to the PNOs of providing them and was universally high. In some countries, the PNO was effectively used as a hidden tax collector, with the government taking advantage of its PNO's surpluses to reduce the amount they would otherwise have to collect through some more overt form of taxation.

Dealing with user requirements was not high on the PNOs' priority list. Although an indication of delivery delay might be given, one PNO could not be expected to take responsibility for failure by one of its partner PNOs to deliver by a fixed date. When customers, including those in the research community, demanded higher circuit capacity or other services which a PNO was not providing, the standard response was along the lines of "We don't believe that you need this, therefore we will not provide it; and since it is not available, you cannot prove your need". The PNOs were primarily concerned with protecting their lucrative monopoly of voice traffic and were reluctant to make available what they considered to be the basic elements of their infrastructure to organizations which might find a way of exploiting these elements in competition with them.

The liberalization of European telecommunications took effect on 1 January 1999 following several years planning and legislation managed by the EC and it had a dramatic effect. Restrictions on the provision and use of leased circuits were abolished, existing PNOs were free to provide services outside their former national territory and new PNOs (in many cases, companies which had already exploited the possibilities opened up by earlier liberalization within individual countries) were able to expand and extend their coverage internationally.

Under the new regime, customers can acquire a set of leased circuits between several countries from a single supplier and all the major European PNOs can now cover all the countries of the EU with equipment and circuit capacity that they control. In practice, the redundancy and duplication of resources which this implies is not as great as might be expected. Although the newcomers and the established national PNOs had taken steps in the years immediately preceding liberalization to extend their networks, no single organization owns infrastructure that covers the whole of Europe and there is a considerable amount of trading at different levels.

Installing a vandal-proof cable between two cities which are several hundred kilometers apart is a major exercise. There may be civil engineering problems in finding a suitable route, burying the duct which carries the cable, and crossing rivers and other obstacles; there are legal and administrative issues, particularly concerning rights-of-way and access to the repeater stations that are needed along the route.

A PNO which has already dug trenches across one country, installed ducts in the trenches and laid a group of optical fibers in the ducts is in a position to trade on several levels. Such a PNO can make a swap arrangement with a PNO in another country ("you can put your fibers in my ducts if you let me put my fibers in yours"). More commonly, there will be an exchange of fibers, leaving each PNO free to decide what use to make of the fiber's capacity and which type of equipment to control and manage the services for which it is used. In some cases, one PNO might simply lease a fully equipped fiber from another PNO. Through some combination of these arrangements, an organization can claim to have Europe-wide coverage.

Since liberalization, a new facilities management industry has been created. Specialist property development companies (often formed by a consortium of PNOs) have constructed buildings which are designed to meet the needs of operators who wish to interconnect their services. The buildings are equipped with highly reliable power supplies (including back-up in case of failure of the mains supply), tight access control systems and security procedures, and ducts which allow cables to be installed easily between any two points in the building. PNOs can rent space, install their own equipment and use the location as an interconnection point for both their own circuits and for exchanging traffic with other PNOs (such a location is commonly referred to as a "point of presence" or PoP).

The effect of the competition between PNOs which was introduced by liberalization has been to reduce prices (in terms of cost per unit of transmission capacity) by several orders of magnitude, to provide a better match between price and cost of provision, and to allow PNOs and their customers to introduce new services which go far beyond the voice telephony which was traditionally supplied.

It may be noted that although DANTE provides services to only a relatively small but distinct community and does not act as a PNO, it operates by leasing circuits or fibers from a number of PNOs and, since the installation of the GÉANT (gigabit European academic network technology) service, has a network which is more extensive and which has a higher aggregate capacity than any of the commercial network operators in Europe.

2
The Role of Funding Bodies

In order to create a pan-European research and education network, a number of management groups are required. Some of these may already exist but others may have to be created. Country specific requirements often need to be taken into account. This chapter explains how the major European groups emerged and developed, how they needed to interact with government agencies to gain recognition, and how they got the necessary funding for their operation. It focuses mainly on the years from the mid-1980s to the mid-1990s.

2.1
EUREKA and COSINE

As a result of the discussions during the EUREKA (European Research Coordination Agency) meetings in November 1985 and February 1986, it was accepted that the newly established RARE organization was to elaborate a plan for a 1-year COSINE specification phase but it took some time to get things organized. Some countries, and the EC, did not subscribe to the German view that, in essence, the function of COSINE (cooperation for open systems interconnection networking in Europe) was to collect money for RARE to do whatever it felt should be done. Some of the deliberations were informal. For example, Horst Hünke from the EC arrived one night in Zoetermeer (where the Dutch Ministry of Education and Science was located) for discussions with Peter Tindemans, Karel Vietsch, Frank van Iersel and Hans Rosenberg; the last of these had been instrumental in getting RARE going financially and legally. Similar discussions took place later with Johan Martin-Löf from Sweden, who played a key role in this early phase, together with Birgitta Carlson.

Two meetings of what was to be the CPG with standardization bodies were necessary before the ground was sufficiently cleared to make the actual start in Stockholm in January 1987. Eventually 19 countries plus the EC were to participate. A COSINE Policy Bureau (CPB) was elected, consisting of Peter Tindemans as President, Keith Bartlett from the United Kingdom Department of Trade and Industry and Arne Moi of the Norwegian Ministry of Education, Research and Church Affairs as Vice-Presidents. Nicholas Newman was made available by the EC as more or less full-time secretary, and John Beale was to be the EC's first project

A History of International Research Networking. Edited by Howard Davies and Beatrice Bressan
Copyright © 2010 WILEY-VCH Verlag GmbH & Co. KGaA, Weinheim
ISBN: 978-3-527-32710-2

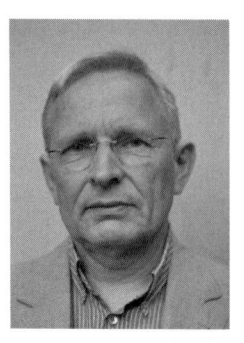

Figure 2.1 Chairmen, COSINE policy group: Peter Tindemans, Horst Hünke (no photo).

officer, a necessary role because the formal contracts would be concluded by the EC on behalf of the COSINE partner countries. Horst Hünke in whose unit all the relevant EC officials actually worked became a member of the CPB as well. Regular CPB-RARE liaison meetings were set up not only to ensure a closer overview of ongoing work, but also to discuss the more political aspects of an emerging European networking infrastructure (Figure 2.1).

The funding arrangement for the COSINE specification phase, costing 2 MECU (Millions of ECU, the European currency unit) of which 0.8 MECU would come from COSINE participants and the rest as in-kind input from RARE) entered into force on July 1 1987. The contract between the EC and RARE was signed and RARE started on the task of defining standards, operational, migration and other requirements for key information services to be provided during the subsequent COSINE implementation phase. RARE delivered its technical work on the COSINE specification phase in June 1988; it was reviewed in September 1988 in Brussels.

In the meantime, preparations had started for contracting the first operational service, IXI, a pilot pan-European service based on X.25. In anticipation of a another funding arrangement between the COSINE partners, now for a 3-year CIP, an MoU (memorandum of understanding) was concluded between the EC and RARE to create an interim COSINE project management unit (iCPMU) to continue work on the X.25 backbone and to make detailed plans for other activities. The final CPMU (COSINE project management unit) would not be established until after some tough discussions both with RARE and within the CPG, but eventually the view prevailed that COSINE needed a dedicated CPMU as a central technical and operational team instead of merely relying on the existing RARE bodies. The new funding arrangement was agreed in June 1989 together with the CIP execution contract with RARE, in which a distinction was made between a core package (X.25, gateways to the United States, X.400 message service, directory services, FTAM (file transfer and access management) and additional and future services. The funding arrangement required 30 MECU of which 20 MECU, mostly for IXI, came from the EU.

One might say that the view of a separate management unit was vindicated later when DANTE was established in 1993 as an incorporated company to take over operational responsibilities for the successive backbone networks in Europe. RARE, now evolved into TERENA (Trans-European Research and Education Networking

Association), has successfully focused on development, dissemination, training, and exchanges of views and so on. The CIP was completed in 1993 and the CPG, chaired by Arne Moi since May 1991, continued in the form of the High Level Officials Group for Computer Networking for Research and Technological Development.

The story told so far is straightforward from the OSI perspective on networking. However, it was not an undisputed view of how things would best be organized, and turned out to be an increasingly disputed one. Of course COSINE had not come out of the blue. On the official side (EC, CEPT and European industry) there was the European Harmonisation Activity (the so-called Zander initiative). In the science community a variety of, usually company-backed, practical networking initiatives had been set up, such as EARN, EUnet (European UNIX network) and HEPnet with varying allegiance to OSI.

Thus a parallel track was pursued within COSINE, especially by the CPB, though it was a source of significant contention: how to create a European networking infrastructure for the benefit of all, and one that would be supported by all. The CPG, the CPB (though less so) and RARE were divided on how strongly to adhere to OSI, on what to think of TCP/IP and other issues. With hindsight, it seems fair to say that the CPB and pragmatists within RARE were instrumental in making the community of scientists, politicians and industry accept a much more flexible approach, which then led up to a dominance of IP-based services.

One critical development was a Joint Statement reluctantly agreed upon by RARE, EARN and EUnet in the spring of 1988, though it was never "ratified". But it did lead to Joint Working Group A comprising RARE, EARN, EUnet, CERN/HEPnet and the EC information exchange system (IES) facilitating communication between the partners of ESPRIT with CEPT as an observer to work out the details of an X.25 (1984) backbone linking all the national and international inter-research networks. No doubt the prospect of the EU paying a considerable part of the cost of future infrastructure contributed strongly to the willingness of the various parties to participate, given the financial problems faced by all the research networks at the time. (It should be noted that the government of Norway was not only willing to co-fund but gave the good example of how governments and the EU could have acted). As a further aside: Joint Working Groups B (on messaging) and C (on directory services) were soon to be incorporated in the RARE WGs.

Another development was the 1991 ECFRN (European consultative forum on research networking) initiative taken by the Chairman of the CPG outside the formal scope of COSINE, but with the explicit encouragement of the CPB. The ECFRN meeting took place in Paris on March 8 1991 in an environment which was by then much less marred by ideological controversies. It was meant to lay the foundations for the post-COSINE era without the restrictions that COSINE was formally tied to (OSI, no high bandwidth services yet, difficulties with involving organizations such as CERN or ESA, the European space agency, etc). Agreement on two general basic principles, namely "serve the users first and foremost" and "standardization after implementation" was followed by the identification of crucial areas for further work.

An ECFRN Steering Group chaired by the EC was established, and it has certainly been instrumental in improving the European situation, amongst others by helping into existence a policy body to take over eventually from the CPG. The lines along which to work were no longer contentious. Creating a pan-European organization for planning, implementing and running communication services, more central funding for operational services and not only for research, as well as the need for longer-term planning covering successive generations in terms of speed and quality were agreed upon, while concern was raised about the competitive disadvantages of pan-European carrier services and the reluctance of European manufacturers to engage in product development and to use research networks as test-beds for this purpose. RARE's decision in principle in January 1991 to set up an operational unit, later spun off in the form of DANTE, has met the organizational challenge. Large amounts of EC funding, the need for which was no longer disputed, responded to the second one and enabled longer-term planning, while liberalization has created a much more dynamic European market for network services.

It took a long time for COSINE to deliver, too long, and it did not deliver the OSI world as it was supposed to do. Yet COSINE has been an important step in European research networking. One may always speculate whether the European scene would have drastically improved in any case without COSINE: the answer is "most likely". But it is equally true that COSINE was the crucible from which emerged the crucial ingredients for a European networking infrastructure for R&E (research and education), today a pillar of the European research area.

Though IXI itself suffered from some teething troubles and was relatively slow in attracting large amounts of traffic, it did set the stage for all successive generations of pan-European networking backbones. No serious discussion that Europe did need such an infrastructure was necessary afterwards.

The emphasis in COSINE on having a professional and dedicated unit responsible for defining the specifications of the various services, and especially for implementing and providing those services, has been a major factor, first in establishing the CPMU, and later in RARE's creation of the operational unit and DANTE. That was also the basis on which RARE's, and later TERENA's, role could be defined more clearly and to the great advantage of European users, and later many more users in other continents as well. Against significant initial reluctance to bring together the various networking communities with their separate networks, traditions, standards, financing mechanisms and so on, it was already clear early in the COSINE implementation phase, that is, in 1990 and 1991, that this was the way to go. Subsequent developments have borne out this reality.

Finally, through the discussions in the CPG and through preparing for the post-COSINE world via, for example, the ECFRN initiative, COSINE has considerably enhanced the awareness among policy makers, both at the national and the European level, that a research networking infrastructure is worthy of policy interest, and that significant central European funding is indispensable, together with the contributions of research networks and/or governments. The rapid succession of pan-European networks shows that a funding model and a parallel policy track have developed to ensure an astounding increase in bandwidth, quality and connectivity of networking services in Europe in less than 15 years.

2.2
EC and National Governments

COSINE was, in many respects, the odd man out, as it was a EUREKA project and not an EC (European Commission) one. EUREKA projects were supposed to be near-to-the-market and industry-driven. However, COSINE was set up by several governments, namely, all the EC member states, all the EFTA (European Free Trade Association) countries and Yugoslavia. Whilst a number of people involved clearly saw it as a project with a high political profile, others considered it largely as a technical project.

It was not surprising that Germany came up with COSINE under the EUREKA umbrella. Many countries, primarily the United Kingdom, stressed the bottom-up nature of EUREKA meaning that companies or, if necessary, research centers would be its primary drivers. However, Germany saw EUREKA as a vehicle not only for industrial cooperation in high technology areas, but also for projects that improved European infrastructure (e g. for research, transport or communication) as well as for projects focusing on cross-border problems. These three categories were even incorporated into the so-called Hanover declaration of 1985 which formed one of the founding documents of EUREKA.

Peter Tindemans, the Chairman of the CPG during its most turbulent phase, agreed with this vision. He went even further than the IT (information technology) research directorate-general of the German ministry in emphasising the crucial role of government in creating, or at least enabling, an advanced computer communications infrastructure for research as a European requirement, and for research cooperation in particular. Today, one would say that such an infrastructure is vital for the "European Research Area". In fact, that is exactly how the GÉANT (gigabit European academic network technology) infrastructure is now described in official policy documents from the EU.

EUREKA projects provided a good way of involving policy decision makers in the project; the bi-annual meetings of the EUREKA High Level Group were an excellent platform to present progress and discuss requirements with those responsible for science and technology policy in EUREKA member states. However, being a EUREKA project created problems as well. The relationship between the EC services and EUREKA has always been strained. From the German perspective an active and financially high profile role for the EC was thought normal. The programs were meant to be complementary but in reality it was not that simple. In the specification phase of COSINE the EC role was financially restricted. However, the EC was still visibly present, for example, during the important contribution made by Nicholas Newman. He was made available by the EC and appointed secretary of the CPG to deal with all contractual aspects. We must not forget the close involvement of Horst Hünke. Yet, it was clear that the relationship between COSINE and the EC was not always without conflict. ESPRIT, the successful R&D programme in information technology was up and running and the telecommunications R&D programme RACE (research for advanced communications in Europe) was already defined and about to start in late 1987.

As part of ESPRIT, several services had been set up to facilitate collaboration amongst participating companies and research institutes. It was not easy for the EC to accept that the goal of COSINE was all-encompassing, in the sense that it was to create an infrastructure serving all of Europe's research, making dedicated international communication services which targeted only a specific user group redundant. When the EC was willing to pay a substantial share of the cost (eventually two thirds of the budget of COSINE's implementation phase) an attitude of "who pays the piper calls the tune" compounded the confusion. During the summer of 1989, the rumors about two EC-supported network projects, X-net and later Y-net, (at the time when the final details of IXI were being elaborated) were often shrouded in mystery. This illustrated the mixed feelings of some members of the EC. The protracted procedures and the complexity of the EC organization were then, as now, formidable barriers. These were perhaps nicely illustrated when Peter Tindemans arranged a meeting one night in February 1989 with Director-General Michel Carpentier to try and solve some hiccups when he found himself opposed by officials from six layers of the EC hierarchy: Carpentier, Parajón-Collada, Cadiou, Hünke, Sanderson and Newman. Overall, however, the EC played a very constructive and indispensable role.

EUREKA and its relationship with the EC was not the only instance where COSINE both benefited and suffered from a rather complex situation. That was even more apparent in the 1980s when the world of ICT (information and communication technology) was in a permanent state of flux. As the interest of national governments and the EC in networking had started to grow, the promises of benefits for economies and societies were extravagant. National policies in the area of information or information technology abounded and covered broad areas of government responsibilities. These were not only in R&D, but also in education as well as applications for government and other important sectors of society. The initiative of EC Commissioner Davignon to bring together Europe's twelve largest IT manufacturers and have them cooperate "pre-competitively" under the ESPRIT banner proved very successful. The budget for what was supposed to be a five year program had run out after three years. Hence the wide support amongst governments for COSINE was not surprising. However, the institutional environment was changing rapidly.

The privatization of British Telecom and the liberalization of the United Kingdom telecoms market in the early 1980s set in motion a Europe-wide drive to create a market for telecoms services that would operate under more standardized conditions. The EC took the lead in trying to enforce this, but obviously this only started in the mid-1980s, so COSINE saw life in a period of considerable antagonism.

The EC wore many hats and not all of them were easy to reconcile. Pushing for legislation to abandon the telecom monopolies that existed in most countries (in some Scandinavian countries the situation was different) was one of those hats; strengthening the European telecom industry another one. They went hand in hand in theory but, in practice, the monopoly power of the telecom operators proved to be very challenging.

RACE had been defined by the same twelve companies that were at the origin of ESPRIT. Difficult compromises made at the inception of RACE in order to accommodate the companies' ideas about future broadband networks were supported by the EC but the ideas were not always shared by the telecom operators who still wielded considerable power. The strategic games played between the PTTs, manufacturers and EC had an impact on COSINE and one result was delay.

COSINE's second objective, (the first one being the provision of a user service), was to provide an early opportunity for vendors to demonstrate their OSI products and to create a market interest for those products. The EC strongly supported this aim, and this resulted in many discussions and a number of attempts to bring European industry on board. For industry, however, COSINE largely seemed to be another opportunity to get EU funding for development work, and this sometimes translated into an attitude that came close to saying "just give us the project and the money".

On the other hand, the PTTs were trying to organise themselves to offer Europe-wide MDNS through a joint venture set up by national PTTs under the aegis of CEPT. Such efforts took time, but were eventually abandoned. All these factors were perhaps partly responsible for what turned out to be a major bone of contention (viz. the commitment to OSI standards on the part of the EC and some national governments, notably the United Kingdom and Germany, but equally amongst PTTs and companies). Not that the latter were front runners in offering OSI-based services and products. That would have made a difference, because a fairly widespread agreement existed that an OSI world on paper looked beautiful, if only it had been demonstrated quickly and on a large scale.

The funding system for research networking in Europe was another factor that was very different from the situation in the United States. The research networks were funded on a national basis and they were not in a position to fund international connectivity on the scale required. Up to and including the 5th Framework Programme, the EC's mandate was limited to research, development and some demonstrations, and did not extend to funding operational services. The only exception was the IES which offered a number of communication support services to partners of ESPRIT projects. This is where the funding for COSINE originated, but getting it was no easy matter.

It is fair to say that the United States context differed substantially in several ways. The large defense efforts not only created a very early demand, but also provided funding and the freedom to come up with solutions.

2.2.1
Impact on the Internal COSINE Debates

COSINE was not immune to the debates taking place in the world at large over standards and the organization of the new data communications world, as the outside world was not totally in agreement with OSI. Organising pan-European research networking was another issue that divided both COSINE and RARE, and hence had a considerable influence on their relations over time. The initial debate on the organisation of the COSINE project, starting at the beginning of 1986, was in reality prolonged until the CIP documents neared completion in early 1990. In the German COSINE proponents' view, RARE was to rule the waves, with the governments and the EU supplying the funding. Most countries did not agree, nor did the EC. The result was a much more formal customer-contractor relationship. The country representatives in the CPG were the customers and RARE was the contractor.

On a few occasions, most notably at a CPG meeting in Paris in December 1988, it was even considered to opt for an open tender and not automatically give the COSINE contract to RARE. That was not, of course, a real option but the reasoning was serious. The CPB was strongly convinced of the need to create a professional, business-like organizational model for pan-European computer networking. At that time, RARE was not only new but very much organized as a platform for technical discussions and exchanges of views between research networking organizations. COSINE was there to establish an operational network.

The debate flared up time and again. It took a full year, until early 1987, to get the foundation documents on COSINE agreed, especially those concerning the structure of the project and the role of RARE. True, RARE had nothing much to do with this, it was an internal discussion between government representatives. However, other developments did concern RARE. The CPB-RARE liaison meetings were set up right from the beginning to discuss progress on the COSINE work and the best way to organize the implementation phase.

After completion, in the summer of 1988, of the specification phase deliverables and the documented results of studies carried out according to the terms of the contract, the CPB felt that the planning and the organization of the CIP needed much more input from the governments. The result was that a joint CPB-RARE task force was established in November 1988 to produce the outlines for the CIP. A few of the concerns of the CPB focused on the need to establish a dedicated unit inside RARE to deal with COSINE but one that did not conflict with the existing organizational units (the secretary-general and the working groups). In the summer of 1989 an interim CPMU was established and this was soon followed by the real CPMU. The debate inside RARE continued and led to a decision in January 1991 to create an independent operational unit which eventually, in 1993, became DANTE. All of this required some walking on thin ice, and was one of the reasons why obtaining agreement on the CIP funding arrangement and the CIP execution contract turned out to be so difficult.

The other major reason concerned the financial aspects. Germany wanted the EU to pay 100%, others did not want an exclusively EU-funded implementation phase and the EC itself had difficulties in reaching a conclusion and deciding on the conditions under which the EU would contribute. Within the CPG the debate on standards was not always a debate about technical merits. This was partly due to the policy focus of the group: the CPG was always a somewhat eclectic mix of people, some coming with an overall science policy perspective and others with a background in networking. Some members were very strict in adhering to the OSI basis, whilst others were inclined to be more relaxed. In all outside presentations and in the perception of the outside world, COSINE has always been an OSI-based project. Of course, in the later stages it became clear that a pure OSI view was no longer tenable and the multiprotocol backbone that was to be specified (it became part of the CIP) was one manifestation of this shifting position.

The real debate in COSINE was on reaching out to other networking communities, EARN in the first place, and to a lesser extent EUnet, or for example the CERN/HEPnet community. EARN was vociferous and put itself forward with the aim of establishing a different network model. It was not limited to one specific discipline, as most of the others were.

Based on the conviction that a truly European solution, which COSINE wanted to create, needed to encompass everyone, Peter Tindemans started, in the middle of 1987, to explore what basis cooperation was possible; first with Dennis Jennings and next with both Dennis Jennings and Peter Linington. This initiative was supported by some members of the CPG, tolerated by most and rather fiercely opposed by a few. By the end of 1987 RARE, EARN, EUnet, CERN/HEPnet and the IES were drafting a joint statement concerning the principles of cooperation in networking. It was to be approved by their various governing bodies in the spring of 1998 but when that turned out to be difficult, the substance of the statement was acted upon and three Joint Working Groups were established. Joint WG A took on the task of specifying an X.25 backbone which was eventually the basis for IXI. The two others, on messaging and on naming and directories, were soon incorporated into the existing RARE WGs.

It was not long after this, from 1990 onwards, that the big "unification" gradually took place. Yet, late in 1990, the CPB was still concerned that more effort was needed as part of a broader attempt to ensure that Europe drastically improved its networking situation and that it would have to do so in a more pragmatic way than COSINE could pursue.

This was the basis of the ECFRN initiative. Discussed many times in the CPB and the CPB-RARE liaison meetings, the CPB did not feel free to take the same initiatives that a COSINE body could. It stimulated the chairman, Peter Tindemans, to organize this in a personal capacity. In the end, some 70 people representing all the organizations involved in one way or another in networking in Europe accepted his invitation for a meeting on March 8 1991 at Charles de Gaulle airport in Paris. RARE, national and EU policy makers, industry, PTTs, organisations such as CERN and ESA, research networks and so on, were all represented. Two documents had been prepared, one on the European situation and another on North America.

In the changing atmosphere of 1991, it was no longer necessary to follow the formal limitations and opposing policy requirements that characterized COSINE. The dominance of TCP/IP was becoming evident, the need for high bandwidth services was growing fast and it was evident that CERN, ESA and the other multilateral research organizations had an important role to play. As a result, two basic principles were agreed, namely "serve the users first and foremost" and "standardization after implementation".

Everybody agreed that several crucial steps had to be taken to put European research networking on a par with that of North America. Creating a pan-European organization for planning, implementing and running communication services was one such step. Reference was made to the ongoing efforts in RARE which resulted in the operational unit and afterwards DANTE.

It was also concluded that more central funding was required, not only for research but also for operational services. Emphasis was put on longer-term planning covering successive generations in terms of speed and quality. The short-term focus should be on a 2 Mbps multiprotocol backbone on which work had already started but a 34 Mbps pilot would soon be necessary as well as Gbps migration pilots for local and research networks. The EC accepted to chair an ECFRN Steering Group that was set up to raise awareness at a high political level and to make sure that after the CPG ceased, a policy forum would still exist. In addition, it would engage in discussions with PTTs on the competitive disadvantages of pan-European carrier services and with industry for greater involvement. Large amounts of EU funding, the need for which was no longer disputed, provided a response to industry, and enabled longer-term planning. Liberalization created a more dynamic European market for network services.

The ECFRN Steering Group met several times and it interacted with the successor to the CPG, the High Level Officials Group. This group largely spawned EuroCAIRN (European cooperation for academic and industrial research networking) which would lead to TEN-34 (trans-European network at 34 Mbps) and to the European Networking Policy Group, ENPG. As a result of liberalization, tariffs have been reduced and performance has increased. The concerns about usage-based charges were already laid to rest with IXI. Most of the wishes of the ECFRN participants have thus been fulfilled and even European industry is doing much better.

Throughout the period of the development of European research networking, the biggest single source of funds has been the EU. Collectively, however, national governments have funded more than 50% of the total costs through payments for services by the research networks. Other sources of funds have acted on a smaller scale and have supported specific projects which have resulted in significant developments in a number of cases. During the early years, when the COSINE project was in operation, the EC had the responsibility of managing the financial aspects of the project which was funded by the EUREKA programme; in the later stages of the project the EC also provided the chairman of the CPG, Horst Hünke. The IXI network was part of the COSINE project and the cost of its operation was the subject of a contract directly between the EC and PTT Telecom of the Netherlands; payments under the contract were made directly to PTT Telecom and were not visible to the research networks.

This situation changed when EMPB started operating. The research networks became responsible for paying PTT Telecom charges and were then partially reimbursed from COSINE funds, which covered roughly 50% of the cost. For later generations of European networks, the EC itself provided funds from the Fourth and subsequent Framework Programmes. A series of projects followed the same sequence of steps: submission of the project proposal, approval of the project (often with minor changes to the proposal), negotiation of a detailed Technical Annex to a standard EC contract, signature of the contract, EC payments – an advance payment and further payments which were dependent on acceptance of defined deliverables – to the Coordinating Partner within the project, distribution of EU funds to individual project partners by the Coordinating Partner according to the terms of a Consortium Agreement. In all cases, the research networks were ultimately responsible for paying the total cost of the services provided, even though the EC contribution was more or less guaranteed.

The administrative procedures associated with this sequence of steps were at times laborious and many engineers were often frustrated by the requirements imposed by a large and complex bureaucracy. A particular difficulty in the early years was that the EC funding was provided from projects whose mandate was to fund research, and the EC had no authority to fund infrastructure in support of research. Although the work carried out by the research networks involved a large element of R&D, there was a clear mismatch between the objectives of the national research networks, which were primarily to provide services, and the ability of the EC to supply funds within the constraints imposed by the terms of its budget approvals. Project proposals had to be "dressed up" with emphasis on the R&D aspects of the work program in order to get past the EC's project evaluation procedures. Too many engineers felt that it was self-evident that their ideas and proposals deserved funding and were unwilling to understand or even to find out about the constraints under which EC officials were working. This sometimes resulted in mutual irritation between both groups.

As time went on, there was a greater appreciation on both sides of what needed to be done and how best to present requirements to higher authorities. By the Sixth Framework Programme, provision of infrastructure was an authorized activity for the EC, and both the funders and the recipients had gained valuable experience in working together. Funding of new developments still had to be justified and was subject to strict evaluation procedures, but the roles of both parties were better understood and had led to a smoother working relationship.

The bulk of the EU funds came through the Telematics program of DG XIII, but other EU programs have made significant contributions. The most notable of these was the PHARE program, which provided support for the introduction and improvement of network services to the Central and Eastern European countries following the collapse of the Soviet bloc. PHARE was a program of DG I which handled the EU's relations with countries outside the European Union (the equivalent of the Foreign Ministry in a national government). Although the activities undertaken in relation to research networks were ultimately successful, the early stages provided a textbook example of what can go wrong when funding bodies and recipients do not communicate effectively.

The EC's first step in 1993 was to provide equipment and connections which were the same as had been provided through IXI to the Western European networks two years earlier without realising that technology preferences had radically changed. As a result, the equipment remained largely unused until DANTE arrived on the scene and, via a management contract with the EC, acted as a bridge between the funders and recipients.

Even then, matters were not straightforward. DG I's lack of staff with relevant technical expertise, its caution in dealing with outsiders who might have something to contribute and, for a long time, the absence of anyone in the EC who felt the obligation to understand and to disentangle the components of a complex situation, led to extreme slowness by the EC in making payments. These payment delays (which, in DANTE's opinion, represented a clear breach of contract) added to DANTE's already considerable cash flow difficulties and also put the reputations of DANTE and PTT Telecom in jeopardy. It was only with the appointment by the EC of an effective Project Officer that order was slowly restored, and the relationship between DG I officials and the CEEC (Central and Eastern European Countries) research networks became smoother.

With hindsight, DANTE might have approached the situation differently, for example by cooperating more closely with PTT Telecom at an earlier stage, but its experience of the PHARE program underscores the need for recipients of funds to take the trouble to understand the aims and procedures of the funding body.

3
Organized Cooperation

This chapter looks at the various governing organizations that had been established and, where necessary, replaced. It explains the interactions between them and the conflicts of interest that arose leading up to the new millennium. DANTE and TERENA are two such organizations that exist today. The origins, differences and problems arriving at this point in time are looked at from a TERENA viewpoint.

3.1
The Activities of RARE

As the association of European research networking organizations and their users, RARE's aim was to foster cooperation between both national and international research network organizations in order to develop a harmonized international communications infrastructure. RARE merged with EARN to form TERENA in 1994, but there are a number of other organizations and initiatives that RARE established which are still active today. Perhaps the best known of these are the Operational Unit, which was then transformed into DANTE, and RIPE (Réseaux IP Européens). In both cases RARE acted as midwife and provided an early home to allow these organizations to grow and flourish on their own.

The annual RARE Networkshop was held in May each year. In 1990 in Killarney, Ireland this became the RARE EARN Joint Conference, continuing as the annual TERENA Networking Conference following the RARE/EARN merger. The 1994 Joint European Networking Conference, which was held jointly with the Internet Society's Annual Conference (INET), had over 1100 participants from some 100 different countries – a significant increase from the 60 or so participants from perhaps 15 countries at the first European Networkshop held in Luxembourg in 1985.

The RARE Secretariat was established in NIKHEF (Nationaal Instituut voor Kernfysica en Hoge Energie Fysica) which provided its first permanent home at the WCW (Wetenschappelijk Centrum Watergraafsmeer) in Amsterdam in June 1987 (Figure 3.1). In 1991 RARE took over responsibility for employing its own staff, and at the end of the year the office moved to a central location in Amsterdam on the Singel, which remains the TERENA office today.

A History of International Research Networking. Edited by Howard Davies and Beatrice Bressan
Copyright © 2010 WILEY-VCH Verlag GmbH & Co. KGaA, Weinheim
ISBN: 978-3-527-32710-2

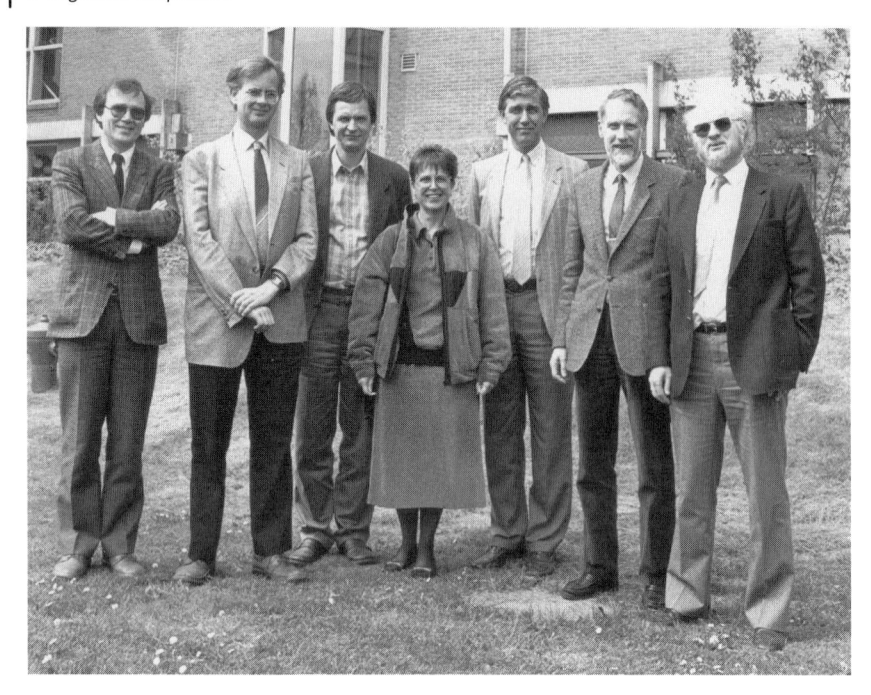

Figure 3.1 The RARE executive committee, 1988. Left to right: Kees Neggers, Peter Linington, Klaus Ullmann, Birgitta Carlson, Rob Brinkhuijsen, Jürgen Harms, James Hutton.

RARE's first service activity was the Pilot MHS (message handling service), which was operated by staff of the Norwegian Research Foundation SINTEF (Selskapet for INdustriell og TEknisk Forskning ved norges tekniske hoegskole) in Trondheim. This project supported users of the X.400 protocol including access to non-X.400 mail systems through gateways. The project was funded by the EU, France and Norway.

At the end of 1989, 20 countries were participating in this project. There were more than 100 000 users connected through 530 installations with 15 different X.400 implementations. At this stage all international traffic was carried over the public X.25 network. The IXI network was used once it became available. In 1991, the MHS project was moved under the COSINE umbrella and was subcontracted to SWITCH, the NREN in Switzerland.

The work for the COSINE specification phase was the major activity of RARE and its Working Groups in the period up to 1988. The overall reports based on these detailed studies were produced by RARE's COSINE project management team.

RARE and its members were also active outside Europe. In October 1987, a meeting was held between those involved in European and United States networking at which it was resolved to create the CCIRN, the coordinating committee for intercontinental research networking. At this stage the United States federal departments undertaking research each had their own network or networks, often running different protocols. Thus NSFnet and ARPAnet were using TCP/IP whereas NASA (National Aeronautics and Space Administration) and the DoE (Department of

Energy) Energy Sciences Network (ESnet) were mostly using DECnet. For the first few years, two meetings per year were held and other regions joined. It proved a valuable forum to enhance the mutual understanding of the differing approaches and structures in different areas of the globe. The CCIRN saw its role as providing a forum where policy level problems could be discussed and resolved. In 1990, the CCIRN created the IEPG, the Intercontinental Engineering and Planning Group, to give technical support to its activities. The IEPG continues as an informal gathering that meets on the Sunday prior to IETF (Internet Engineering Task Force) meetings. The intended theme of these meetings is essentially one of operational relevance in some form.

The RARE Working Group meetings allowed technical experts from across Europe to meet together and exchange ideas and thus develop a strong collaborative basis for the provision of pan-European services. These meetings were funded by the EU separately from the COSINE project.

The Working Groups each operated according to the technical requirements of the area concerned. For example, WG6 organized a number of symposia to promote higher speed services for the research community (Figure 3.2).

In 1991 it was realised that the activities of the Working Groups established in 1986 no longer matched the priorities of the research networks and that a new structure was needed. The RARE Technical Committee was created to oversee the ongoing technical programme. Working Groups were established in areas where there was seen to be a long-term technical interest, whereas a Task Force was established where a specific, and relatively short-term activity was to be undertaken. Following the 1991 reorganization, the RARE Working Groups were as follows:

- International character sets
- Interactive multimedia
- Information services and user support
- Lower layers technology
- Mail and messaging
- Network applications support
- Network operations
- Security technology

3.2
The Gestation of DANTE

In early 1991 there were a number of activities going on in parallel. Consensus was growing within RARE that a new organization, a dedicated operational unit, was needed to take on operational tasks resulting from projects like IXI and COSINE.

In May 1991, the EEPG (European Engineering and Planning Group) stressed the advantages of developing a multiprotocol backbone. Furthermore, the COSINE services had been running for some time and there was a need to plan for their continuation. RARE, as the contract holder for the COSINE implementation phase,

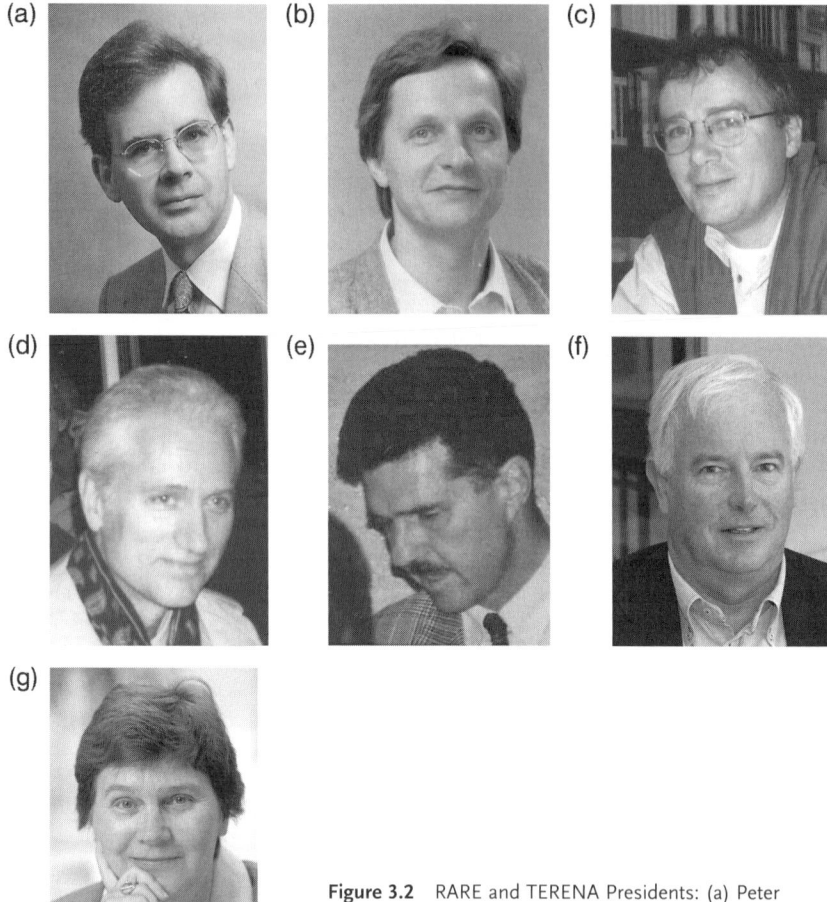

Figure 3.2 RARE and TERENA Presidents: (a) Peter Linington, (b) Klaus Ullmann, (c) Kees Neggers, (d) Frode Greisen, (e) Stefano Trumpy, (f) David Williams, (g) Dorte Olesen.

had addressed the question of future service provision for the education and research community, and at its CoA (Council of Administration) meeting in Blois in May 1991 it established a task force to examine the possibility of creating a new entity to take responsibility for the provision of pan-European backbone and value-added networking services. ("OU" was quickly adopted as the working name for whatever organization the task force would eventually propose.)

The task force was established with the following mandate: "To propose to the CoA the organization of an OU under the guiding principle of a single OU for all services". These services should include X.25 (IXI), IP (Ebone, i.e. European backbone), e-mail and directory services, any other services which had been initiated by COSINE and EARN, and even the RIPE NCC (Réseaux IP Européens Network Co-ordination

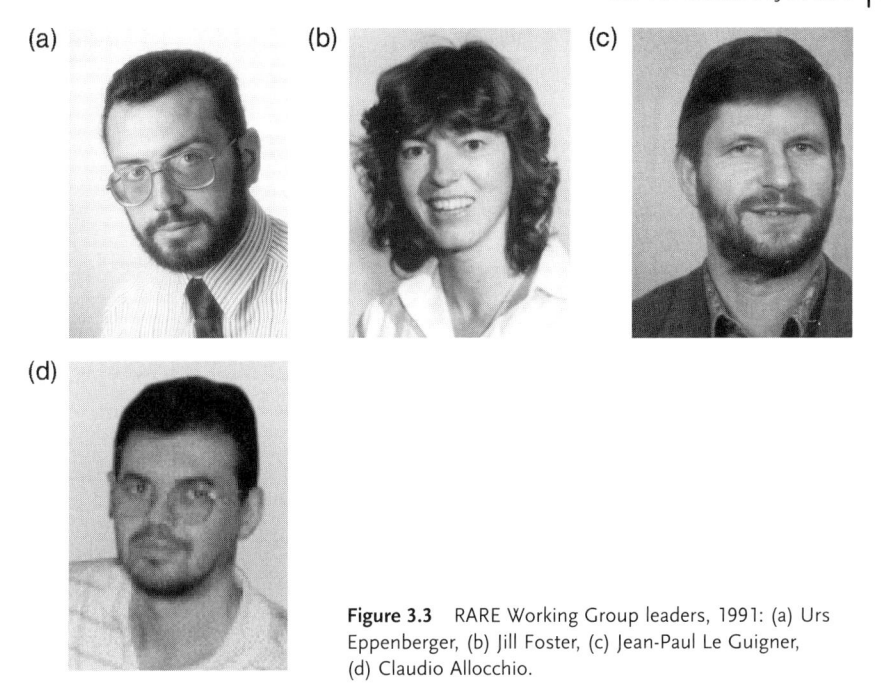

Figure 3.3 RARE Working Group leaders, 1991: (a) Urs Eppenberger, (b) Jill Foster, (c) Jean-Paul Le Guigner, (d) Claudio Allocchio.

Centre). The task force was formed with Dai Davies (CPMU) as chair, Frode Greisen (EARN), Klaus-Eckart Maass (DFN), Christian Michau (CNRS, Centre National de la Recherche Scientifique and UREC, Unité Réseaux du CNRS), Boudewijn Nederkoorn (SURFnet, the NREN in the Netherlands) and Bernard Delcourt (previously Secretary-General of RARE) as secretary.

3.2.1
The Process and the Structure

The gestation of what became DANTE (delivery of advanced network technology to Europe) was a process of several steps. The TF-OU (task force operational unit) held its first meeting on June 28 1991 and produced its final report six months later on January 16 1992, after ten meetings and after issuing two interim reports. The final report (in a yellow cover but normally referred to as the "Green Report") presented the objectives of the OU, the organizational options, ownership issues and establishment planning, governing principles and an initial business case. The task force recommended the CoA to proceed with the formation of an OU based on a Collaboration Agreement between interested parties involved (i.e., the research networks). The task force report also presented a first draft of the main elements of such an agreement (the "Heads of Agreement") based on the recommendation that the OU would be set up as a conventional company limited by shares. Once the

Collaboration Agreement (later: Shareholders Agreement) came into effect, the new body would appoint temporary management to set up the OU. RARE would approach the EC and COSINE to seek financial and political support for the unit. The task force presented a launch and start-up plan lasting one year (1992) to get the OU fully established. That timetable turned out to be too optimistic. The bootstrapping process required another two steps, the establishment of a constituting Shareholders Meeting with all interested parties involved and an OUSC (operational unit steering committee) of seven people reporting to the Shareholders Meeting. The three major tasks were:

- Further refinement and eventual conclusion of first the Heads of Agreement and then the full Shareholders Agreement.
- Further development of the initial business case and preparation of policy decisions related to it.
- Step by step implementation of the OU along the lines described in the Heads of Agreement.

The first Shareholders Meeting was held on April 10, 1992. The Heads of Agreement were finalized in mid-August 1992 and presented to the research networks for signatures. By 1993 a sufficient number of signatures had been collected to justify the setting up of a private company in Cambridge, United Kingdom, limited by shares and called OU Ltd, for the time being fully owned by RARE. This step was taken on March 30 1993, after another 6 Shareholders Meetings and 17 meetings of the OUSC. Initially, the OU Ltd was only a vehicle to facilitate the start-up of the real OU. Until that time, all commercial and operational activities remained where they were (with COSINE, EARN, etc.).

The final step was a transformation of the empty OU Ltd owned by RARE into a fully implemented and operational company as proposed by the task force, owned by the interested research networks. That implied collection of start-up money from the future shareholders, employment of two General Managers, renting premises in Cambridge, hiring staff, changing the name to DANTE and gradually taking over service provision from RARE/COSINE. The Shareholder Agreement came into effect on March 17 1994 after another 3 Shareholders Meetings and 8 OUSC meetings. At this date research networks representing more than 50% of the total share capital had signed the Shareholder Agreement. Finally, on March 25 1994, the first Shareholder Meeting of a fully established DANTE took place.

The gestation of DANTE has to be seen against the background of the so-called protocol war between OSI and IP. Most of the problems and conflicts that caused delays can be explained by the influence of the protocol war. The troubled relationship between COSINE and the Ebone initiative was a clear example. The Ebone integration into the OU failed and the late entrance (or even non-entrance) of some research networks as shareholders had its roots in this protocol war. The company had to start from scratch with respect to funding. The need to collect and to attract enough working capital was the major issue that determined the legal form of the company, the timing for taking over services from COSINE and even the location of DANTE in the United Kingdom (which offered tax exempt status). The working capital issue was on the agenda of all meetings of (future) shareholders and the OUSC. Finding the right legal and governing structure with many parties involved and many degrees of freedom took a lot of time and effort. The proposals from the initial task force had not been modified drastically and the final result did not differ much from the original proposals.

3.2.2
Relationships with Other Bodies

The EC was expected to contribute to the start-up money but these funds did not materialize and in the end COSINE funds were used only for co-funding of services. RARE was the legal body that operated on behalf of the shareholders until DANTE was fully established and, as such, was indispensable. The wish to have one single provider for all services also did not materialize. After the planned integration with Ebone failed in September 1992, Ebone became a commercial IP-provider; integration of EARN only took place two years later, when RARE and EARN merged; the RIPE NCC became an independent organization. DANTE was fully built upon the results of COSINE (EMPB and its successors). Nevertheless, DANTE became the major provider of pan-European backbone services for the research networks in Europe. The implementation of the company required close attention in order to resolve the problems that arose unexpectedly, but involved the resolution of a large number of minor issues rather than of one major issue.

At the time of the initial task force, where and under which legislation the OU would be established was not yet known. Lawyers advised that the Unit should be established as a private company under the law of an EC member state. The OU would increasingly be dependent upon dealing with the private sector and most contractors understood the limited company format. It was also expected that a private company could easily be established and there might be some tax advantages in doing this. After the United Kingdom had been chosen as the location of the OU, two possible structures were considered:

- a company limited by shares
- a company limited by guarantees.

The second choice would normally be considered the most appropriate for a not-for-profit environment and the choice of the first option was based on the need to collect working capital and to address the question of voting weights that had become an issue within RARE.

To deal with these two matters, issuing shares was a necessary ingredient (next to the building of reserves by some profit making). Voting rights of the owners would be weighted according to financial commitment. (With hindsight, the choice of the company limited by guarantee might have been better. The DANTE structure was the source of a number of difficulties in the ensuing years, and, in 2007, the first steps were taken to transform the company into a company limited by guarantee).

The free and unlimited issue of shares to every interested research network was a step too far. It could create a distribution of voting rights that would destabilize the cooperation between the research networks. For that reason, a scheme was developed where the biggest shareholders (like DFN) would have 15 times as many shares as the smallest (like RESTENA, Réseau Téléinformatique de l'Education Nationale et de la Recherche). There are restrictions on the ownership and transfer of shares. The initial set of shareholders and the allocation of shares to them was specified as part of the procedure setting up the company. It is possible for a shareholder to transfer its shares to another organization but this organization must be located in the same country as the transferor, it must perform roughly the same functions as the transferor, and the transfer must take the form of a gift for which the transferor receives no payment. This scheme has essentially not changed over the lifetime of DANTE. In a second round of share issuing (doubling) the take-up was optional; not all research networks used the opportunity to buy additional shares.

There was a clear choice for the "continental" model for the governing structure: General Meeting of Shareholders, a Board of (non-executive) Directors and the Management. This choice was not contested after the establishment of DANTE in the United Kingdom; the structure with three levels was still preferred, even though the Anglo-Saxon model with only two levels (shareholders and executive directors) is much more common there. During the second and third steps of the establishment, RARE was exclusive owner of the company. The decision-making process was, nevertheless, in the hands of the Shareholders Meetings and the OUSC. A MoU and indemnification contract was signed between RARE and the (future) shareholders, and it implied that the shareholders were carrying full responsibility for all actions.

In the first interim report of the TF-OU in September 1991 a first draft of the business case was presented. It forecast that the turnover would grow to €15.5 M in 1996 and that working capital of at least €2 M was needed initially, growing to a comfortable level of €6 M. In the final report of the task force (January 1992), these figures were refined to a level of €16.8 M revenues in 1996, but the minimum level of working capital was raised to €4 M. Collecting capital turned out to be very cumbersome, and it was agreed that the minimum level to be able to run backbone services could be lowered to a more risky level of €3 M.

At the end of 1992, those who had signed the Heads of Agreement were asked to contribute some start-up money to finance the preparation of the OU. There were different opinions on the status of that money (was it a loan, prepayment of shares or prepayment for services?) but the financial problems were so persistent that it was agreed that "the invoices will be "customized" if necessary, so as to meet specific shareholders' requirements". In fact, the company capital at the start in March 1994 was only €0.5 M, causing many difficulties. The employment of the General Managers in 1993 was only possible on the basis of a guarantee of the salary costs of one of them by DFN, and with the use of COSINE money for the salary of the other. Building up further capital was only possible by making profits and/or by issuing more shares.

The real figures in 1996 turned out to be a turnover of €18.1 M and a capital level of €2.8 M (€1.1 M share capital and €1.7 M accumulated profits). In 2006 these levels had grown to €55.8 M turnover and €7 M (€1.6 M share capital, €5.4 M accumulated profits). In later years, EC procedures for the funding of projects helped to relieve the working capital problem. The EC contribution generally covered 40–50% of total project costs and as much as 50% of the budgeted cost might be paid in advance. (At one stage, being used to dealing with large corporations which had reserves counted in hundreds of millions of euro, EC accountants were worried about handing over several million euro to a small company in Cambridge. What was there to stop the General Managers from disappearing with the money? The banks were not prepared to offer the EC any financial guarantee since they had no control over the company's actions; the Directors, being non-executive, were not in a position to check the day-to-day operation of the company's bank accounts over which the General Managers had total control. It was only after hard work on the part of the EC Project Officer and his immediate colleagues that the accountants were persuaded that there was no alternative to simply trusting the General Managers.)

Back in the early days, however, after the launch of the first services in the second half of 1993, the General Managers complained about the payment behavior of several research networks which added to the difficulties they already faced. It was mainly because of shortage of working capital that backbone services could only be taken over in 1994. The final report of the TF-OU in January 1992 targeted three types of shareholder: 19 members of RARE (European research networks), seven associate members of RARE (four Central European research networks and three from other continents), and nine international organizations, giving a total of 35 potential shareholders. In the final Heads of Agreement six months later, the figures had changed drastically.

Five Nordic research networks decided to operate under one umbrella, NOR-DUnet; there was no real interest from the international organizations and the research networks decided to keep it simple. According to the Heads of Agreement, 15 European research networks plus NORDUnet were allowed to buy shares. If approved by the signatories of the Heads of Agreement, this could be extended to research networks from the Czech and Slovak Republics, Hungary and Poland.

On October 22 1992 signatures of the Heads of Agreement were received from France, Germany, Greece, the Netherlands, Portugal, Spain and Switzerland. Further signatures were expected from Belgium, Italy, Slovenia and the United Kingdom. Ireland formally announced on October 19 1992 it would not sign the Heads of Agreement. Its position was the following: "The Network Management Committee (NMC) of HEAnet requires seeing clear definitions of:

- how the shortfall of capital will be obtained
- what the minimum services will be
- the cost structure of these services.

The NMC also feels that no artificial acceptable-use restrictions should be placed on any IP backbone infrastructure for Europe, and that such an infrastructure should be able to carry both commercial and research traffic. In addition, the NMC feels that the scale of the RARE OU is inappropriate at this time, and that a less costly model for an OU which focuses on coordination and management of existing on-going research networking activities would be more appropriate. Lastly, the NMC is concerned at the haste with which the OU is being put together, and with the control orientation of the OU, and fears that this will result in inappropriate decisions on the appointments of the OU Management."

On February 17, 1994 the Shareholder Agreement was presented for signature to the following 12 countries: Belgium, Switzerland, Germany, Spain, Greece, Hungary, Italy, the Netherlands, Nordic countries (NORDUnet), Portugal, Slovenia, and United Kingdom. These countries were entitled to buy shares of £1 each, up to a total amount of 610 500, according to a distribution scheme that had already been presented by the TF-OU in early 1992. A number of countries were missing: Ireland (no change in position since 1992), France that had had an active role until early 1993, but became more or less detached from the mainstream European cooperation in research networking (despite having been represented in the task force and in the OUSC) when there was a change of Director at RENATER (Réseau National de Télécommunications pour la Technologie, l'Enseignement et la Recherche); and Austria (a strong supporter of Ebone and disappointed by COSINE). Croatia, Luxembourg, Poland and the Czech and Slovak Republics were candidates as shareholders but were not yet ready to join.

As soon as Shareholders applying for 305 250 Shares in aggregate (50% of the possible total) had executed the Agreement, it would come into full force and effect. On March 17 1994 signatures were received from Germany, Hungary, Italy, the Netherlands, NORDUnet and the United Kingdom and the Shareholder agreement came into full force. However, the signature of NORDUnet was presented with some reservations. The message on March 16 was: "the NORDUnet board yesterday confirmed its intention to sign the Shareholders Agreement and the application for shares. We found, however, that we would not propose a candidate for the new Direction to be elected." NORDUnet had expected "more openness in the technical field and a more open attitude to collaboration with Ebone."

On March 25, 1994 the first Shareholder meeting under the Shareholder Agreement took place. All the signatories were present except Belgium. At a late stage, the Belgian representatives felt that the value of participation did not justify the costs or the time and effort needed to convince government officials to allow them to sign the agreement. Until 1999, the remaining 11 countries were the only shareholders. In that year France and the Czech Republic also became shareholders, later followed by Luxembourg and Ireland. Belgium and Austria remained outside. At the first Shareholder Meeting under the Shareholder Agreement (March 1994), a Board of Directors was elected. Klaus Ullmann, Fernando Liello and Boudewijn Nederkoorn had all been members of the OUSC. Juergen Harms from SWITCH was also elected and the position that had been reserved for Peter Villemoes was left open for some time. At its second meeting, in September 1994, the shareholders elected Geert Hoffmann from the Centre for Medium Range Weather Forecasting as a Director. Geert Hoffmann was the only Director without an affiliation with a research network.

Backbone services as of August 1994 were provided to many more countries than those which held shares in DANTE (Table 3.1). Research network organizations

Table 3.1 EuropaNET (backbone) access ports (July 1994).

Country	Research network	Public data network	Capacity (kbps)	Service
Austria	ACOnet		64	IP
Belgium	BELNET-IP		1984	IP
	EC		64	X.25
		DCS	64	X.25
	JRC-Geel		64	X.25
	RESULB		64	X.25, IP
Czech Republic	CESNET		512	IP
Denmark		DATAPAK	64	X.25
Germany	WIN		2048	X.25, IP, CLNS
Greece	ARIADnet		64	X.25, IP, CLNS
		HELLASPAC	64	X.25
Hungary	HUNGARNET		64	IP
	BMEnet		64	IP
	PLEASE		64	X.25
Ireland	HEAnet		64	X.25, IP
Italy	GARR-IP		2048	X.25
	GARR		64	X.25
	JRC/Ispra		64	X.25
Luxembourg	RESTENA		64	X.25, IP
		LUXPAC	64	X.25
Netherlands	SURFnet-IP		1984	IP
	SURFnet		64	X.25, CLNS
		AMS-GWY (to commercial ISPs)	1984	IP
		DN1	64	X.25
	ESAPAC		64	X.25
Portugal	RCCN-IP		64	IP
	RCCN		64	X.25, IP, CLNS
		TELEPAC	64	X.25
Romania	ICI		9.6	X.25
	PUB		9.6	X.25, IP
Slovenia	ARNES		128	X.25, IP
		SIPAX.25	64	X.25
Spain	REDIRIS		2048	X.25, IP, CLNS
	IBERPAC		64	X.25
Sweden	NORD-IP		1984	IP
	NORDUnet		64	X.25, CLNS
Switzerland	SWITCH-IP		1024	IP
	SWITCH		128	X.25, IP, CLNS
	CERN		1024	IP
	Gateway EuropaNET-Ebone		512	IP
UK	JANET-IP		2048	IP
	JANET		2048	X.25, IP

3 Organized Cooperation

Table 3.2 EuropaNET Intercontinental Connectivity (July 1994).

Circuit	Capacity (kbps)
Amsterdam-Washington	2048
Geneva/CERN-Washington	1536
London-Korea	64

which were not share holders could also use the intercontinental capacity shown in Table 3.2.

3.2.3
Management and Staff

In April 1992, the first Shareholder Meeting issued a request for proposals for the location of the OU. Six proposals were received and two months later an evaluation group was formed: Alexis Arvilias (Greece), Jose Barbera (Spain), Juergen Harms (Switzerland) and Fernando Liello (Italy). Proposals were received for locations in Amsterdam, Bonn, Brussels, Cambridge, Copenhagen and Paris. The evaluation group shortlisted Bonn and Cambridge. These two locations received similar assessments in terms of quality and availability of office accommodation and staff housing (good) and accessibility (by car and rail – at best fair) but then the evaluation group realized that the issue of corporate taxes had not been mentioned in the initial guidelines. Enquiries with the United Kingdom government showed it was likely that the company would be granted the status of a "Research Association" which meant that it would not be subject to corporation tax on any surpluses it generated. This was the deciding factor in the choice of location and, in November, the shareholders decided in favor of Cambridge with five votes for Cambridge, two for Bonn and three abstentions.

A first call for applications for the post of Managing Director of the OU had been issued in August 1992. Soon thereafter, the procedure was postponed until a decision on DANTE's location was taken as this would influence the attractiveness of the job for a candidate. After the choice of Cambridge, a second call was issued at the end of November 1992. The call asked for candidates with a sound experience in operational data networking, a proven management track record, sensitivity to customer needs and the ability to deal with governmental funding bodies. Salaries would be appropriate to an international job with high managerial responsibilities.

Six applications were received and three shortlisted by the OUSC. On January 19/20 interviews were held in Copenhagen and two candidates ended more or less ex aequo: Howard Davies and Dai Davies. Both were well known by the OUSC and while the OUSC was contemplating which one to choose, the two candidates jointly presented a proposal to form a management structure with two General Managers.

The idea was accepted and the "Davies twins" would become General Managers of the OU. Financial problems prohibited direct employment of the General Managers. Dai Davies became interim General Manager from April until September 1993 (still paid by COSINE) and Howard Davies could only be contracted from September 1993 on the basis of a guarantee by DFN of continuation of employment until May 1995 should the OU become insolvent.

The OU TF-OU had proposed an international organization with a headcount of 12. With two General Managers from the United Kingdom and the company location in Cambridge, the General Managers were asked to attract staff members as far as possible from countries other than the United Kingdom. On March 31, 1994 a first call for staff (four positions) was issued. The first staff members came from Spain, the Netherlands, Germany and Finland.

Finding a name for the company turned out to be difficult. In the course of 1992 several names were suggested but none received any real support. By spring 1993, the issue had become urgent and Howard Davies came up with the name DANTE: as an acronym, it could be expanded to the officially registered name "Delivery of Advanced Network Technology To Europe Limited" (he actually had no other explanation for the name other than that he liked it!). Nobody had a better proposal, so in July 1993 the OU became DANTE.

In the minds of the founding fathers of DANTE, the OU would become the single provider of pan-European services for the national research networks; its governing structure and business model were based on that. DANTE would invest in connections, equipment and people, and would deliver services at its own risk. Income would come from tariffs set by the company, supported by EC funding, and business would be carried out with a liability limited to the level of the shareholder capital.

In practice, EC funding of up to 50% of costs became paramount for the development of the consecutive generations of the backbone network (EuropaNET, TEN-34, TEN-155, GÉANT and GÉANT2). The whole provisioning of services, investments to be made and tariffs to be set (in the form of cost-sharing agreements) became part of the EU projects. The role of DANTE became more and more a coordinator of EC projects rather than a self-governed organization providing services on demand and on behalf of the founders (shareholders). Related to these projects, parallel governing structures were developed (NREN Policy Committee, GÉANT Executive). Decisions about investments are now taken by all 30 research networks united in the NREN Policy Committee, tariffs are also set there in a sometimes cumbersome process and all risks are carried by the research networks.

This has led to sub-optimal decision-making processes and a disputed view on the ownership of assets. Things could improve if all research networks became shareholders. Only half of the 30 European research networks using DANTE services are shareholders. It has turned out that the structure of DANTE as a company limited by shares presents a serious obstacle to joining for research networks with close ties to their government and a restructuring is being considered. We could say what the Irishman was supposed to have said: "If I wanted to get to there, I wouldn't have started from here." However, the need to collect initial capital obliged DANTE to start from where it did.

The difference between the plan for the OU and the reality of DANTE has contributed to confusion over its role. Two basic issues underlie this confusion: is DANTE a commercial organization? Yes, in relation to its suppliers; no, it is part of the research community in relation to the research networks. And are the research networks customers, partners or controllers of DANTE? The answer is "all three, at different times". These two issues can never be completely reconciled and the confusion is compounded when the company is viewed from different perspectives. Some people take the trouble to understand why DANTE acts as it does, and judge it by results measured against realistic criteria. Others still think of it as it was planned, and a third group ignore the actual position and express their views on the basis of what they think the company should be doing, something that may be quite different from both the plan and the reality. No wonder newcomers to the scene have difficulty understanding how all the pieces fit together.

3.3
RARE and EARN: the Merger

During the first part of 1993, with the EMPB and Ebone networks in operation and the community committed to the use of manufacturer independent protocols, it was becoming increasingly obvious that the EARN network service, and consequently the EARN Association, had no long-term future. With some reluctance, the EARN Board of Directors concluded that some action was needed to maintain those activities that were still of value. Some of the research networks realized that services were being increasingly duplicated at the European level and felt they were paying twice for the same thing. They sought ways of reducing expenditure at a time when budgets were under strain, and intensified their efforts to find economies. The research networks, through RARE, were establishing the OU as a vehicle for providing international services and there was little scope for EARN to take new initiatives in that direction.

The alternative to simply closing down the EARN Association was to find a way of continuing the services that were still in demand, in collaboration with some other organization so, in May 1993, a joint meeting of the EARN Board of Directors and the RARE Executive Committee agreed that they would start negotiations with a view to merging the two organizations. The issues that the EARN Board of Directors wished to see resolved if the EARN Association was to be closed down were: continuation of the operational services which were still of value to end-users, fair treatment of EARN employees who would be affected by any change in the organization, the disposition of the reserve funds that the EARN Association had built up during its lifetime and, last but not least, recognition of the role that EARN had played in the early development of European research networking.

The two services which EARN were particularly concerned about were NJE and coordination and maintenance of LISTSERV software. (NJE is a protocol and a set of tools, originally developed by IBM, for managing the sharing of resources and the distribution of tasks between several machines in a network. A coordination function is necessary for the administration of machine names and addresses, user access control and so on. LISTSERV is an applications package which permits users to set up and manage their own mailing lists).

Terms of employment seemed likely to be a difficult issue since RARE was based in Amsterdam while the EARN Association had offices in Paris. Given the pressure to reduce costs, concentrating staff in a single location would have to be considered.

The negotiations extended over several months. At an early stage, the two options of closing down both organizations and starting from scratch with a new one (which would require a complex set of legal steps), and for RARE to take over the functions and responsibilities of EARN which would then be closed down (which would be administratively simple) were rejected in favor of a third option. This was to merge the two organizations by adapting the statutes of RARE to take account of changes in its role, and by changing its name in order to emphasize the revised nature of its functions.

Further detailed negotiations concluded with a proposed set of statutes and rules of procedure for the new organization. They specified, amongst other things, that the organization and its secretariat were to be based in Amsterdam and set up as an Association under Dutch law, the conditions for membership, overall control was to rest with a General Assembly composed of all members, an Executive Committee with nine members, including the President of the organization, a number of Vice-Presidents and several ordinary members. The size of the Executive Committee was deliberately large so that both parent organizations could be well represented, a choice of voting schemes, one of which provided for members to be assigned to one of seven categories according to the GNP (gross national product) of their country, the number of votes allocated to members of a given category being greater than those in lower categories, and less than those in higher categories.

At a meeting of the RARE Council of Administration on October 24 1994, to which EARN representatives were invited as observers, RARE members unanimously approved the amendments to the statutes and the accompanying regulations, the changes became official, and the meeting continued as the first General Assembly of TERENA.

The first tasks of the General Assembly were to agree changes to the membership list which arose as a consequence of the merger, to confirm approval of the proposed regulations, to decide on the voting system to be used in decision-making and to use this voting system to elect the first President, three Vice-Presidents and five ordinary members of the Executive Committee.

The voting scheme that was selected was the GNP-based banded scheme mentioned earlier. The smallest countries in terms of GNP (and international members) were allocated one vote each; the largest countries were allocated seven votes. The General Assembly also decided that the same categories would be used to define individual membership fees, but with a broader range of values: members in Category 1 would pay one unit per year while those in Category 7 would pay 16 units per year.

3 Organized Cooperation

The first vote was for the position of President and there were two candidates for this position, one of them (Frode Greisen) previously associated primarily with EARN, the other (Kees Neggers) with RARE. It was generally accepted that Kees Neggers as the outgoing President of RARE would go on to lead the new organization and that the election would be little more than a formality. The actual result was very close, with the "EARN" candidate receiving 56 votes and the "RARE" candidate 53. The individual members appear to have voted according to their previous allegiance to one or other of the parent organizations, and the result came as a big surprise to many people, not least the two candidates.

The new Executive (Figure 3.4) inherited the responsibility of ensuring that steps were taken to deal with the practical issues that arose from the merger. Decisions were needed on staffing levels, on the matching of staff numbers to the activities that had to be performed, on the organization of those members of staff who were retained, and treatment of staff who would be affected if the Paris office were closed, as well as arrangements for continuation of the NJE and LISTSERV services.

The research network members were already concerned that although €1 M had been set as a guideline for the total budget of TERENA in 1995, the cost of running the organization based on existing staffing levels would be €1.5 M and it was not clear how the gap between these two figures would be bridged. While it was possible that additional income might be gained by finding new projects, the lack of specific examples, the absence of a transition plan for moving to a more cost-effective organization and a lack of

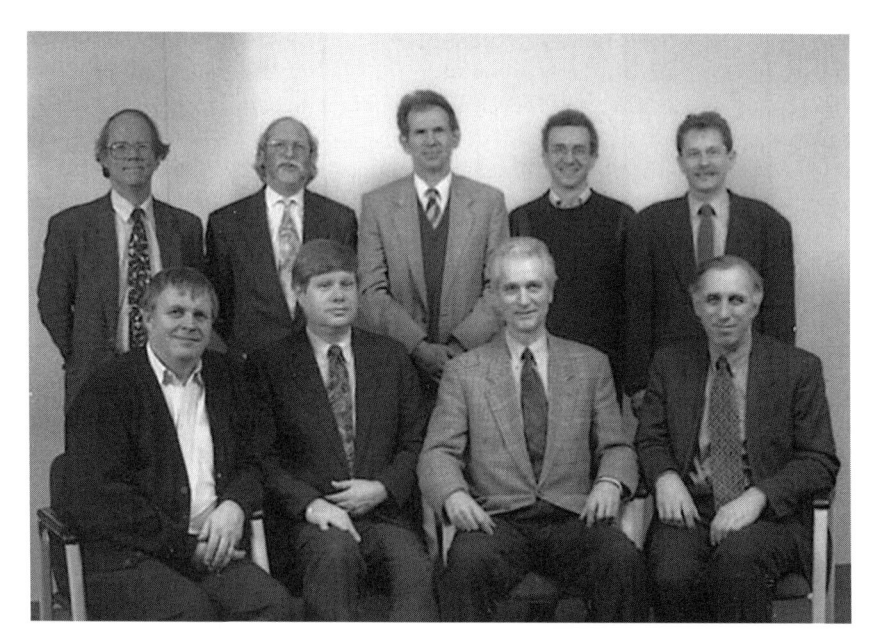

Figure 3.4 TERENA Executive Committee, 1995. Back row, left to right: Brian Gilmore, Paul Van Binst, Peter Bakonyi, Marco Sommani, Bernhard Plattner; front row, left to right: Sven Tafvelin, Steve Druck, Frode Greisen, Peter Rastl.

clarity about its financial viability, led members to ask for a special meeting of the General Assembly in December 1994 for the specific purpose of discussing financial matters.

At the December meeting there were ominous signs that the new organization was not working well. There was still no plan for a transition to a lower budget and no date had been fixed for the closure of the Paris office. Several members expressed the view that, because of the low level of benefit they were getting from TERENA, they could justify only Associate Membership rather than full membership in 1995. TERENA was also experiencing cash-flow difficulties, in part because the EARN reserves had not yet been transferred to the new organization. In order to keep TERENA alive, the meeting approved a six-month budget for the first half of 1995. The Executive was asked to produce a revised budget for the year, in time for discussion at the May 1995 meeting of the General Assembly, and to take immediate steps to close the Paris office to cut costs.

By May 1995, however, the situation had gone from bad to worse. One member of the Executive had resigned in April 1995, pleading too heavy a workload; three more members resigned just before the General Assembly meeting started. It was clear that there were serious disagreements within the Executive, within the Secretariat, (i.e., the group of full-time employees who administered the organization) and between the Executive and the Secretariat. The General Assembly was presented with three different business plans, none of which was acceptable. Several members threatened to leave TERENA altogether if these management problems were not resolved. The conclusion of a long discussion was that the remaining members of the Executive should be asked to resign, leaving the field clear for the election of a new Executive with a more manageable size of five members. In the elections that then took place, Stefano Trumpy, who after holding office in EARN had been the representative of the Italian government in the CPG, was elected President. The two 1994 candidates for President were appointed as special advisors to the Executive so as to maintain continuity of approach in areas which were working well. Twelve months later, the Executive (Figure 3.5) was able to show that decisions vital to the

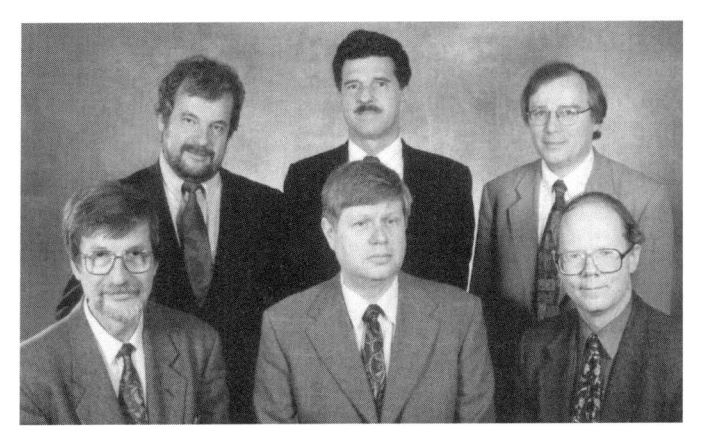

Figure 3.5 TERENA Executive Committee, 1996. Back row, left to right: Wulf Bauerfeld, Stefano Trumpy, Kees Neggers; front row, left to right: Lajos Balint, Steve Druck, Brian Gilmore.

good health of TERENA had been implemented and that a large degree of consensus over the activities of the organization had been restored: TERENA was "back on track".

3.4
RARE, EARN and TERENA

In March 1996, a year and a half after the merger of RARE and EARN, TERENA was still in a difficult situation. The merger of RARE and EARN had been a marriage of convenience, imposed by the difficult problems that both organizations were experiencing. EARN's problem was that basically it no longer had a purpose. EARN used to run a network, but that activity had been taken over by the successive generations of the pan-European network, now run by DANTE. But EARN still had a lot of funds – around €1 M. For RARE it was the other way around. Its members wanted RARE to continue organizing many activities, and there were many additional plans, but RARE did not have the money to fund them. Many research networks were members of both EARN and RARE and were increasingly concerned about the cost of subscribing to two organizations. The RARE-EARN merger was, therefore, inevitable. It was a classic marriage of convenience, with one partner bringing in the plans and ambitions, and the other partner bringing in the money.

In the years before the merger, RARE's financial situation had been really desperate. From 1991 until 1994, income had been less than essential expenditure and the organization had been living off its reserves. By 1995, these would have been exhausted and the organization would have been bankrupt. When EARN and RARE merged, RARE – now called TERENA – received some €800 000 from EARN which, when combined with RARE's own funds, brought the total reserves of the new organization to more than €1 M. However, not all the reserves were money in the bank: some of the reserves were long-standing debts of the member organizations and others – no use for paying bills. Even in the beginning of 1995, every month the TERENA bookkeeper would first pay the staff's salaries and then see how much money was left to pay other bills.

Although TERENA had been put back on track at the May 1995 meeting of its General Assembly, a new complication arose when towards the end of the year its Secretary General, Tomaz Kalin, resigned. The TERENA Executive Committee appointed Karel Vietsch to take over the job, initially for an interim period, on the basis of a secondment from the Dutch Ministry of Education, Culture and Sciences. In 1984–1987, Karel Vietsch had been involved from the government side in the creation of SURFnet. He had also represented the Dutch government in the CPG and was therefore familiar with the European research networking environment (Figure 3.6).

When Karel Vietsch arrived at the TERENA Secretariat in March 1996, the situation was still very difficult. Money had come in and the financial situation was no longer an urgent problem, but there were still a lot of outstanding debts and Karel

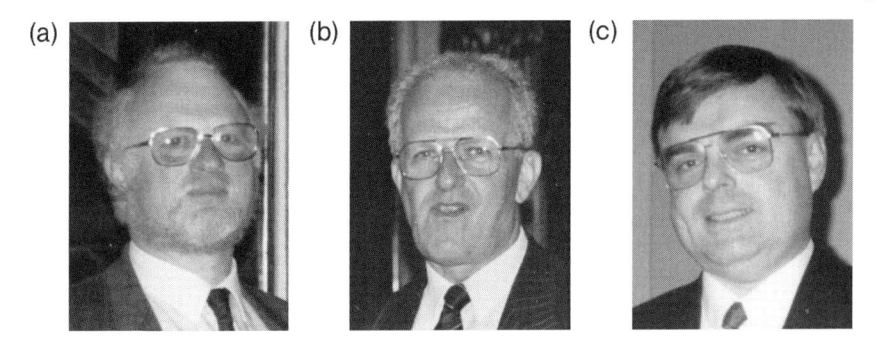

Figure 3.6 RARE and TERENA Secretaries-General: (a) James Hutton, Bernard Delcourt (no photo), (b) Tomaz Kalin, (c) Karel Vietsch.

Vietsch made it one of his first priorities to try collecting them. However, the major problems were the overall image of the TERENA organization and the functioning of its Secretariat. Most of the goodwill built up by RARE and EARN over many years had evaporated because of the chaos in the 1994–1995 period, staff members had left and the organization as a whole was in a bad shape. During the next two years, Karel Vietsch spent much of his time introducing conventional management structures and administrative procedures in the TERENA Secretariat, while travelling around Europe to re-establish the organization's reputation with its members, DANTE, the EC, representatives of national governments, industry and other important stakeholders of European research and education networking.

Since those days, the number of TERENA activities has grown enormously. TERENA organizes many workshops and seminars, as well as the annual TERENA Networking Conference. The long tradition of RARE Networkshops (dating back to the event in Luxembourg in May 1985) and EARN conferences (dating back to 1986) was continued in those TERENA conferences, and, nowadays, they are organized in a much more professional manner than in the past. All in all, TERENA has turned into a much more professional organization, better run and with a large range of activities.

Of course, technology has changed a lot in the last ten years and consequently there have been many new challenges. Many of the anecdotes that have been submitted for this book reflect disputes over, and differences between, different network technologies and network generations. In the 1980s and early 1990s, research networking was very much about the networks themselves, but nowadays much of the work is about services that are offered via the network – for example, videoconferencing – and about middleware: authentication to provide users access to the network or to other services. Middleware is a completely new area that first came up in the United States in the final years of the twentieth century and that is now a major part of European research networking activities. TERENA has been able to take the lead in this. In June 2000, TERENA organized the very first European middleware workshop, which took place in Leiden, the Netherlands. Since then, middleware has been the focus of attention, with much work being undertaken in TERENA task forces and in projects.

Currently, Europe is recognized as a world leader in the middleware area, and the task force meetings and other events attract participation from the United States, Canada, Australia and Japan.

The major advance since 1996 has been the enormous increase in available bandwidth in the wake of the liberalization of the European telecommunications markets, and the opening up of new markets in component equipment and services needed to build a network. For many years, the concept of customer-owned darkfiber was just an impractical dream. Bill St.Arnaud of the Canadian national research networking organization CANARIE (Canadian Network for the Advancement of Research, Industry and Education) was one of the early evangelists of the concept. In 2001 he gave a keynote presentation at the TERENA Networking Conference that really opened Europeans' eyes to the possibility of owning – or long-term leasing – one's own fiber and lighting it oneself. Just a few years later, most of the national research networks in Europe were based on the darkfiber concept, and the same holds for the GÉANT2 network, which was rolled out starting in 2005.

The transition to dark-fiber networks was heavily promoted by the SERENATE (Study into European Research and Education Networking As Targeted by eEurope) reports. SERENATE (2002–2003) was a foresight study funded by the European Union that aimed to look 5–10 years ahead into where research networking was going. The study was coordinated by TERENA under the charismatic leadership of its President, David Williams, but it also involved DANTE and some other organizations. When, in 2000, the EC approached TERENA with the request to coordinate such a study, the organizations assembled in the GÉANT project consortium were almost unanimously strongly opposed to the plan for such a study to be carried out. David Williams spent more than a year convincing the TERENA member organizations one by one of the potential benefits of a foresight study, and, as a consequence, SERENATE started in July 2002.

The SERENATE Summary Report, which was published in December 2003, was very influential on the developments in research networking in Europe nationally, and also on the plans for GÉANT2. An important element in that report was the concept of hybrid networking. If a networking organization owns or leases darkfiber, it can use the fiber in two ways. On the one hand, the transport infrastructure can be used to offer classic IP-based networks: the data streams are split in packets and each packet is routed to its destination. IP networks are robust and ideal for relatively small transfers of data from many different sources to many different destinations. However, they are offered on a best-efforts basis and without additional, sometimes complicated, measures, service quality cannot be guaranteed. On the other hand, there are applications that require very predictable network performance or that generate very large data streams between just a small number of locations. In these cases one requires a permanent connection through the network between two locations: a dedicated circuit, or, as it is called nowadays, a lightpath. Thanks to self-owned dark-fiber networks, classic best-effort IP networks and lightpaths can be combined using a single network infrastructure: a hybrid network.

The concepts of dark-fiber networks and hybrid networking were promoted by the SERENATE reports. But at that time – towards the end of 2003 – no-one would have guessed that these concepts would be implemented so quickly at the national and European level. It shows that the time has to be ripe for new ideas to be accepted. Customer-empowered networks could be established only after the liberalization of the telecommunications markets, which enabled customers to buy or lease their own fiber. Of course, one needs money to do that, so in itself the new concept required a pretty well-organized world of research networking organizations. And of course industry, in this case telecommunications operators and vendors of switches and routers, must be willing to play its part. There are too many examples in history where potentially good ideas did not come to fruition because of lack of industrial support.

Since the late 1990s, TERENA member organizations have brought forward many initiatives for studies, workshops, task forces and small projects that TERENA could undertake or coordinate. Almost all of these initiatives have been very successful although there are a few that were not, at least not immediately. One example is the coordination of activities of CERTs (computer emergency response teams), where – as described elsewhere in this book – a number of different approaches were tried before the current set-up was established with a very active task force CSIRT (computer security incident response team) in combination with training activities and a Trusted Introducer service. A second example is the portal initiative that TERENA prepared in the 1999–2000 period at the request of IBM and some of the national TERENA member organizations. The idea was to create a single portal on the Web that would provide access to all kinds of information about research in Europe. In those days, portals were very much in fashion, but with the advent of much more sophisticated search engines like Google, initiatives of this kind disappeared – the IBM–TERENA initiative never got off the ground.

A few words should be said about the relation between TERENA and the Grids community. A few years after Ian Foster and Carl Kesselman published their book which made "Grid" a well-known concept in the data processing and data communications world, the concept became popular in Europe and ranked high on the European Union's list of areas to be supported. TERENA's President David Williams felt strongly that Grids were of strategic importance to research networks, and that the research networking community should work closely with the Grids community. Both in the network transport area and in the middleware area the two communities are very much interested in the same things, and without good communication between the two communities there is a real danger of different solutions to the same problems being developed, which would be detrimental to the scientific community as a whole. There was, therefore, – and there still is – a role for TERENA to bridge the gap between these two worlds.

Initially, TERENA took up the challenge by becoming a partner in the largest Grid project funded by the European Union, EGEE (enabling Grids for e-science), which ran from 2004 until 2006. The idea was that by being in a project consortium with some 70 other organizations active in the European Grid community, TERENA would be able to establish many contacts and pursue its bridging role with the networking community. Unfortunately, it turned out that with such a very large number of project participants, establishing contacts was no easier for a project participant than for an outside organization. Moreover, only 50% of the costs of that work was reimbursed by the European Union, and consequently participation in EGEE brought TERENA a yearly net cost of some €200 000. Therefore TERENA decided in 2006 not to continue as a partner in the successor project EGEE-II, but to try bringing the Grids and research networking communities together through different initiatives. These have taken the form of the semi-annual "research networks and Grids" workshops, which are very successful and are still being organized by TERENA until this day.

3.5
DANTE and TERENA

When Karel Vietsch took up the duties of TERENA Secretary General in 1996, his first trip was to Cambridge to discuss with DANTE's General Managers, Dai Davies and Howard Davies (Figure 3.7), possibilities for collaboration between the two organizations. Because of his background in the Dutch civil service, Karel Vietsch had had many contacts with the European research networking community but he had little knowledge of the relations inside that community. He was therefore very surprised to find that the reception in Cambridge was less than friendly.

In the first years of DANTE's existence, there had been much confusion about the organization's role. Despite the fact that DANTE was merely carrying out the task that only a short time earlier had been identified as necessary, there were people who complained that DANTE now had a monopoly on the provision of services and that this was unacceptable. They felt that any new services should be managed by a different organization, with TERENA as the obvious candidate. In DANTE's view, TERENA was only too willing to support and encourage this approach. At the same time, the TERENA Executive Committee and the TERENA Secretariat staff were blissfully unaware of this latent conflict.

For the DANTE General Managers, the main bone of contention was that the TERENA Secretariat was continuing to provide administrative support to Ebone. Although the participants in Ebone92 had said that they would connect to the EMPB network when it provided an adequate multi-protocol service, they held back their commitment until the very last minute, and even then some of the national research networking organizations maintained connections to both EMPB and Ebone, leaving open their choice of supplier for future increases in capacity. Ebone was also offering new incentives, for example, in the form of relatively cheap connectivity to the United States. DANTE may have been unduly sensitive because of its precarious financial position, but it saw Ebone as a serious competitor. Its General Managers therefore found it surprising that TERENA, as the successor to the organization that had created DANTE, should now be supporting Ebone by providing secretariat functions and a financial clearing house.

A further concern was that Ebone operated as a barter trade organization. It neither paid VAT (value added tax) on its supplies nor charged VAT on the services that it

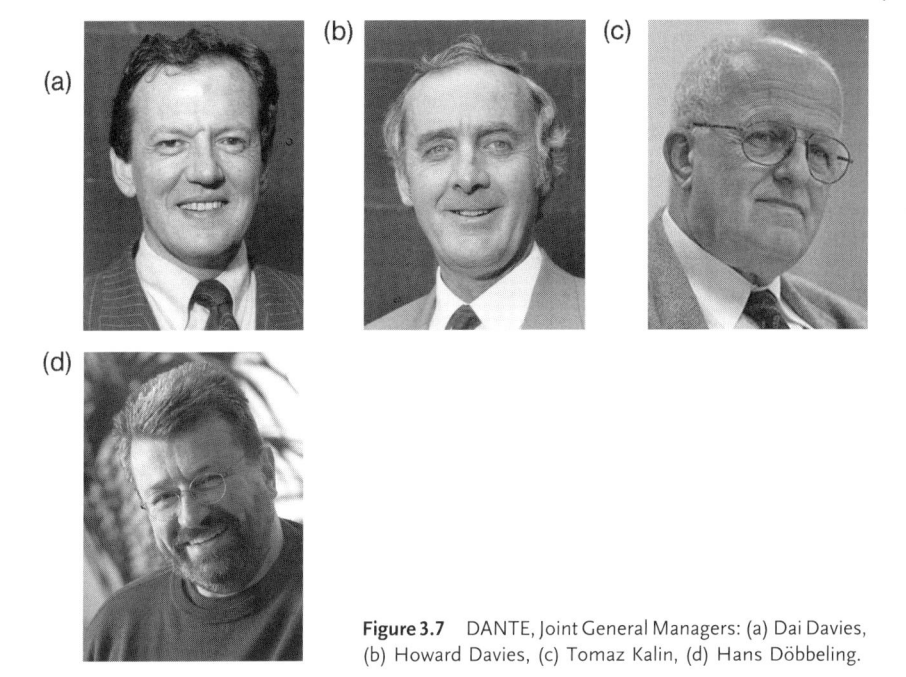

Figure 3.7 DANTE, Joint General Managers: (a) Dai Davies, (b) Howard Davies, (c) Tomaz Kalin, (d) Hans Döbbeling.

provided. For those national research networking organizations that were not in a position to reclaim the VAT that they had to pay if they used DANTE's services, this gave Ebone a 17.5% price advantage over EMPB. In fact TERENA, worried about possible legal liabilities, was not very comfortable with the situation either. Soon after the Secretary General's visit to the DANTE offices, TERENA announced that it would discontinue its provision of administrative support to Ebone and this was effected in July 1996.

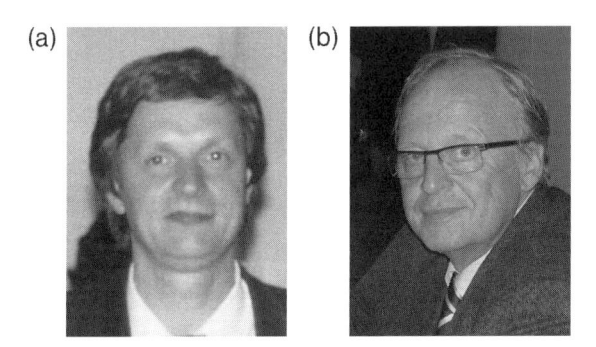

Figure 3.8 Chairmen, DANTE Board of Directors: (a) Klaus Ullmann, (b) Dany Vandromme.

TERENA, being released from its Ebone burden, did not immediately transform the relationship with DANTE. As a new organization, DANTE was gradually working towards a more stable financial situation and trying to define more clearly its role and the services that it would provide. At the same time, TERENA was regaining the ground which it had inherited from RARE and EARN but which had been neglected during the 1994–1995 crisis. Obviously, this made TERENA-DANTE relations sometimes unclear. Nevertheless, things improved gradually. The role of the TERENA Secretary General as an observer in the DANTE Board of Directors was instrumental in this, as were the efforts of TERENA's President, David Williams, in frequent meetings with DANTE Directors (Figure 3.8). The breakthrough came early in 2002, when changing circumstances made it clear to the DANTE and TERENA managers how much the two organizations could benefit from each other as allies. Soon after, TERENA and DANTE joined forces in the SERENATE foresight study (July 2002– December 2003), and the two organizations collaborated in many other EU-funded projects. In 2004, TERENA became a member of the GÉANT2 project consortium, taking on a number of responsibilities in that project alongside the leading role of DANTE for the provision of the GÉANT2 network.

Even now, DANTE feels that it suffers from a certain degree of mistrust from among the national research and education networking organizations. Those organizations are members of TERENA and at the same time they use GÉANT2 connectivity organized by DANTE. Some of them are DANTE shareholders but others are not. DANTE is a limited company and operates commercially. Because of its company structure, the ways in which even its shareholders can influence its activities in the short term are limited; non-shareholders have no formal channel for expressing their views on the way DANTE operates. In contrast, TERENA is an association and is perceived to be more democratic, with decisions on TERENA activities and financing being taken directly by the TERENA member organizations.

3.6
The Future of TERENA

Tensions have existed within the European research networking community ever since collaboration started in 1984 and they are still present. This is because there have been two different philosophies being followed. Some people like to do things as quickly as possible and to demonstrate that something works, without worrying initially about management or financing. Others want to have long-term planning and pay much attention to hierarchical management and finances. Ever since 1984, Europe has been divided into these two camps, and radicals and conservatives have been battling about many issues. As an example: in the protocol wars of the late 1980s, the conservatives supported OSI for as long as possible, while the radicals turned to IP at an early date. Although the topics of disagreement have changed over the years as technologies developed, it appears that most often it is the same set of national research networking organizations that can be found in one camp, and the same different set of organizations that can be found in the other. For example, Germany and Italy usually opt for a careful approach with long-term planning, while the Netherlands and the Nordic countries tend to find themselves in the radical camp, trying to benefit from new opportunities as soon as possible.

It is helpful for pan-European research networking organizations to have a balanced representation of both points of view in their management. Unfortunately, that has not always been achieved. In the case of DANTE, its company structure, with its attendant legal obligations concerning financial reporting and accounting, tends to enforce a conservative approach. The initial set of DANTE Directors was selected with the intention of providing balance but the more radical members of the DANTE Board found it difficult to work within the constraints imposed by a strict interpretation by their colleagues of the company's legal obligations and for some years after the creation of DANTE, its Board of Directors was seen to be largely dominated by conservative members. At the same time, the TERENA Executive Committee had a large number of members from the radical camp. This polarization was not beneficial for the European research networking community as a whole. The situation was much improved around the turn of the century, when members from France and Italy were elected to the TERENA Executive Committee, and members from the Czech Republic, the United Kingdom and Ireland to the DANTE Board of Directors.

The strength of an organization is built on its reputation and its track record. Today, TERENA has a good name. Consequently, whenever people come with new initiatives, they very soon think of TERENA as a body that can play a coordinating or organizing role. TERENA is often asked to organize a meeting or workshop about such new ideas, and when the initiative evolves into a more permanent activity, it can be organized under the TERENA umbrella. The TERENA Secretariat is a small group of people, but there is a large community of hundreds of technical experts all over Europe who attend TERENA conferences and workshops, and who participate in TERENA task forces. They can be mobilized when new ideas need further discussion and investigation. This makes TERENA lean and flexible, and, at the same time, effective.

Of course TERENA also has its vulnerabilities. The modus operandi of the organization depends very much on the ability to recruit good staff for the TERENA Secretariat. This can sometimes be a problem, as is the case for other local, national and international organizations in the research networking environment.

Another built-in vulnerability – but at the same time a strength – is that TERENA is an open organization. Its activities and meetings are open to anyone who can contribute, whether they are employed by a TERENA member organization or not. Results from TERENA work are placed in the public domain. TERENA receives half of its income from the annual fees paid by its members. The membership fee to be paid by a national research networking organization depends on the GNP of the country, but both for large and for small research networking organizations it can be a not insignificant amount. For this payment, the TERENA members do not receive a quid-pro-quo. They see their financial and other contributions to the TERENA activities as a token of solidarity and a contribution to the general good. This view is supported by the TERENA membership, but the openness of TERENA always carries the risk that an organization in financial difficulties might discontinue its membership, while continuing to benefit from the TERENA activities as a free-rider.

There is a large need for international collaboration in research networking, and TERENA is an instrument to achieve that collaboration. Consensus building is necessary in the face of all the financial and political issues. Looking at the European history of research networking and the often conflicting interests and opinions, it is something of a miracle that the European research networking community and its collaborative organization TERENA have survived for all these years. It is necessary to work hard to build consensus and support democratic decision taking without falling into the trap of acting on majority decisions that are not supported by an influential minority.

It is difficult to predict where TERENA will stand a number of years from now. No doubt one of its main roles, namely the rapid provision of support to new initiatives that may lead to the adoption of new technologies and directions, will remain. TERENA's activities, the topics and the technologies are bound to change a lot, but the TERENA structure and the way in which things are organized are stable and probably future-proof. An association as a democratic organization is a stable set-up. Having a small TERENA Secretariat and limiting it to providing support for people from the community who want to get together and do something together, is a stable formula.

This also illustrates the difference between TERENA and DANTE. The latter has an operational role and a much larger staff. Recently it has been decided to in-source the GÉANT Network Operations Centre which will make the number of the DANTE staff grow even more and will reinforce the operational nature of its activities. That is quite different from the sort of things that TERENA would ever want to do. TERENA's core business is and remains to bring people together and to support them in working together.

3.7
The Value of COSINE

Although COSINE did not meet its principal goal of creating an OSI world it nevertheless had some substantial achievements in technical, organizational and political areas. These achievements laid the foundations of the top-level infrastructure which is available today through the research networks on the national level and GÉANT2 organized by DANTE on the European level. The main COSINE concepts have survived dramatic technological changes and they have been adapted to new boundary conditions created by the market revolution which was initiated by deregulation. All those concepts survived a major market crisis which saw a great many companies collapse in the 1990s. COSINE was more than just another technical project. After the creation of RARE some years before as the organizational vehicle for the European research networks, it was very much a second "big bang" for the research network community in Europe, as it created a stable framework by means of which research networks and DANTE have since organized top-quality data network services for the R&E community.

The main achievement of the COSINE project is that it created a stable environment for collaboration in the technical, the economic/organizational and the political/public-financing domains. This is no small achievement as the dimensions of the research networks in Europe are very different. There are smaller and larger research networks and the organizational set-up of each research network has always been adapted to its country's needs. Indeed, there are not many similarities in the formal organization between any pair of research networks in Europe.

3.7.1
The Importance of the Achievements

The basic technical concept, which survived all later technological changes, was to add a European layer to the existing hierarchy of group (or departmental) LAN, campus network, and national network services: one example of this, and the most important one, is the data network commonly referred to as an "overlay network" which provides to research networks in Europe – and only to them – those international services that national research networks need. The underlying assumption is that research networks keep contact with their end-users and take care of all the contractual obligations with end-users. Moreover, the overlay network was intended to be used for connections to other world regions, especially to the research networks in the United States and Canada, rather than letting the research networks build their own links to North America and other world regions. This technical concept unloads this essential task from the research networks and remains valid today, even though the underlying technology has changed completely several times and has covered an impressive sequence of network generations from the first network IXI, the X.25 64 kbps network already started in the COSINE project, to the present GÉANT2.

These networks were developed through other EC co-funded projects after COSINE had come to an end. The developments were carried out by a research network consortium, basically a copy of the COSINE set-up, but after 1990 extended to new research networks from Central and Eastern Europe and with DANTE as the consortium coordinator. The major difference from the COSINE era is that the research network Policy Committee controls the consortium, and there is no direct influence (for example through members of a government) on the development path of the research network consortium.

Application developments took place within COSINE as well. One prominent development dealt with open directories. But compared to the network-related work, the importance of these developments is lower as far as concrete results are concerned. The research network community did learn through these sub-projects to collaborate closely on a European scale, for the benefit of all project participants.

At that time there was a heavy debate on how to organize research networking in Europe. As there was nothing to copy worldwide, the conclusion was open. The basic economic/organizational concept built through the COSINE project is called today a "federated approach". This means that there should be one research network per country, or at least only one interface to the set of networks if there is more than one, and only one European entity responsible for the European overlay network and other services needed to interconnect national research network-provided data services. Moreover, national and European activities in this field should mainly be organized in a complementary and collaborative fashion. This differs in a lot of aspects from other more centralized approaches which were debated at that time. In several areas, a huge economy of scale effect made this organizational approach even more attractive. One prominent example of this kind, where benefits were immediately visible, was the provision of links to the United States research networks.

The European entity, DANTE, is a direct consequence of the COSINE project. For several reasons, most of them of an economic or organizational nature, it was clear that RARE, as the body carrying out the project organization, could not be used as the organization for service provision after COSINE's end. The problem therefore was to organise a sustainable framework, i.e. to create a new organization, which could fulfill this task. This organization was named DANTE and is a real success story: it serves the same general goals and had to adapt to upcoming new technologies, ongoing technical challenges and, especially in the beginning, a bigger economic challenge. DANTE still serves European research network's needs by providing the overlay network to the research networks on behalf of the consortium, and DANTE is acting as the coordinator for the research network consortium in the EU framework programs.

It is interesting to see that the European model of organizing research networks, which was pushed and finally created through the COSINE project, namely having research networks as the basic structure and the "federated model" on top of it, has a lot of successors worldwide. The most prominent one is Internet2, which the United States R&E community set up in the late 1990s after the leading-edge (in terms of technology) and successful NSFnet had been closed by the United States government. Contrary to what the United States government had expected, the market was unable to offer appropriate services to the United States research community, so they created their research network, Internet2. Today, adapted versions of the European (COSINE) model can be found in other world regions such as South America.

At the beginning of the COSINE project it was not at all clear how to finance data networking for the research community on both national and European levels and how to steer this process politically. Most people in ministries or public funding agencies with political responsibilities for research budgets judged data networking in the 1980s (before COSINE started) as a relatively expensive tool. They felt they were, in the best case, useful only to a few research groups from "the big sciences" such as particle physics, and only a few people already had the vision that networked services would become an indispensable tool for all researchers and people in the higher education environment.

Moreover, on the higher political European level there was no mandate to fund anything which had to do with infrastructure. Unlike in the Sixth Framework Programme, EC officials had to be creative in order to spend money on a data network which had the main goal of interconnecting research networks as an infrastructure. This was a substantial burden at the time and the COSINE project created the awareness that this should be changed. It was quite a slow process involving a lot of people, but the problem was eventually solved largely thanks to the COSINE project findings.

The same holds for the even bigger financing problems at the national level. Bringing together people involved in funding from all participating countries automatically triggers an inherent process of mutual-influencing. Fortunately this process ended with a consensus that research networks would be the vital tool for researchers in all European countries, and that all national ministries should engage in funding these activities.

One of the more political reasons why COSINE had been created was an increasing awareness that a top-level data network infrastructure for the R&E community would enable similar processes of technical developments in and for society at large. During this period the United States research networks, especially the NSFnet, funded with public money through the NSF but also agency-funded networks like ESnet, were several years ahead of the developments taking place in Europe and there was a feeling that Europe was at risk of becoming completely uncompetitive in the IT field, particularly in telecommunications, where European vendors had traditionally a quite comfortable position on the worldwide markets.

This problem was strongly interlinked with another high level political problem: the problem of deregulation. The national telecoms monopolies hindered an appropriate (in the sense of using existing and proven technologies) development of any data communication infrastructure and, moreover, made any networking – but especially networking on a European or worldwide scale – extremely expensive. The problem was first raised within the scientific community, as this community would have liked to be one of the first users of such new technical options – their demand was clearly formulated. Raising the issue and solving it are two distinct topics. The CPG was more than useful in conveying this problem to top-level political circles, which took up this general issue and finally created a much more relaxed regulatory environment which in turn pushed the data communication market in the right direction. Except for the EC there was no other "political body" than the CPG which could take up these issues as a spokesman for the R&E community and contribute to resolving them.

3.7.2
COSINE Epilogue

While the COSINE project was alive, a lot of criticism was formulated in respect of its technical concepts, but also in respect of its organizational concepts. This criticism came from people who sometimes claimed they were "pragmatists", in contrast to what they thought were "theorists". It is always difficult to offer a final judgment within the lifetime of projects. However, considering that the basic concepts have survived for more than a decade, which has included both a technical and a market revolution, the main conceptual findings of COSINE were obviously on target.

Most of these accomplishments are more or less closely tied to specific people. Success is always a collective achievement, especially in such a consensus-building environment, but at least two among the acting "political" people in the CPG deserve to be mentioned: Peter Tindemans, the Dutch representative and Chairman of the CPG; and Horst Hünke, the EC representative and Vice-Chairman of that group. Both worked very hard (and successfully) together with their colleagues in the CPG to make COSINE both a political and an organizational success, and both of them have contributed substantially to the progress of European research networking.

3.8
RIPE and the RIPE NCC

RIPE (Réseaux IP Européens) was established towards the end of 1989 as there was a growing recognition of the importance of IP for research networking in Europe (Figure 3.9). Following energetic discussion, it was agreed that RIPE would operate under the RARE umbrella. RARE had originally focused on the use of international standards based on the OSI model and its working groups were structured accordingly. However, it was accepted that the IP protocol suite was vendor independent and provided a much fuller set of facilities than were available from OSI at this time and these were urgently needed by the academic and research community. From the beginning, the regular RIPE meetings provided a valuable forum for the exchange of technical information, to enhance expertise and to establish the necessary technical coordination for those operating or planning to operate IP networks. Until then all the IP activities had been predominantly United States based. In the light of the political changes in Central and Eastern Europe, advice and assistance was provided for the use of IP in these countries. United States export restrictions relating to advanced technologies became more relaxed in this period.

It soon became clear that it was necessary to establish the RIPE NCC (RIPE network coordination center), to support those activities which were best handled by

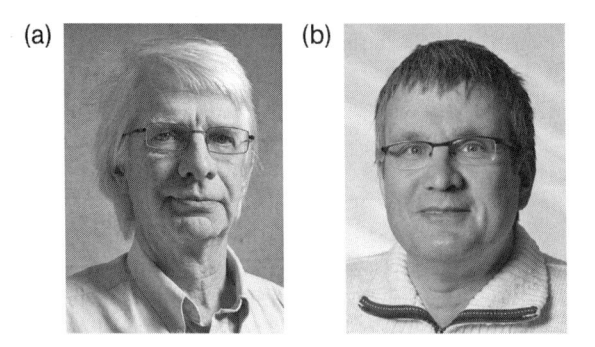

Figure 3.9 RIPE and RIPE NCC officials: (a) Rob Blokzijl, (b) Daniel Karrenberg.

full time staff. These activities included the establishment and maintenance of the RIPE network management database, which contained information needed for the coordination of the European IP networks, and operating the European Internet Registry. The RIPE NCC started in April 1992 under the RARE umbrella and for the first two years was funded by the RARE members, the National Research and Education networks, EARN and EUnet. RARE reorganized its technical activities in 1992 and RIPE decided that it would become an independent body to coordinate IP activities in Europe, providing advice to the RARE technical program as necessary. The RIPE NCC was rapidly established as an important center for IP in Europe due to the skill and expertise of the staff. It was the first regional Internet registry (RIR). Originally IP addresses and other IP resources, such as autonomous system numbers, were all allocated centrally from the United States. However, it was recognized that to ensure that the allocation of IP address space would be fair and efficient that RIRs would be needed in each geographical region of the world. Each RIR then allocated address space to local Internet registries, which were mostly IP service providers. This structure remains today.

In 1993, the first IETF meeting held outside North America was held in Amsterdam, the home of both RARE and the RIPE NCC. The RIPE NCC undertook a number of technical projects that were funded by individual RARE members, in particular SURFnet. The Internet was not just a resource for the academic and research community and from 1994 subscription funding was introduced, with each member ISP (Internet service provider) paying according to its size. Initially the subscription funding was on a voluntary basis. However, it was soon clear that this was unworkable and it was decided that priority to responding to queries, including the allocation of more IP address space, would be given to organizations that had paid a subscription. Other queries were dealt with "as time permitted". This approach had the desired effect, although it was up to each organization to decide whether it was a large medium or small ISP for the purpose of determining the amount of its subscription.

In 1998 the RIPE NCC started to operate as a legal entity in its own right, instead of sitting under the TERENA umbrella. TERENA was then already formed from the merger of EARN and RARE. The RIPE NCC has certainly now outgrown its original host, having some 100 staff and using a complex algorithm to ensure that ISPs pay according to their use of the RIPE NCC services. There are currently more than 500 members, covering Europe, the Middle East and parts of Central Asia, and the annual budget is about €12.5 M.

The priority of the RIPE NCC has always been service provision. By being firm but fair, the RIPE NCC, and the other RIRs, have ensured that IP address space continues to be available for those who need it, despite the expectation that address space would run out. Innovation has also always been an important aspect of the RIPE NCC's work, both in the development of tools to enable the staff to work more efficiently and also in technical development, such as the Internet routing registry. The Internet has always required new ideas to be developed to ensure it remained an innovative means of communication and the members of staff of the RIPE NCC have actively contributed to this over its lifetime.

Points of Presence

A point of presence (PoP) is a physical location where a telecoms operator or a major telecoms user installs line termination, switching and other equipment needed to support the services it provides to its customers. An ancestor of the PoP from the days of monopoly telephone operators is the telephone exchange.

The building which houses a PoP has a number of special characteristics. Details depend on the size and importance of the PoP and on the operator's policies, but in general the following description applies to all PoPs.

There is tight security with rigorous controlled access procedures, in order to protect the equipment and to deter attacks by vandals or terrorists (damage to a PoP which houses international circuits could cause a major disruption of services, including emergency services, and be very costly).

There is a stable power supply and electrical earthing to protect equipment from "spikes" in the mains supply caused, for example, by lightning strikes. Backup power is provided in two ways: by batteries which can maintain power levels for at least a few seconds, and usually a few minutes, and a motor generator which provides power in case of a more prolonged failure of the mains supply. A false floor and false ceiling allow for the interconnection of equipment in adjacent racks and for environment control, in particular the dissipation of heat generated by the equipment. Extensive cable ducts (and holes in the walls between rooms) are provided, so that new connections between equipment in different parts of the building can be installed easily. There are at least two separate entry points for cables entering the building, so that it is possible for two circuits with the same destination to follow completely independent paths.

Many PoP sites are owned and occupied by a single telecoms operator. For many years, the owners of such premises would not allow other telecoms operators to use them. They might permit major customers to install their own equipment (i.e., to establish a PoP of their own at that location) but the arrangement would almost always be conditional on customers continuing to use the telecoms operator's transmission services. Hosting PoPs belonging to other organizations was not a service offered by the traditional telecoms operators.

With the advent of telecoms liberalization in Europe, the growth in the number of ISPs and their need to exchange data in order to provide global coverage for their customers, this exclusivity has diminished. Increasingly, it has been in the interest (sometimes imposed by a national telecoms regulator) of a telecoms operator to allow the installation of competitors' equipment in order to allow fair competition. A side-effect of liberalization has been the creation of a new service industry based on "telecoms hotels". Independent companies, sometimes with several telecoms operators as major shareholders, have set up new buildings expressly designed to house PoPs for several operators. Physical space, building services including power supplies, empty equipment racks, access control and other security services are available for telecoms operators and their customers to rent.

Customers of a telecoms hotel remain responsible for the installation and operation of their equipment which is controlled remotely from the customer's

NMC. Control instructions, new configuration tables, software updates, and so on, for equipment in the PoP, as well as performance data and diagnostic information are exchanged over the network itself. "Out-of-band" access in the form of a dial-up ISDN (integrated services digital network) connection or a simple telephone line are included in the equipment configuration, so that management functions can still be used if the PoP becomes otherwise inaccessible as a result of network failure. Operational services provided by the building's owner are usually limited to "Press the restart button" at the request of the owner of a piece of equipment.

For large telecoms users, decisions on where to locate PoPs can be difficult to make. Many factors have to be taken into account and each case needs to be judged on its merits. Usually, the main criterion used in making a choice is the total cost over the expected lifetime of the project being supported. Given the structure of European research networks, with one research network in each country, interconnected with the others by a pan-European network, the European level needs one PoP in each country, the only possible exceptions being countries served by a single international circuit which can be connected directly to the research network's equipment.

In principle, there are three alternatives which need to be considered for the location of the PoP. First, the installation of a PoP on the premises of the principal provider of international circuits in the country concerned. These circuits can be connected directly to the research network's equipment and the telecoms operator can recover the costs of providing space, power, and so on, through the charges it makes for international circuits. The research network concerned has to procure and pay for a local loop (or two if resilience is required) from its own PoP.

Since the research networks operate complex configurations of circuits and have their own PoPs distributed around their country, the second alternative for the European PoP is co-location in one of the national PoPs. In this case research networks can connect directly to the European network, but local loops are needed for each of the international circuits that terminate in the country concerned. Since in most cases there will be two or three (or more) of these, the overall cost will be higher than for the first alternative. The overall reliability of an end-to-end international circuit is also reduced if it has to include a local loop at one or both ends, especially if the local loop is provided by a different supplier. Nevertheless, each research network has a clear interest in seeing this alternative adopted for its country, especially where local loops are particularly expensive. Several research networks have pursued this interest consistently and aggressively for many years.

The third alternative for the location of the European level PoP is for it, and one of the research network's PoPs, to be installed in the same telecoms hotel. There will be rental and other recurrent charges to be paid, but if the international circuit supplier is also present in the same telecoms hotel, the local loops that are needed are reduced to interconnections within a single building and the cost to all parties is minimized.

Over the years, telecoms operators have increasingly established themselves in multiple PoPs within large cities, connected by a set of high-capacity circuits often configured as a dual ring, so that any of their PoPs can be selected as the termination point of an international circuit, and their customers have an element of choice in deciding where to make the interconnection.

4
Different Approaches

This chapter looks at the networks that already existed before the European collaboration was initiated, how these networks needed merging together and the management processes which were created in order to achieve this. In addition, the methods used to acquire funding are discussed. There were shortcomings both in the very beginning and even more recently. It discusses how the different countries that required the service gradually got together to make decisions. Different protocols were in use and predicting where the future might go and hence what would be the best choices presented many dilemmas. EMPB and Ebone were two such networks and the contentions between them are presented from an EMPB perspective. DANTE is an organization that offers networks and services and this chapter also looks at their offerings, upgrade paths, operational problems and how different network protocols affected these offerings.

4.1
HEPnet

The particle physics community, which is also known as the high energy physics, HEP, community, undertakes most of its research at large research centers; in Europe, examples are CERN and DESY (Deutsches Elektronen Synchrotron). The teams working on experiments are usually large international groups, and although the scientists and engineers are sometimes able to work on secondment at the research centres, they also have to spend time at their universities or home research laboratories.

ECFA is a high level coordination group for European particle physics. In 1979, ECFA established a Working Group on Data Processing Standards. With the building of the LEP (large electron positron collider) at CERN, it became obvious that a coordinated approach was necessary to address the computer networking needs of the community. In 1981 the decision was taken to establish ECFA Sub-group 5 on Links and Networks as part of this Working Group. Sub-group 5 was created under the leadership of Mike Sendall of CERN. His role was key in getting the group started – he later encouraged Tim Berners-Lee in his work creating the World Wide

Web (WWW). Sub-group 5 coined the term HEPnet to describe the required set of technical services needed to support/meet the required user facilities.

Sub-group 5 had members from the many European countries undertaking research at CERN and DESY, and sought to agree on what practical actions would enable the community to use the developing technologies in wide area networking to support their research programs. Sub-group 5 meetings were held every 3 to 4 months, at different centers so as to encourage the involvement of local experts. The group reported directly to the senior management in European particle physics, including both CERN and DESY, which ensured that those involved in the organizations concerned gave increasing support for international communications services.

In the initial 1982 Sub-group 5 report, it was recommended that HEP institutes should be connected to the emerging national public X.25 networks and that the international standard known as X.29 should be used for interactive terminal access. However, the issue that X.29 had many options and that an appropriate HEP dialect had to be identified was flagged up. International standards tended to have many options from which a sub-set, or profile, had to be chosen by a particular user group, and this was an ongoing problem. Sub-group 5 also developed an international directory of computer systems relevant to particle physics that could be accessed over the public X.25 networks, which at this stage were the only public international networks. (Note that Sub-group 5 left open the option of using leased lines rather than public network services; Figure 4.1 shows a proposed set of links and represents one of the earliest network configuration diagrams.)

In the early 1980s, there were international leased lines to CERN from France, Italy and the United Kingdom. Initially these links were used to enable users in Geneva to use their large computers in their home countries for data processing. Perhaps the most complex set-up at this time was the international leased lines from the United Kingdom to both CERN and DESY for the United Kingdom particle physics community. The leased lines were split so that they were able to provide links to the IBM-based mainframes at the two centers, using IBM's RSCS as was done for EARN, as well as X.25 network connections. Both the Italian and United Kingdom links were then developed to provide network access to the DEC VAX™ machines used as experimental control computers for the four LEP experiments which were still under development. The Italian link used DECnet and the link to the United Kingdom used the JANET Coloured Book protocols over X.25. CERN itself had developed a special file transfer protocol as part of its CERNET project. Hence, a project was established by Sub-group 5 to create a multiprotocol file transfer gateway (known as GIFT, general internetwork file transfer), which allowed files to be exchanged between CERNET, DECnet and the JANET Blue Book FTP in the first instance and, eventually Internet FTP and even (but only on JANET), ISO FTAM.

In 1983, Sub-group 5 undertook a study on electronic mail and computer conferencing. At this time, most users could only access electronic mail services by remote terminal access to a central mail system or computer conferencing system, such as QZ at the University of Stockholm. It was recognized that gateways (protocol converters) were needed between a number of different mail systems; DECnet, EARN and the JANET Grey Book mail protocol were identified in the report.

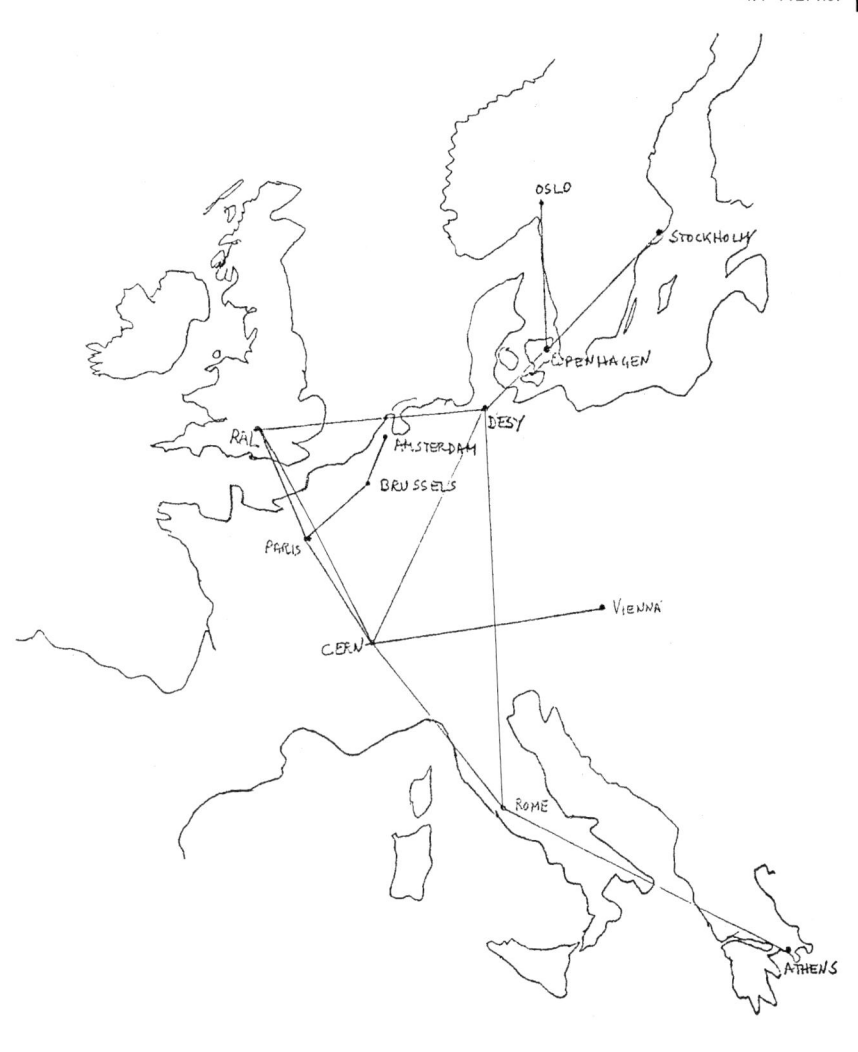

Figure 4.1 HEPnet planned configuration.

Electronic mail systems developed more rapidly than expected. Thus, by early 1985, the CERN study of e-mail services, called COMICS (computer-based message interconnection systems), made its first recommendation that "X.400 compatible electronic mail systems should be installed and used wherever available. All new developments should be done in the context of X.400." Naturally, there was still a widespread need for gateways between the different existing e-mail systems, and over the years these became more reliable and user-friendly.

Initially it had been believed that widespread use of the public X.25 networks would enable the particle physics community to access other centers easily and at reasonable cost. However, it rapidly became clear that the bandwidth available for international X.25 and the incompatibilities between the different implementations made this an inappropriate solution. However, the cost of international leased circuits in Europe and the restrictions imposed on the carrying of "third party traffic" slowed the take-up of international leased lines. In 1984, the wider HEP community was asked to provide input to studies of how to enable and support international collaborative research in better ways. These problems of creating an effective HEP network were among those taken up with the EC Research Directorate as input for the Summit meetings of Heads of State. Sub-group 5 recognized that its concerns were of wider importance than just for the particle physics community.

In the mid 1980s, there was no organization for international collaboration for networking for the wider research community even though there were a number of conferences where such things were discussed. As can be seen from the above, the technology was at an early stage of development and even creating national education and research networks was difficult. International activity was hindered by the restrictive rules and high circuit prices of the public telecommunications operators, PTOs, which exercised their regulatory right at the time and took the view that only they could organize an open international network.

Attendees at he first European Networkshop in May 1985 came from many European countries and included many technical experts from the particle physics community. The establishment of RARE which followed on from this enabled many of the technical and organizational concerns of the particle physics community to be dealt with on a wider basis by involving groups across the academic and research communities in Europe. In addition, with funding from IBM, EARN had been established and enabled many users on a wide range of computer systems to benefit from access to an international network supporting electronic mail and file transfers.

By the second half of 1987, CERN was able to report that it had an understanding based on a "letter of agreement" with the Swiss PTT to allow it to switch traffic between leased lines where some protocol conversion was done at CERN. Explicitly forbidden was the switching of X.25 traffic between the Swiss public network and any of the leased lines, as this would act as an "international tariff bypass". Hence at least for CERN, and thus for the particle physics community, the restrictions were easing. As the real cost of international leased lines also dropped, the number of international leased lines into the CERN site grew, both for particle physics and as part of the EARN configuration.

By the end of 1988, it was clear that a stronger management and support structure was needed for the growing number of international connections operating for the particle physics community. This led to the creation in early 1989 of the HEPnet Requirements Committee to represent the needs of the community and the HEPnet Technical Committee to coordinate the planning and operation of HEPnet, through consensus wherever possible. All formal agreements had to remain bilateral. Although many protocols were still being used, it was already clear that the use of IP was going to grow substantially (RIPE was established towards the end of 1989). By early 1991, the aggregate HEPnet bandwidth had become 11 Mbps over 25 lines, up from 0.65 Mbps over 16 lines two years earlier. 70% of the bandwidth was allocated to IP traffic. Although general purpose research networks were starting to become available, their performance was not yet adequate to support the particle physics community.

In 1992, the HEPnet community made use of Ebone before starting to move to EuropaNET in 1993. It was not until TEN-34 became available (in 1997) that the community started to feel that general purpose network performance was good enough to fully support particle physics. The focus of the community is now on higher level Grid activities, though monitoring of the underlying networks and the use of non-standard settings for IP, where appropriate, continues. With the latest generation of network, GÉANT2, the community can create its own private network, if it needs to.

Many of the members of Sub-group 5 later became leading players in the wider European networking scene. For example, Rob Blokzijl was one of those who led the RIPE initiative, James Hutton was the first Secretary-General of RARE, Enzo Valente is GARR (Gruppo Armonizzazione Reti della Ricerca) Director and Peter Villemoes was General Manager of NORDUnet for many years. Of course, there were many CERN staff who were key to supporting the growing wide area networking needs of the particle physics community. Perhaps the leading person in this period was François Fluckiger who led CERN's external networks team.

4.2
DECnet

DECnet was a proprietary network architecture and set of protocols that nearly became an international standard. DECnet was designed and implemented by the Digital Equipment Corporation, commonly known as "Digital" or "DEC", for use on the range of minicomputers that it manufactured.

Starting in 1974 with supporting the exchange of data via a direct link between two DEC PDP-11 computers (Phase I), DECnet was extended and expanded in a number of distinct phases, the number of DEC hardware platforms and operating systems offering DECnet services being increased with each successive phase.

Phase III (1980) already supported gateways to other proprietary systems including IBM's SNA (systems network architecture) and offered X.25 as one of its link level protocols, but the most widely used version was DECnet Phase IV which was integrated with the VAX/VMS (virtual address extension/virtual memory system) operating system as well as being available for use with DEC's other operating systems. The development of DECnet software was carried out exclusively by DEC engineers but from Phase II onwards DEC made the detailed specifications openly available so that anyone could develop complementary systems. As a consequence, connecting a new computer from another manufacturer to a DECnet network was relatively straightforward; someone, somewhere had probably produced a working gateway already.

Given the success of DECnet Phase IV, expectations for Phase V were high. Phase V was intended to provide a full OSI protocol stack alongside the established DEC proprietary protocols and, for some time, DECnet OSI Phase V was a strong candidate to become the "next generation IP protocol" at the IETF. Eventually, IPv6 (Internet Protocol version 6) took most of the good things from DECnet OSI, leaving aside other features which were difficult to manage. As the focus of development moved from OSI to the Internet protocols, the particular attractions of Phase V faded.

The DEC VAX series of computers was nevertheless very popular in the science research community and there were very many organizations which had a need to intercommunicate with others and which already had one or more (VAX) machines already equipped with hardware and software which made this possible; all that was needed in addition were the circuits to link pairs of VAX sites and some rudimentary coordination to minimize circuit costs and to handle addressing and routing issues. It was only natural that some of these organizations would get together and set up interconnections as an immediate, partial and interim means of meeting their needs. There were even some enthusiasts who believed that DECnet could be developed to provide the complete answer to the need for universal networking. In a few European countries in the late 1980s, the embryo national research network was composed of DECnet capable machines or operated in parallel with such a network. In the end, however, the principle of manufacturer independence was the winner and interest in DECnet declined.

4.3
EUnet

For nearly two decades, EUnet was a vital contributor to European research and academic networking. During the earliest days, EUnet was a primary provider to the research networking community. EUnet was unique due to its origin, motivations, structure, means of funding, style of operation, and membership. It made great contributions as a provider of network services to the research community, as an example of how to organize and operate a network for that community, and by developing broad European expertise in the management and use of modern data networks. EUnet was also an important contributor to Europe's rapid adoption of internetworking (that is, the IP suite) in the 1990s, a contribution that has had wide-reaching and very positive effects on European economies and society.

In 1982, although there were substantial computing facilities at universities across Europe, communication between campuses using services such as email was almost non-existent. What would later become important networks and networking organizations, such as EARN, Ebone, and COSINE, had yet to be founded. The ISO OSI standard had not yet been fully defined.

EUnet began in 1982 in response to a pressing need, by leveraging an available technology and by adopting and transforming an example that came from a far simpler political environment. European computing enthusiasts formed EUnet as an independent, cooperative network based at leading research centers across Western

Europe. It grew rapidly, providing vital services to both the academic and corporate research communities, and would eventually become the leader of commercialization of internetworking in Europe. The story of EUnet begins much earlier however, with the creation of new, powerful, and flexible systems, software, and networking technologies over a decade before.

4.3.1
Precursors

In 1969, researchers at AT&T's (American Telephone & Telegraph Company) famous Bell Laboratories created the UNIX operating system in an *ad hoc* effort. AT&T was precluded by regulation from participating in the computing and software industries. So, AT&T took an unprecedented step: they widely distributed UNIX source code free of charge to universities in the United States, Europe, and elsewhere. UNIX was surprisingly simple, and surprisingly effective as well. UNIX had a highly modular structure, which permitted easy changes to, and replacement of, the many parts that made up the system, in both the operating system itself as well as in its powerful suite of software development and text processing tools. Also, unusually, Bell Labs, on a case-by-case basis, modified the lower layers of UNIX so that the system could run on several different popular computer architectures (a process known as "porting").

UNIX users, usually computer science professors and students, were encouraged to analyze the source code and submit improvements. UNIX was an engineer's dream – modular, simple, and elegant – and many of those who used and modified UNIX grew accustomed to diving into a problem and making fixes directly on their own, asking for neither permission nor substantial support from outside parties. These software engineers also "ported" UNIX to different computers; in time it would run on nearly every major computer architecture of the day. Bell Labs often integrated many of these changes into regular AT&T releases. These actions became the first, and arguably the most important, step in the global computer industry's transition from a manufacturer's proprietary model, to an open, more popular model of technology. UNIX users became a vibrant, self-aware community. They formed the United States UNIX Users' Group, USENIX (a conflation of USEr and uNIX), in 1975 as a technical society for UNIX professionals, engineers, academics, and enthusiasts. This enthusiasm and independence of action was to have a powerful influence on European research and commercial networking.

During the 1970s, AT&T sought a more economical way to distribute the UNIX source code other than postal mailing of large computer tape reels. Bell Labs researcher Mike Lesk subsequently developed a simple networking facility, the UNIX to UNIX copy protocol, or UUCP. UUCP provided communication between pairs of UNIX computers over conventional dial-up telephone lines using modems. Once connected via UUCP, UNIX computers could exchange information using existing network applications such as email, file transfer, and others. Connections could be set up on a regular schedule, or on demand. AT&T bundled UUCP into their standard UNIX distributions.

In 1979, Tom Truscott and Jim Ellis, graduate students at Duke University in North Carolina in the United States, developed a new network based on UUCP. Their approach was simple and powerful: arrange UNIX systems running UUCP into a "store and forward" network, a high-tech "bucket brigade". Pairs of UNIX computers would exchange information, buffer that information, and then forward it to a distant UNIX system that would in turn buffer that information for hand-off to another UNIX system, and so on. The only requirement for interconnection and long-distance hop-by-hop transfer was that each pair of computers agreed to exchange information and that one or both made the phone calls.

UUCPnet (UNIX to UNIX copy protocol network) employed this free, open, voluntary, cooperative structure. After its announcement at the USENIX conference in January, 1980, it quickly grew to trans-continental scope, primarily in United States research and academic environments where UNIX systems were popular. Operating the network was exceptionally economical. In many environments, participating in UUCPnet incurred no additional hardware or communications costs; existing UNIX systems were employed, and many of the telephone calls (the "hops") were made without incremental communications cost thanks to the structure of dial-up tariffs of those days. Networking was so new, and the enthusiasm was so great, that individual system administrators often participated without bothering to seek approval from superior management. The UNIX culture of technical initiative and self-reliance had extended to the field of networking.

Nevertheless, as the size of the network and the level of traffic grew, it began to consume a large fraction of system and administrator time. Major computer manufacturers such as Digital Equipment soon provided systems acting as store-and-forward nodes, and free of charge. USENIX provided coordination and technical guidance, through various committees of UNIX enthusiasts, and by other *ad hoc* means, although USENIX did so without any explicit authority. In fact, there was no central or general control at all. Cooperation ruled the day.

In 1980, Steve Bellovin, then a graduate student at the University of North Carolina at Chapel Hill, developed the first "Network News" software, in the form of UNIX ("shell") scripts. News group content was generated by users and distributed without central control. Many groups were unmoderated. The software was soon re-cast into the C programming language by others, and distributed widely without charge. The service quickly spread throughout the United States, and was known as the USENET (a contraction of user network).

Around that time, national UNIX user groups began to form in Europe, with the same motivations as those that inspired the USENIX Association in the United States. The United Kingdom group (UKUUG, UK UNIX Users Group) was formed in 1977, and the Dutch group (NLUUG, NL UNIX Users Group) in 1978. Each national group usually took as its name the ISO-3166 country code standard followed by "UUG" (i.e., UNIX Users Group) such as NLUUG, UKUUG, and so on. The European UNIX Users Group (EUUG) was formed in 1981. However, being in Europe required a more sophisticated organization than was necessary in the single country, culture, and market environment of the United States' USENIX Association. EUUG was structured as a federation of national chapters, each of which elected representatives to a European coordinating body. National User Groups held regular meetings and annual conferences, and at the annual European-level conference, technical sessions and a trade show were included. The EUUG provided a home for this very creative community of computer scientists, engineers, marketers and other UNIX computing professionals. Their annual meetings were highly enthusiastic gab-fests known for particularly energetic sessions in the conference bar late into the night. They created an institution unique for its time: a self-aware Europe-wide community of computing experts who knew each other well personally.

In the early 1980s, UUCPnet was a topic of great interest in EUUG circles. If they can do this in the United States, why can't we do this in Europe? The usual objections were hauled out: "...phone costs in Europe are prohibitive, particularly international tariffs, the anarchistic United States model won't work here, connecting equipment to the phone systems is technically problem-fraught and often forbidden by national laws, and interconnection across borders is especially difficult...". The genius of EUnet was to find a specifically European solution. They established a UNIX machine to act as an exchange point in each participating country. Users in each country would be responsible for dialing their national center, and for paying for those calls. To minimize international phone costs, each national center would call a single international center (often at night time when phone calls were cheapest) for information exchange. Each national center would be responsible for its dial-up costs, and each would charge a flat rate for each of their subscribers. Teus Hagen and Piet Beertema, in association with the NLUUG, established EUnet's European Center at CWI, the Centrum voor Wiskunde en Informatica (Centre for Mathematics and Computers Science), in Amsterdam. They announced the system at the April, 1982 EUUG meeting at CNAM (Conservatoire National des Arts et Métiers) in Paris. Four countries initially participated: the Netherlands (whose national operation was not initially separate from the European operating centre), the United Kingdom (led by Peter Collinson at the University of Kent at Canterbury), Denmark (led by Keld Jörn Simonsen at DIKU, Datalogisk Institut Københavns Universitet, the Department of Computer Science at the University of Copenhagen), and Sweden (led by Björn Eriksen at KTH, Kungliga Tekniska Högskolan, the Royal Institute of Technology). Like the User Groups, each national EUnet took as its name some variant on the ISO-3166 country code standard, this time followed by "net", such as NLnet, UKnet, and so on. EUnet subscriptions concentrated on research and academic organizations and technology companies.

From its first days, EUnet connected to the United States by transatlantic X.25 to the famous "seismo" server, run by Rick Adams at the University of Maryland's Seismological Institute, and from there to the ARPAnet. Email and USENET news groups were exchanged with the United States. EUnet also distributed European national and pan-European news groups, and was frequently the source of USENET "feeds" to universities throughout Europe.

Although EUnet was created by technologists, it was much more than a technical accomplishment. At that one moment in 1982, three important innovations were realized. First, creating a network architecture that suited the geographic, political, economic, and regulatory environment of European nations. Second, an organizational solution: autonomous national teams working under the umbrella of their national UNIX User Groups, a European-level effort under the umbrella of the European organization, and the participating universities of each national team and of the European International center. Finally, a double-legged economic solution was found. Existing resources and facilities at participating universities, primarily UNIX computers, telephone accounts, and staff were used, representing incremental rather than new costs. Furthermore, although EUnet was often assembled by using borrowed resources, national EUnet organizations and the European EUnet center charged a flat monthly rate for participating in the network right from the start. All fee collection was done at the fine-grain level of the subscribing organization, resulting in great freedom for the national groups – they did not receive money from some large external entity that directed it be used for some specific purpose or in support of some specific policy. It was thus able to find the optimal solutions between user (and eventually, customer) needs and available and emerging technologies. Not only was this "researchy" network able to pay for itself, it made a continuing demonstration of value to customers, it stood on its own practical value proposition – a critical input in the evolution of modern internetworking. This technical and organizational initiative was substantially influenced by the UNIX heritage.

The network and the EUUG established a compelling symbiosis: creating a new national EUnet required the formation of a national User Group, which was a powerful motivator of growth of the organization, and the EUUG functioned as an effective unifying force. Many early EUnet actions were *ad hoc*, and appropriately so. Most decisions and activities were accomplished without resorting to contracts, nor were there any clear or formal processes, or clear agreements regarding authority and ownership. EUnet started off small, operated in support of R&D, and was in a niche in which commercial activity was unknown. These approaches were entirely appropriate at the time and were necessary for the network to succeed in the first place.

During this time, Europe had not yet begun to implement telecommunications deregulation and there was no clear legal or regulatory context for competitive commercial networking. Although there was no thought within EUnet of engaging in commerce per se, and certainly not in profit-making enterprise, EUnet was nevertheless exposed. Providing services to the research community, both academic and commercial, helped keep EUnet from appearing to engage in commercial activity, or in appearing to compete with the PTTs. Furthermore, the requirement that each EUnet subscriber be a member of the national UUG conferred a "closed membership club" status for EUnet, and further reinforced its non-commercial status.

Similarly, EUnet operated without high-level "official" status in the research community. Although it cooperated with, it did not directly participate in the newly emerging academic model of European research networking, nor the official status of government sponsored university networks, national research networks, and pan-European entities. EUnet was instead an entire research networking world unto itself, with end-user (emerging "customer") networks, national EUnets working in conjunction with their respective national European UNIX User Group, and a pan-European operating centre operating in conjunction with the European UNIX User

Group umbrella organization. EUnet legitimacy in the research community derived most importantly from its delivery of vital and effective networking services to research and academic organizations throughout Europe, and its cooperation with leading networking research centers throughout Europe. EUnet's many participants were often leaders within that community.

One of the drivers of EUnet was the youthful enthusiasm of the 1960s. Many of its initial leaders came of age during that time. Rather than being motivated by money or conventional status, EUnet enthusiasts were often driven by the sheer fun of creating this amazing new project. The enthusiasm extended to the act of technical creation, of providing new ways of communicating with one's peers both nationally and abroad, the construction of a vast new technical capability, and the great fun of inventing, step by step, a new European entity and community that one immediately participated in during one's daily work. And it was done with a minimum of bureaucracy and cost.

One of the first machines used to operate EUnet's UUCP mail system, "mcvax", was donated by DEC. Because EUnet predated the Internet's DNS, UUCP mail delivery addresses required routing information as part of each email address, defining the sequence of hops that the email was to take. mcvax was the primary routing node for Europe and became one of the well-known points in the UUCP world. Similarly, the USENET news system used source routing that would contain the name of the central routing machine, mcvax.

4.3.2
The Network Grows Quickly

Once EUnet's structure was established, the network grew quickly. By 1983, EUnet had grown to 10 countries. The original four were joined by France via CNAM in Paris, Germany via Siemens in Munich, Norway via Kongsberg, Scotland via EdCAAD (Edinburgh computer-aided architectural design) Studies in Edinburgh, and Switzerland via CERN in Geneva. By 1985, EUnet had grown to approximately 500 subscribing sites. Additional links had been established to Australia, Canada, Israel, and Japan.

On April 1, 1984, at the height of the cold war, a USENET article was distributed which purported to come from Konstantin Chernenko, the then Soviet leader, supposedly originating from a machine named "kremvax". The author announced that the Soviet Union would be joining USENET to communicate with the West and "hope to have a possibility to make clear to them our intentions and ideas." This April Fool's joke created a great deal of agitation around the network. The entire episode was later attributed to Piet Beertema, head of operations at EUnet's European center in Amsterdam. In an ironic real-world twist to this fantastic joke, years later when mcvax was replaced at the center of EUnet by mcsun, the original mcvax was actually shipped to Moscow to run the emerging network there.

Being UNIX enthusiasts meant that participants in the EUUG were also Internet protocol enthusiasts; IP was soon part of standard UNIX distributions. EUnet began deploying IP throughout Europe in the second half of the 1980s led by EUnet network manager Daniel Karrenberg, who had joined EUnet's European center at CWI from EUnet Germany at the University of Dortmund. EUnet deployed the first transatlantic, open, dedicated IP link between the United States and Europe in November 1988, again to "seismo", and from there to the NSFnet. EUnet received a donation of what was possibly the first Cisco router deployed in Europe. EUnet research networks were often the first users of the DNS in their respective countries, often began their respective national DNS authority, which they frequently operated for many years.

During the 1980s, nearly every remaining country in Western Europe joined EUnet: Austria, Belgium, Finland, Greece, Ireland, Italy, and even Yugoslavia. EUnet was either the first, or among the first Internet service providers in every country in which it operated. EUnet was also first in providing early access to countries in Eastern Europe, even during the cold war, including Bulgaria, Hungary, Czechoslovakia, and the Soviet Union. For a time, EUnet had what was among the widest span of any non-governmental network in the world, from Washington DC to far eastern Russia. EUnet had succeeded in unifying Europe without large-scale governmental sponsorship.

4.3.3
Cooperation with Emerging European Research and Academic Networks

In the meantime, the research networking community evolved and other networks began to be formed, including NORDUnet and EARN. EUnet actively participated in cooperative efforts with these emerging networks, including the establishment of the CERN-Amsterdam link consortium, which included EARN, IBM and EASInet (European academic supercomputing initiative network), CERN, and NORDUnet. It was through this facility that CERN, the birthplace of the World Wide Web, first connected to the Internet.

In 1991, the first discussions were held at CERN regarding the creation of Ebone (Figure 4.2). Ebone was initially a cooperative shared-resource network. EUnet contributed its share of the CERN-Amsterdam link to the Ebone consortium.

By 1990, in some countries such as the United Kingdom, national EUnet activity had grown so large that it could no longer fit within the budgetary practices of an academic organization. The amount of money flowing was sufficiently large (in the United Kingdom, annual turnover was over £500 000) that there was concern that the United Kingdom national tax authority might consider taxing the University of Kent at Canterbury as if it were a commercial business. The EUUG concluded it must determine if a transition to commercial status was viable, or if it would be necessary and appropriate to shut down the network. The EUUG hired a European-level managing director, Glenn Kowack, to perform that evaluation. In 1992, the national EUnets and User Group community came to a consensus that EUnet would be reconstituted as a commercial enterprise. Each of the national EUnets would convert to commercial enterprises, and in so doing move out of their academic environments. A similar transition was to take place in Amsterdam at the European networking center, and European-level operating and holding companies were to be established. Over the next several years, that transition was accomplished, with national User Groups holding various shares of their newly formed commercial companies, and the EUUG (renamed "EurOpen" in the early 1990s) holding a similar position in EUnet's European enterprises. All EUnet national groups made the transition to IP networking, and established leased line connectivity to the Amsterdam operating center. Transalantic bandwidth to the United States grew quickly.

During this period, the growth of internetworking world-wide began to explode just as the European and EU-national regulatory environment was being reconceived. In both the US and Europe, regional (in the US) and national (in Europe) networks were in a murky half-way world. They provided more and more services to external, even commercial research centers, and in some cases to explicitly commercial entities that had no research role. While there had always been exceptional cooperation between EUnet national networks and national research networks, and similar cooperation at the European level, now there began a degree of competition in some countries and at the European level. EUnet was becoming more and more openly commercial, and national research networks were similarly relaxing their criteria for the entities to which they would provide service. The competition was occasionally vigorous. However, it energized the growth and evolution of the European networking industry, both industrial and academic.

Around this time, network service provisioning became better understood, and user understanding and sophistication also grew. Internet access became less "researchy" and more of a commodity. As a consequence, over time EUnet would need to fully embrace a commercial model of service provisioning and operations. The European research networks would similarly focus on their academic and research roles, providing levels of bandwidth, responsiveness, and service not readily available off-the-shelf from commercial entities.

In 1994, the vast majority of EUnet companies agreed to merge into a single, integrated European enterprise, which they completed in 1996. National EUnets and European-level capacity and service continued to grow and develop. EUnet was acquired by Qwest in 1998 for $US156 M. Qwest later merged with KPN to form KPN/Qwest, a leading pan-European network service provider of its time.

EUnet stands as a unique example of the creativity, dedication, adaptability, and technical insightfulness of a generation of researchers and technologists. Their insights were not just technical, they were organizational, economic, and social as well. Driven by technical enthusiasm and the thrill of creation, they adapted very simple technical building blocks to create a world-class, world-spanning network. They did so in the early years without commercial motivation, at exceptionally low-cost, and in a new, open, and participatory manner. They managed to find ways to accomplish all of this in an exceptionally complex, non-supportive and highly uncertain regulatory environment during one of the most uncertain and intense periods of European integration and change. In time, they would redirect their early enthusiasm toward evolving nimbly and rapidly into a major, influential commercial organization. In so doing, they made a great contribution not just to global internetworking and commerce, but also to the character and connectedness of contemporary Europe and the world at large. A contribution that even now continues to evolve rapidly, providing ever greater economic and social value.

4.4 Ebone

At the beginning of the 1990s, one of the most urgent issues was to set up a well-managed pan-European multi-protocol backbone service (MPBS). The recognition of this need was expressed by the RARE CoA in its May 1990 meeting in Killarney and the EEPG was set up to study the issues. The EEPG presented its findings at the next Joint EARN/RARE Conference in May 1991 in Blois. The EEPG recommended the adoption as a matter of urgency of a pan-European multiprotocol approach and the setting up an OU to operate pan-European services. In addition it recommended starting an ATM (asynchronous transfer mode) pilot.

Two options were presented for the backbone technology: either X.25 with embedding of other layer 3 protocols, or TDM (time-division multiplexing) with native support of layer 3 services. For the latter case, an evolutionary scenario was proposed whereby the existing separate X.25, IP and other backbones would migrate towards a common bandwidth-management structure based on TDM. The RARE CoA in Blois concluded that a European backbone and an organization to run it were definitely needed. A task force was set up to make a proposal for an OU for discussion in the next CoA meeting in the autumn of 1991. It was also agreed to progress the idea of an ATM Pilot. But RARE was unable to make a choice with respect to the technical direction of the multi-protocol backbone itself. There was hope that soon more information would be available on the X.25-with-embedding option as a result of the ongoing tender evaluation for the COSINE IXI Production Service. Several members wanted to wait for this outcome before making a choice.

No formal plan to explore the TDM option in more detail was proposed. To fill the gap that was left, SURFnet took the initiative to set up and sponsor an *ad hoc* task force to refine the TDM option, concentrating on the technical and operational aspects of

(a) (b)

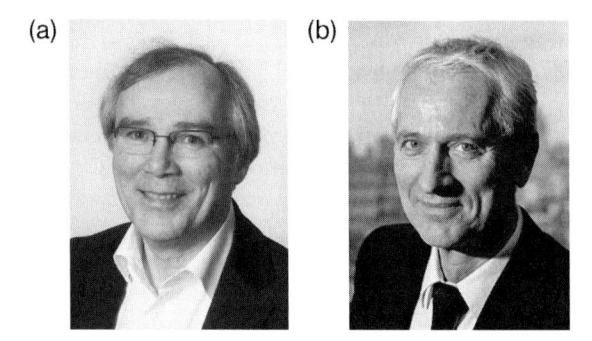

Figure 4.2 Senior Ebone officers: (a) Kees Neggers, Christian Michau (no photo), (b) Frode Greisen.

the backbone. This work was done in parallel with the IXI and OU activities. Initial participants came from CERN, Ireland, NORDUnet, SURFnet and the Chairman of RIPE. The results of the *ad hoc* Task Force were sent to both the RARE CoA and RIPE mailing lists on September 19 1991 and a first meeting of interested organizations took place on September 26 1991 at CERN in Geneva, back to back with a RIPE meeting. The Task Force recommended a two-step approach: creation and growth during 1992 of a kernel backbone by combining and enhancing existing facilities, and merging the resultant backbone into the RARE OU plans for 1993.

The two-step approach recommended two streams of activity: short-term implementation in 1992 and a parallel tender/procurement process aimed at 1993. The short-term approach, named Ebone92, provided for the immediate establishment of a common managed interim pan-European Internet IP backbone based on the existing *ad hoc* Internet IP backbone infrastructure(s). Recommendations also included the provision of pilot CLNS (connectionless network services) in 1992. Developments in technology such as ATM and frame relay were expected to offer increasingly flexible methods of managing bandwidth and sharing of expensive transmission facilities between services in the future. The exclusion of X.25 from the plan was justified because X.25 was considered less important than IP, and because the pan-European provision of X.25 was already well-covered by the current COSINE IXI service and its planned enhancements.

For the second step, RARE was recommended to take immediate action to prepare a draft "Call for Tender" document for a pan-European MPBS Service to be in operation by the beginning of 1993. This step was considered the responsibility of the OU that was being established at that time. The interim backbone was assumed to be integrated into the full multi-protocol services, and operational responsibility would be passed on to the OU in 1993 – hence the name Ebone92, on the assumption that such a body would have been successfully created by that time.

The proposed Ebone92 architecture was based on a model for a network for networks, with clear management boundaries between backbone systems, called Ebone boundary systems (EBS) and regional boundary systems (RBS). Although Ebone92 was initiated by research networks, participation was open to all network providers, including commercial operators. The initial target configuration was a diamond topology around the initial backbone locations Stockholm, Amsterdam and CERN with connections to the United States from CERN and Stockholm. In principle, Ebone92 would have no restrictions on traffic. It would be up to the participating networks to restrict traffic according to their own norms. The proposal was that the interim Ebone92 backbone services operate under responsibility of an *ad hoc* Ebone Consortium of Contributing Organizations (ECCO), with an Ebone management committee for the day-to-day responsibilities, an Ebone action team (EAT) to prepare and implement the Ebone92 kernel, an Ebone operations team (EOT) to provide day-to-day operations and a clearing house to balance out the costs and contributions.

At the meeting in Geneva, 28 organizations were represented and the reactions to the proposal were enthusiastic. The meeting confirmed that managing Layer 3 for IP was an urgent requirement without an alternative solution. Many links were already shared at that time and Ebone92 essentially "renamed" these resources and integrated them to provide a managed Layer 3 IP service. Twelve organizations were already offering specific contributions (in the form of circuit capacity, manpower etc.) and it became clear that the "start-up" backbone configuration could be more extensive than the example given in the proposal. It was agreed to prepare an MoU for the Ebone92 Consortium and to meet again on October 30 in Amsterdam to form the consortium.

The Ebone92 proposal was also discussed a week later at the RARE CoA meeting in Rome on October 3–4 1991. The RARE CoA welcomed the Ebone92 Report and the approach taken to the development of IP services outlined in the report, recognized that its proposals were complementary to the existing IXI service and the 2 Mbps X.25 pilot and were consistent with plans for the establishment of a multiprotocol network and the RARE OU. The CoA then decided to initiate a RARE project to implement the rationalization and upgrade of the European IP and ISO-IP Backbone Services, and to prepare the statement of requirements for the European multiprotocol network services.

The next Ebone92 meeting took place as planned on October 30 in Amsterdam. There were no questions with respect to intent and approach, and the meeting concentrated on discussing a draft Memorandum of Agreement. It was agreed that the Memorandum was to be considered a "Gentleman's Agreement" rather than a legal contract. An *ad hoc* consortium approach was accepted to carry through the initiative, whereby the infrastructure, the services, and the management of them would be provided by temporary no-charge contributions from the interested parties, called Contributing Organizations. Intended contributions were noted, RARE's offer to act as a clearing house was accepted, the EAT team was formed, and an interim Ebone management team was set up. An extensive report of this meeting was published by Carl Malamud in his book "Exploring the Internet".

On November 28 a final draft of the MoU was produced. In December commitments were collected and the Ebone92 network was designed on the basis of the contributions. Initially, the planned backbone configuration was a folded ring: Stockholm, Amsterdam, CERN, Germany, London and back to Stockholm, with an additional EBS in Montpellier connected to CERN. In January 1992, paper copies of the MoU were shipped to 26 organizations interested in becoming a Contributing Organization. Several others did not intend to sign the MoU but preferred to become a so-called Supporting Organization, notably CERN, IBM and NSF, who all contributed considerable resources. IBM's contribution included a T1 (1.5 Mbps) circuit from CERN to the United States, and manpower in Bonn from its EASInet project. KTH in Stockholm was selected as the operational center for Ebone92. The MoU confirmed the principle that Ebone was targeted at research networks, though commercial organizations were welcome to participate. Should their participation result in loading the network to the detriment of the participating research organizations, the commercial organizations were expected to upgrade the network as required. There should be no profit for the participating commercial organizations. The sharing of resources between research networks and commercial networks was considered a genuine source of synergy, both for Ebone92 and for future networking.

4.4 Ebone

At the end of February 1992 the initial backbone design was finalized. A German EBS could not be included for political reasons and the Ebone92 backbone was agreed to be a ring connecting Stockholm-Amsterdam-CERN at 512 kbps and CERN-Montpellier-London-Stockholm at 256 kbps, with 512 k connections to the United States from Stockholm and London, and a T1 connection to the United States from CERN. In Amsterdam a connection to the IXI network was implemented at NIKHEF to allow networks to connect with embedded IP over X.25 (pending approval by the EC of an offer by PTT Telecom to provide a managed connection between IXI and Ebone92 at its own premises in Amsterdam). The initial backbone configuration and the planned connections to participating organizations is shown in Figure 4.3. In March 1992, the backbone Stockholm-Amsterdam-CERN was up and running and 15 organizations had signed on as Contributing Organizations. The connection from Stockholm to London was added in June 1992 and the number of MoU signatories was increased to 20. On September 26 1992, exactly a year after the presentation of the Ebone92 initiative, the final link between Montpellier and London completed the ring, and the full resilient pan-European IP backbone was in operation. This major achievement was only made possible because it was needed, and it benefited from the active involvement and enthusiasm of many, both at the management and at the engineering level.

At the same time, less progress was being made on the COSINE/OU front. Progress was slow on plans to replace the 64 kbps initial IXI service by a higher capacity IXI production service, as well as on setting up the OU. A tentative proposal for a 2 Mbps X.25 pilot service named TRIXI between a sub-set of the COSINE

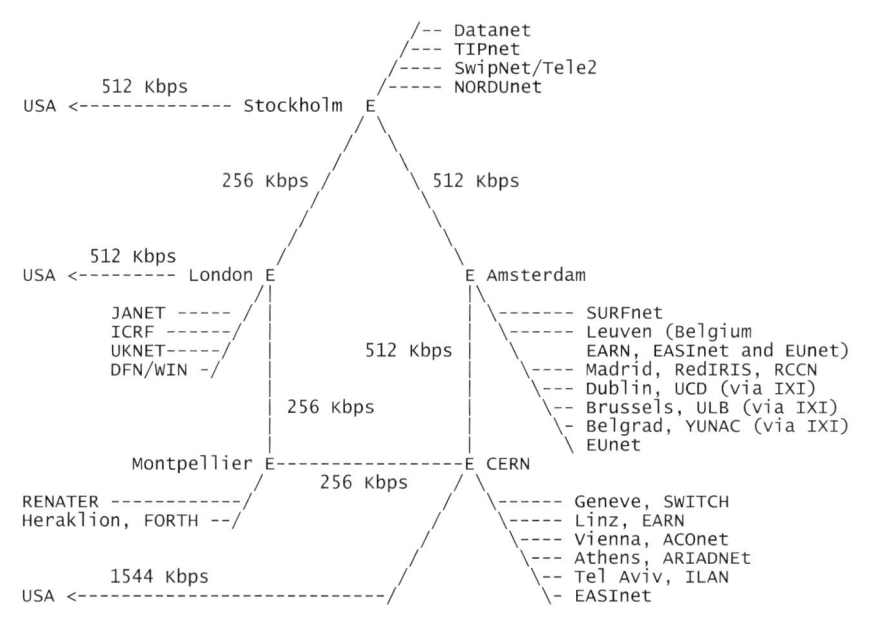

```
                                     /-- Datanet
                                    /--- TIPnet
                                   /---- SwipNet/Tele2
         512 Kbps                 /----- NORDUnet
USA <-------------- Stockholm   E
                              /|\
                             / | \
                            /  |  \
                  256 Kbps /   |   \ 512 Kbps
                          /    |    \
                         /     |     \
         512 Kbps       /      |      \
USA <--------- London E        |       E Amsterdam
              /|             |       |\
         JANET ----- /|             |       | \------- SURFnet
         ICRF ------/ |             |       |  \------ Leuven (Belgium
         UKNET-----/  |     512 Kbps|       |   \       EARN, EASInet and EUnet)
         DFN/WIN -/   |             |       |    \---- Madrid, RedIRIS, RCCN
                      |             |       |     \--- Dublin, UCD (via IXI)
                      |    256 Kbps |       |      \-- Brussels, ULB (via IXI)
                      |             |       |       \- Belgrad, YUNAC (via IXI)
              Montpellier E----------------E CERN      \ EUnet
                      /     256 Kbps      /|\
RENATER -----------/                     / | \------ Geneve, SWITCH
Heraklion, FORTH --/                    /  |  \----- Linz, EARN
                                       /   |   \---- Vienna, ACOnet
                                      /    |    \--- Athens, ARIADNEt
              1544 Kbps              /     |     \-- Tel Aviv, ILAN
USA <-------------------------------/      |      \- EASInet
```

Figure 4.3 Initial Ebone 92 configuration.

countries was discussed with a major operator but the discussions lapsed when it became clear that an IP service was also an essential requirement.

Negotiations with the bidders for the IXI production service were kept confidential by the CPMU and there was no open consultation of the European IP experts who had created Ebone92. Ebone92 began to be concerned about the continuation of the IP service in 1993. The task of identifying an integration scenario for Ebone92 into the planned MPBS rested with the OUSC, and in July 1992 the following message was sent by the Ebone Management Committee to the OUSC.

"The Ebone Management Committee has addressed the continuation of the Ebone92 IP service for 1993. Ebone Management Committee has noted the plans and progress in setting up the OU and the OU's intention to provide a pan-European MPBS. Ebone Management Committee has concluded that to be able to secure a proper continuation of IP backbone services in Europe it will be necessary to continue the current IP services at least until mid 1993. The Ebone Management Committee is keen on optimising the transition process from the current situation to a single pan-European MPBS and on minimising the organizational overhead involved. Therefore, the Ebone Management Committee offers to propose to the Ebone participants that the OU takes up full organizational and commercial control over the Ebone93 IP services as soon as possible. This proposal is conditional to the OU being prepared to continue the operation of the Ebone IP technical infrastructure until the intended MPBS has demonstrated its operational capabilities to replace it."

On August 31 1992, the OUSC distributed an Ebone integration scenario. The proposal was to start the MPBS based on two so-called Boxes: An EMPP (European 2 Mbps multi-protocol pilot) box to be provided by PTT Telecom for X.25, and native IP access points and an Ebone box for native IP based on the Ebone92 kernel. No details were provided on how the EMPP IP service would be implemented, and no pilot implementation was available to test the service. After an initial period, the OU would base its IP service offering on one system, and it would take the results of the EMPP evaluation into account in its choice of system. Until the intended single system had demonstrated its operational capabilities, customers would be free to choose which IP services they wanted to buy, EMPP and/or Ebone. However, Ebone customers would have to respect the OU acceptable use policy (AUP), and to facilitate quick exits from Ebone services, cancellation periods of 3 months were suggested for Ebone lines. The OU would sell all services on a contractual basis, and next to the EMPP subcontract, it would subcontract all necessary elements of the Ebone kernel network. A pricing scheme based on access capacity was included in the scenario. It is also interesting to note that while Ebone consistently talked about Ebone92, the OUSC only referred to Ebone in their proposal.

This scenario did not allay the doubts expressed by the Ebone Management Committee in its July message to the OUSC. In their September consortium meeting, the Ebone participants concluded that no suitable umbrella organization was yet available to take over the management of Ebone. An Ebone93 was needed as a continuation and improvement of Ebone92. October 1 1993 was set as a new checkpoint for a possible handover decision. The open and neutral nature of Ebone was reaffirmed; there should be no restrictions on third party traffic. It was emphasized that the main feature of Ebone93 was to act as a neutral interconnect with strict technical and organizational boundaries between the EBS backbone and the RBS of the connected networks. Thus no peer relations – except with the United States – would be possible. The organization would be reinforced by appointing a general manager and technical staff, to be financed by the contributing organizations. A fairer cost-sharing model would be developed and would now include transatlantic activity; RARE would continue to play the role of administrative support and clearing house. GMD (Gesellschaft für Mathematik und Datenverarbeitung) Bonn offered to house a new EBS in Germany and the offer was included in the new Ebone93 topology planning. At the end of September, a couple of days after the successful closing of the Ebone92 ring, a press release announced the 1993 plans.

In early February 1993, a new topology was agreed. It included Bonn as an EBS; the French EBS moved from Montpellier to Paris. The Stockholm-Amsterdam-Geneva-Paris path was upgraded to T1 speed and a new T1 Paris-United States circuit was added as illustrated in Figure 4.4. Access costs were set as a function of capacity, in a similar way to the model developed for the OU, with a 64 kbps port costing 64 k ECU/year. To facilitate participation of Central and East European Countries, the possibilities for an EBS in Vienna were to be investigated.

Most European research networks and several commercial IP providers were among the Ebone93 partners. Although the IXI production service, now re-named European multi-protocol backbone (EMPB), had started operation in October 1992, at the beginning of 1993 the IP component of the service was in operation only as a pilot and the OU was still not in place so no agreements for a direct interconnect of Ebone93 to the IP services provided by the OU had yet been reached.

During 1993, the OU was incorporated in the form of DANTE. After difficult negotiations, DANTE and Ebone agreed to connect the EMPB to Ebone93 in London and Amsterdam with two 512 kbps connections based on embedded IP over X.25. The compromise reached was beneficial for both parties and was valid for 1993.

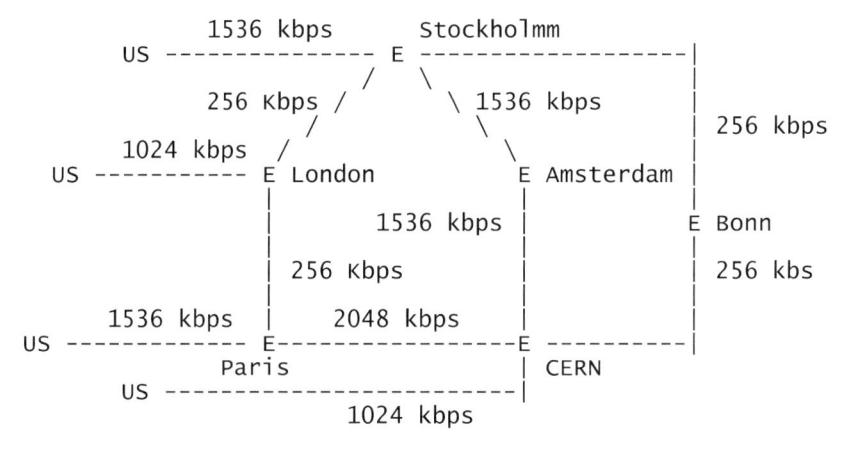

```
                  1536 kbps       Stockholmm
            US --------------- E --------------------|
                            / \                      |
                 256 Kbps /    \ 1536 kbps           |
                        /       \                    | 256 kbps
        1024 kbps      /         \                   |
    US ----------- E London       E Amsterdam        |
                   |              |                  |
                   |   1536 kbps  |                  E Bonn
                   |              |                  |
                   |   256 Kbps   |                  | 256 kbs
                   |              |                  |
      1536 kbps    |   2048 kbps  |                  |
US ------------- E----------------E ---------|
               Paris              | CERN
        US ----------------------|
                  1024 kbps
```

Figure 4.4 Ebone 93 configuration.

However, each party explained the resulting agreement differently. DANTE viewed it as a peering of EMPB with Ebone for European traffic and for the purchase of transatlantic services from Ebone. Ebone saw the arrangement as two regular RBS to EBS connections. In Ebone's view, this was important so as to be able to avoid erosion of the neutral interconnect principle which was considered a main feature of Ebone93. As its RBS connections were based on embedded IP over X.25, this would prevent DANTE using the full capacity of the lines. As a result, DANTE was given a discount. In the Ebone93 cost-sharing model, 75% of the cost of the access lines had to be absorbed in the central backbone cost and it was clear that the shared EMPB connections saved money on the Ebone side. Both parties had realized that not connecting EMPB and Ebone would have been very difficult to explain to the European users. DANTE relabeled the resulting combined EMPB plus service "EuropaNET".

By mid-1993, Ebone had become one of the major IP backbones worldwide. During the summer, Ebone engineers had successfully tested BGP-4 (border gateway protocol, version 4) and subsequently introduced it in Ebone93, making Ebone93 one of the first major IP backbones running BGP-4. CIDR (classless inter-domain routing) was already introduced in the beginning of 1994.

A number of the European research networks participating in Ebone93 became shareholders of DANTE. Others, notably RENATER and ACOnet, did not. The latter proposed a more permanent continuation of Ebone, not just planning for an Ebone94. An investigation was started together with the commercial participants in Ebone93. The strategic discussion about the future direction focused on whether Ebone should become a backbone provider or a neutral interconnect – or both, as it had been in 1992 and 1993.

Because many of the Ebone members were not confident that the native IP service of EMPB would be ready on the contracted date, future planning for Ebone was a difficult exercise. How many of the DANTE research networks would like to use Ebone services and for how long, was not known for a long time. (This uncertainty also made DANTE's planning more difficult, especially because its lack of working capital meant that it could order any additional capacity needed to provide service to a particular research network only after receiving a formal commitment to pay for EMPB service by the research network concerned.) To facilitate the transition process, the Ebone partners agreed that, during 1994, any of them could end their subscription by giving six month's notice to take effect from the end of a quarter.

After the EMPB native IP service had demonstrated its capabilities, some research networks, including Ebone initiator SURFnet, decided quickly to move to the EMPB as of January 1 1994. Some others decided in late December to cancel their commitments with a 6-month notice for July 1994.

The strategic discussion within the Ebone consortium concluded in favor of the RENATER proposal to split the Ebone function of backbone provider and neutral interconnect. For the neutral interconnect it was proposed to extend the Washington-based (GIX, global Internet exchange) by the adoption of a distributed model which allowed network operators to connect at the most convenient of several locations. The extended system was named D-GIX (Distributed GIX). For Europe, Stockholm and Paris were suggested as candidate connection points. All pan-European IP providers were assumed to exchange traffic in these two locations. It was suggested that the Ebone backbone become a triangle between Paris, Stockholm and Vienna.

Due to the cancelations at the end of 1993, NORDUnet's in particular, the future of the Ebone backbone after 1 July 1994 became uncertain. The decision was taken to secure continuation of Ebone only for the first half of 1994, more or less on the same basis as in 1992 and 1993 and to start a new investigation to decide what to do with the backbone services after 1 July 1994. In addition, a pilot for the D-GIX model was agreed on. During this first half year, DANTE would connect with a 1 Mbps connection in Amsterdam.

At the consortium meeting in February 1994, a proposal from RENATER, ACOnet and ECRC (European computer-industry research centre) was accepted: to continue Ebone after July 1994, based on a two node structure (Paris–Vienna). All networks needed to pay the full costs of their access lines. In the June meeting of ECCO it was decided to incorporate Ebone in the form of an association. In the June meeting it was also decided to allow peerings with other major networks, and an agreement was reached with DANTE to peer at 512 kbps in Geneva. On November 2 1994 the Ebone Association was formed under French law. Despite the cancelations at the end of 1993, the Ebone membership count increased in 1994 from 21 in January to 27 in December.

During 1995, Ebone continued to grow and it was decided to upgrade the backbone links to 34 Mbps. In early 1996, over 50 participants were connected to Ebone. In July 1996, TERENA stopped providing secretariat services for Ebone. In September 1996, Ebone set up a limited company to allow it to expand more quickly, so as to improve its service and cost-effectiveness whilst maintaining its not-for-profit basis of operation. Ebone developed into one of Europe's leading IP network service providers. On July 12 1999, Global TeleSystems Group, Inc. (GTS) became full owner and operator of Ebone.

In October 2001, KPN/Qwest acquired Ebone. Unfortunately, following the dot.com crash and various investigations, KPN/Qwest had to declare bankruptcy in May 2002. At that time KPN/Qwest's network was carrying a quarter of the European Internet traffic, and Ebone was serving over 4000 customers. Liquidators allowed the company to operate for a short period while they searched for some way of rescuing the service. Employees in the Ebone Network Operations Centre attempted to keep the Ebone network running even longer – at their own expense – in a heroic fight against time. Eventually, they were told to shut down the network and abandon the building on July 2 2002. Ebone demonstrated how European engineers could make a contribution to the development of the Internet. Prominent Europeans who have made a more general contribution are shown in Figure 4.5.

4.5
EMPB, European Multi-Protocol Backbone

Even before the IXI network had been brought fully into service, some research networks were convinced that the TCP/IP protocols which were already being used extensively in LANs, would also prove to be superior to X.25 in the wide area and were pressing for services based on these protocols to be introduced. Other research

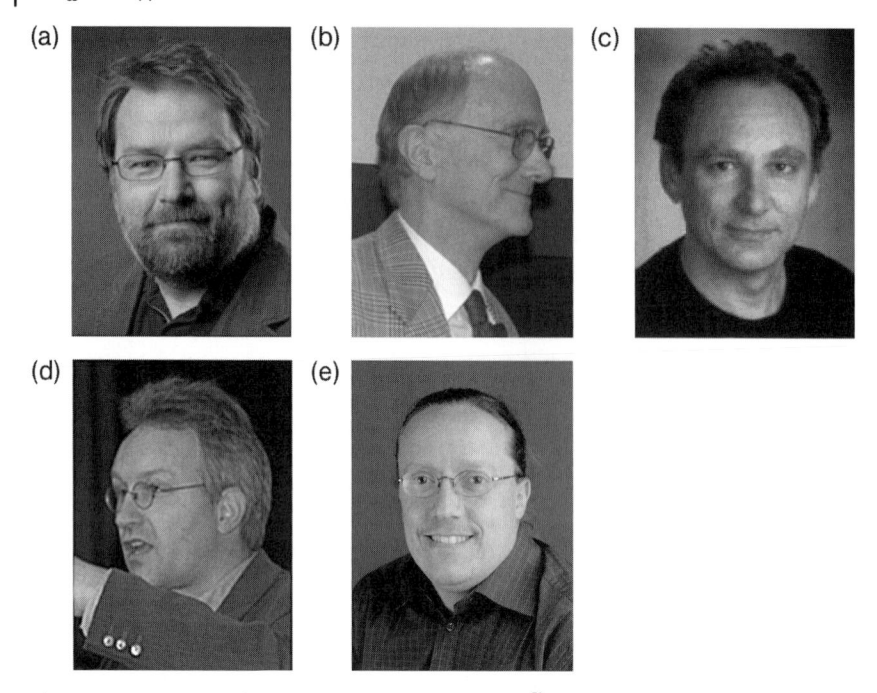

Figure 4.5 Major contributors to IETF and related bodies[1] (a) Harald Alvestrand, (b) Brian Carpenter, (c) Jon Crowcroft, Christian Huitema (no photo), (d) Erik Huizer, (e) Patrik Fältström

networks had recently purchased X.25 equipment as part of a long-term strategy, and had good reasons to support and conform to OSI standards; in any case, their budgeting procedures might not allow for major changes to their equipment at the "wrong" part of the budget cycle.

Since the overall aim at the international level was to interconnect all participating research networks, the European infrastructure had to be adapted to deal with multiple protocol suites and to provide a conversion facility between them so that any pair of end users could communicate with each other, independently of the protocol used by their research networks.

Before the start of the IXI service, it also seemed likely that line capacities of 64 kbps would not be sufficient to cope with demand once the general user community discovered the possibilities offered by new services such as electronic mail. By October 1990, when the IXI service finally came into operation, European PNOs were starting to supply 2 Mbps international circuits (still based on the provision of a half circuit by each of the PNOs at the two ends). Both of these issues were addressed in parallel with the implementation of IXI.

1) A large number of engineers from Europe have made significant contributions to the development of research networking through their participation in the work of the IETF and its associated bodies. The set of individuals pictured is limited to those who before 1997 have been Chair of the IETF (Alvestrand, Carpenter), a member of the IESG (Internet Engineering Steering Group: Huizer), or a member of the IAB (Internet Architecture Board: all those shown).

Telebit, the supplier of the switches used by IXI, was already developing interfaces to support line speeds higher than 64 kbps and the use of IP, as well as the software needed for a gateway between X.25 and IP-based services. As a result, IXI started as an X.25-based network with access capacities of 64 kbps in 14 countries but the switches were already equipped with 2 Mbps access ports and the first of these was brought into service (for WIN – WissenchaftsNetz – in Germany) before the end of 1992. In the first months of 1993, a new IP pilot service supported the carriage of IP packets by the X.25 service. The first native IP port was installed in Amsterdam for SURFnet in the second quarter of 1993. During the third quarter of 1993, the first 2 Mbps circuits were installed in the backbone and the first 2 Mbps access port was brought into service for JANET in the United Kingdom. This implementation was very different from what had originally been planned as the continuation of IXI and the operational service was renamed EMPB (European multi-protocol backbone).

The planning and implementation of IXI was carried out as part of the COSINE project, according to the terms of a contract between PTT Telecom and the EC. The original intention had been that the OU would supervise the operational service that followed IXI but the OU had still not been set up when the service started so alternative arrangements had to be made. Instead, EMPB service was provided according to the terms of a framework contract, initially between PTT Telecom and RARE, but with provision for RARE to hand over responsibility to the OU once it was established. It also gave PTT Telecom the option of assigning the contract to any of its subsidiaries or to one of the companies in the Unisource group. (Unisource was set up jointly by PTT Telecom, Telia of Sweden and Swisscom – joined later by Telefonica of Spain – to manage multinational services). This option was exercised very quickly, and Unisource Business Networks was given the responsibility of operating the network.

The framework contract specified the services that Unisource would provide, including the options available to research networks in terms of access capacity, cost of that access capacity, and quality of service. Quality of service, as measured by access port availability, monthly and yearly service availability, end-to-end (E2E) transit delay and E2E throughput (between any two access ports on an otherwise unloaded network), was "guaranteed" in the sense that provision was made for compensation if specified limits on the values of these parameters were exceeded. It also spelled out the technical requirements that research networks would have to meet in order to make a connection and imposed obligations on them to forecast increases in traffic levels so that Unisource had time to increase the network configuration to cope with the increased load and to maintain the specified quality of service. The contract also obliged the research networks to upgrade their access capacity (or to reduce their traffic) if their traffic levels exceeded defined limits when measured over a three-month rolling period.

It is important to note that the contract was for the provision of a network service at a number of access ports. Although it had the obligation to ensure that the network was configured adequately to meet the service specifications, Unisource was, in principle, free to use the same infrastructure to provide services to other customers. This concept was not fully understood by some of the research networks' engineers and, when it was understood, was disliked by those who would have preferred to look after the "nuts and bolts" of the network themselves.

EMPB access charges were set as a function of access capacity, following the pattern used by many of the PNOs for the provision of leased circuits at that time. A 2 Mbps access cost 11.4 times that of a 64 kbps access, for a factor 32 increase in access capacity. Access charges were independent of geography, that is, the total network cost was shared between the research networks exclusively on the basis of access capacity and no account was taken of particularly high or particularly low line costs for connections to any particular country. In contrast with the practice adopted by the PNOs for their own national services, there were no explicit volume charges (but note the commitment to upgrade if traffic exceeded certain levels).

Many of the IXI switches were also connected to the X.25 service operated by the national PNO, the PNOs' assumption being that the public X.25 service would soon become the standard means by which individual users would intercommunicate and that traffic could then pass easily between a researcher connected to IXI and a collaborator who was connected to the public X.25 service elsewhere in Europe. No charge would be made for traffic passing between a research network and an organization connected to the public X.25 service in the same country. According to the contract, charges for traffic between the research network and a private network in another country were subject to negotiation between the research network and the telecoms operator in the country concerned. In practice, there was little or no such traffic, so no charges were ever defined.

During 37 months of operation between October 1992 and October 1995 several upgrades were made to the initial configuration. The changes can be seen by comparing Figures 4.6 and 4.7. Four Central European countries joined the network with funding support from the EC's PHARE program. Research networks upgraded their access capacity to 2 Mbps, trunk circuits on the busiest routes were upgraded to 8 Mbps and 4 Mbps access ports were made available and became operational. The monthly availability fell below the contracted value of 99.7% in four out of 36 months (performance data collected during the last month of operation was never processed); the annual availability never fell below the guaranteed value of 99.8%.

During this period, there were three external factors which had a significant influence on the operation of EMPB: the extension to Central Europe, the research networks' requirement for connectivity to the United States and the relationship with Ebone.

Following the collapse of the Soviet bloc in 1989, universities and research institutions in the CEEC looked for advice and assistance in setting up network services which were comparable with those in the West. Under its PHARE program for supporting these countries, the EC took the initial step of contracting PTT Telecom to install IXI switches in 3–4 countries and to connect them to EMPB via 64 bps circuits. Although the switches were installed quickly, they were only provided with X.25 connections which were of little interest to the CEEC research networks. These research networks had also been offered IP connections from different sources, including Ebone and the government of Austria. With very limited resources

4.5 EMPB, European Multi-Protocol Backbone

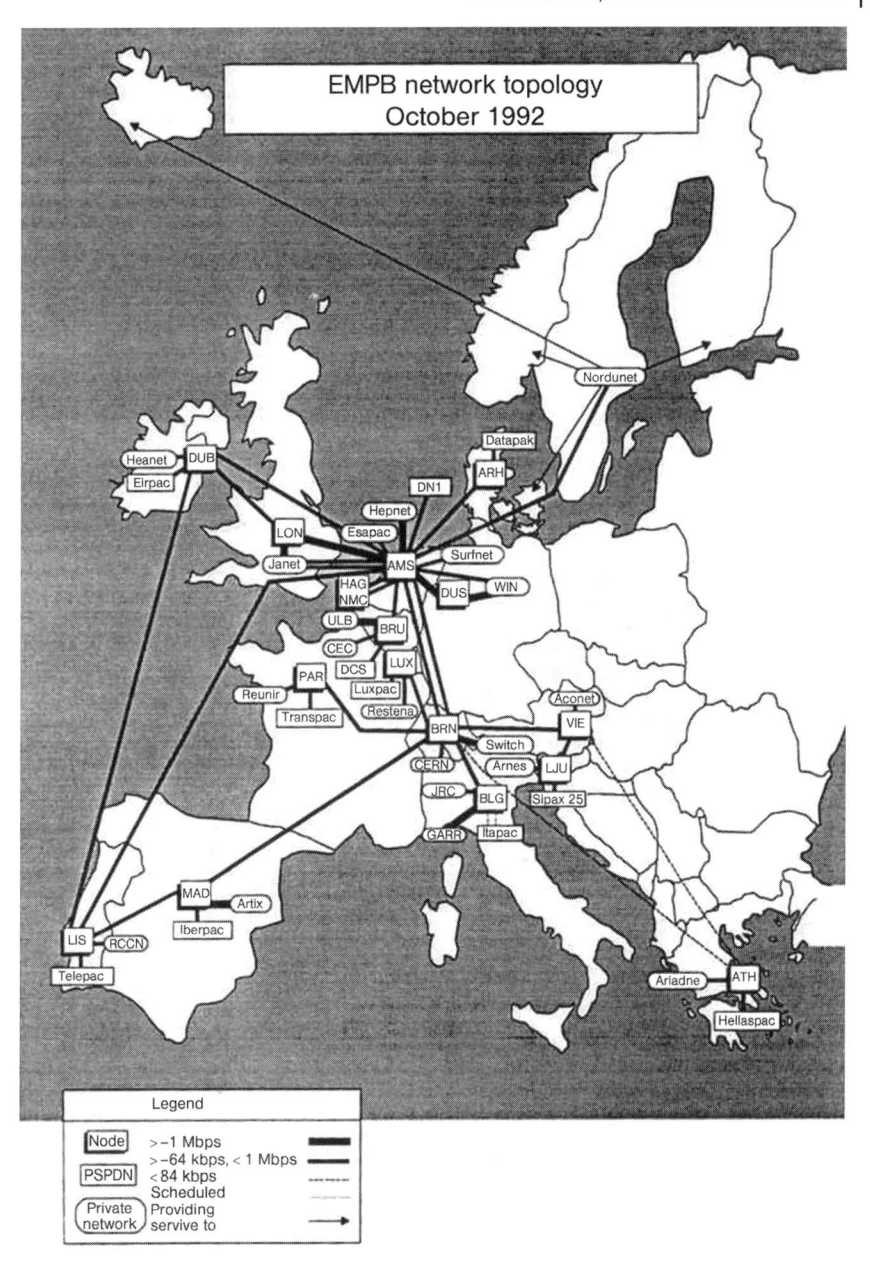

Figure 4.6 EMPB topology, October 1992.

for buying equipment, they could not justify supporting two parallel infrastructures, and had decided that an IP service was a better basis on which to build. The usage of the IXI switches was, therefore, very limited. Then, in a second phase of the PHARE program, and following an invitation to tender by the EC, DANTE was contracted to

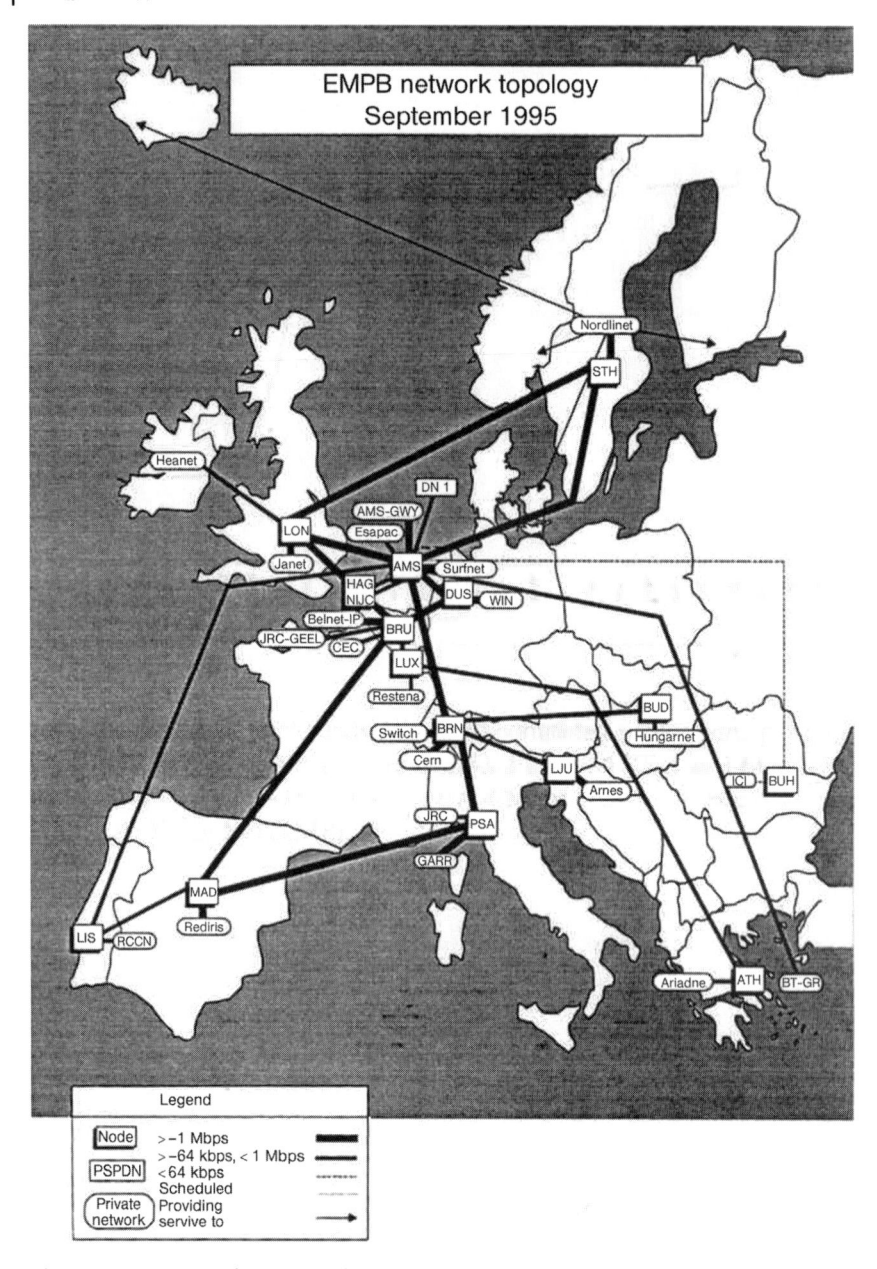

Figure 4.7 EMPB topology, September 1995.

provide support to the CEEC research networks in the form of management of the PHARE funds that were made available. Even before this management contract was in place, DANTE arranged for the switches to be made capable of handling native IP traffic and the four countries that had switches were connected to EMPB's IP service during the fourth quarter of 1993. The connection to Prague was upgraded to 512 kbps to provide Internet connectivity to attendees of the INET/RARE networking conference that was held there in May 1994. The Czech research network was successful in persuading its Ministry of Education to fund the cost of maintaining the circuit in place after the conference, an important step in bringing the capabilities of the research networks of the region into line with those found elsewhere in Europe.

The pattern of traffic to and from the CEEC was different from that in Western Europe. Information resources were lacking in these countries, and there were few research collaborations to generate large amounts of international traffic. Students, teachers and researchers nevertheless took advantage of these new communication systems to access services in the West, and particularly in the United States. The demand was primarily for access to sites on the commercial Internet in the United States, and for several years the capacity of transatlantic circuits (in the West–East direction) was a significant bottleneck. When new circuits were installed, the load would increase, typically within minutes, to absorb over 80% of the additional capacity. Several of the research networks in Western Europe had their own links to the United States which they operated separately from their European connection to EMPB. Others were willing to use EMPB as a transit network to carry United States traffic to and from a shared transatlantic line if this reduced the overall cost (or gave greater capacity for the same budgeted amount).

The use of EMPB to carry traffic to and from commercial organizations was a difficult area and the subject of much discussion. Funding from the EC could be used only for academic and research purposes, and the EMPB contract excluded the use of the network for "commercial activities". This term is not, however, precisely defined, and the exclusion was in conflict with an explicit permission for the network to be used for "administration and direct support" of research activities. For example, if a researcher makes enquiries about an item of equipment with several potential suppliers and subsequently places an order by e-mail, is this "commercial activity" (forbidden) or "administration support"? It is now generally accepted that any network communication which has an academic or research organization at either the receiving or the transmitting end is acceptable, and that it is only communications unrelated to any research activity between two commercial organizations that are not acceptable. For many years, uncertainty about where to draw the line between acceptable and unacceptable use was the cause of much confusion.

At the same time as the IXI/EMPB network was being implemented, a group of research networks together with a number of commercial service providers were establishing Ebone as an alternative IP-based backbone network. For those research networks that had decided to base their service on IP, a connection to Ebone was attractive as a way of making progress while waiting for IP services to be available from EMPB. Another attraction was that there were no restrictions on the type of traffic it would carry, and thus research networks which did not have their own transatlantic capacity could use it without worrying about possible AUP infringements.

By the time the EMPB service became available in October 1992, several research networks had already joined Ebone and had taken out a subscription which committed them to pay Ebone charges until August 1993. In order to fulfill the objective of providing connectivity between any pair of research networks, a gateway between EMPB and Ebone was essential. The technical difficulties of establishing such a gateway were complex but were overcome thanks to positive collaboration between engineers from the two networks (e.g. specifying routing plans which ensured that traffic passed across the appropriate network). Agreement on the financial aspects of the gateway service proved more difficult.

Many research networks joined Ebone simply because it was there (and the IP service of EMPB was not). They saw this as a useful interim measure but as the end of the period of their initial commitment approached, Ebone had been in operation for some months and had acquired a momentum of its own. The research networks were therefore presented with a real choice between EMPB and Ebone (or subscribing to both).

Even though the research networks had set up DANTE specifically to provide them with international services, they had no obligation to use the services that DANTE now offered, and could therefore choose the service they wished to use on the basis of their respective merits. DANTE and Ebone were in open competition to acquire research networks as customers.

As might be expected, different research networks used different criteria in making their choices, and there was no consensus on the way forward. Some of the research networks had never joined Ebone and simply stayed with EMPB, some had good reasons – and sufficient funds – to be able to connect to both networks. Two research networks decided to use Ebone exclusively and not to connect to EMPB.

One of the attractions of Ebone relative to EMPB was its lack of restrictions on traffic exchanged with commercial organizations, including those in the United States. Having accepted that any restrictive AUP was likely to be a condition of any government funding – including EC funding – there was little that DANTE could do about these restrictions apart from setting down clear and precise rules and trying to ensure that their implementation was as simple as possible.

A gateway between Ebone and EMPB was essential to provide connectivity between EMPB customers on the one hand, and the commercial networks and the research networks that had stayed on Ebone on the other. Ebone insisted that DANTE should pay its standard subscription rate for the use of these gateways. Because it did not have the financial resources to sustain a long dispute, DANTE's negotiating position was weak, so it reluctantly agreed to pay Ebone subscription charges for six months from July 1994 and three gateways were set up, in Amsterdam, Geneva and Stockholm.

Connectivity to the United States raised a different set of issues and although it was possible to address some of them there were difficulties that had to be overcome. In particular, many of the research networks in Western Europe had their own circuits to the United States and were unwilling to see EMPB capacity being used to carry CEEC traffic to and from the United States. (Direct connections between Central European countries and the United States were made up of circuits across Europe to a country with an Atlantic coast circuit combined with a transatlantic circuit and were hideously expensive). DANTE could arrange the provision of the United States connectivity and offered it to all EMPB customers for an additional charge on top of the tariff for traffic within Europe. It labeled this combined Europe/ United States service as EuropaNET.

With a view to seeking support from the EC's Fourth Framework Program, the EuroCAIRN project contracted DANTE in 1994 to make a study of the high-speed networking requirements of the research networks and to produce a plan for the setting up of high-speed services as soon as possible. In March 1995, the EuroCAIRN committee approved DANTE's report on the study. The report concluded that growing demand for network connectivity, the availability of new applications requiring high bandwidth and the introduction of new technology to support them were driving an increasing demand for bandwidth. A pan-European infrastructure was needed to keep pace with the higher capacities which were already available in the more advanced European countries. ATM technology was being introduced by the PNOs but was not yet stable enough for services at an international level. It was to be studied further, in parallel with planning for a 34 Mbps structure based on IP technology. Cooperation between the networking community and the telecoms operators should be sought as a way of overcoming the reluctance of the PNOs to make available the 34 Mbps technology and circuits that they already had in place. The report also included an implementation plan for the establishment of a 34 Mbps backbone.

Smooth progress towards implementation of the plan was hindered by two things. The first was that the PNOs were preparing to face the consequences of telecommunications liberalization which the EC was enforcing from January 1998. They knew that they would be competing with each other from that date, and that they would have to abandon the cosy cooperation arrangements that had been in place for so long – at their customers' expense. They were especially reluctant to reveal their own plans for the more advanced services that they would need to have in place when competition took hold. If anything, it was more difficult to arrange positive collaboration with any of the PNOs during the 12 to 18-month period before liberalization than it had been earlier. Access to 34 Mbps capacity was going to be impossible for some time.

The second factor was Unisource's announcement that it was not prepared to extend the contract for the provision of the EMPB service beyond the termination date of its contract in October 1995. Unisource did offer to provide an alternative IP service based on the use of Cisco routers and frame relay connections between international connection points. A close examination of the proposed alternative showed that it would not even provide an adequate replacement for EMPB as well as being unsuitable as the basis for moving towards the use of 34 Mbps and higher speeds.

DANTE was therefore faced with a choice between two alternatives: to negotiate with Unisource to take over the EMPB network (which served no other Unisource customers despite Unisource's original intention) and to operate it itself, or to issue a tender for the supply of an alternative service. The first of these alternatives was not considered a sound way of continuing the service offered to the research networks, and the decision was therefore made to seek a new service provider and to set up a new network service which would have the same features as EuropaNET and would continue to carry the EuropaNET name.

4.6
EuropaNET

Enhancement of the 2 Mbps EMPB service and introduction of advanced (34–155 Mbps) services were seen as distinct activities which would be developed separately and which would almost certainly use different sets of contractors. Linkage was the vital element and there would be a "seamless" integration procedure, so that research networks connected only to EMPB could exchange IP traffic with those connected to the advanced network.

The contract with PTT Telecom for the provision of EMPB terminated on September 30 1995. A replacement for EMPB had to be in place by October 1 1995 at the latest, but in fact some time earlier in order to allow for a smooth transition. Several forms of the replacement were considered: a sub-set of the existing EMPB equipment or lines could be taken over and operated directly by DANTE (the cost of taking over the complete set of lines was prohibitive); as a variant of this, a 4–8 Mbps overlay network could be set up between the research networks for which 2 Mbps access was no longer sufficient, with the use of some EMPB lines and equipment being retained to provide service to the remaining networks; acceptance of the UBN (Unisource Business Networks) offer to move the EMPB service on to its own commercial network (based on Cisco routers connected by frame relay links with a separate set of Northern Telecom switches carrying X.25 traffic); a completely new network might be created and operated by DANTE in collaboration with the research networks using purchased routers and individual leased lines; or a new service could be acquired as a result of a new Invitation to Tender to potential service providers. In addition to technical adequacy and the need to meet the installation deadline, proposals for any new network had to retain all the essential functionality of the EMPB service which was in place, to address the question of providing access speeds of 4 and 8 Mbps and to provide for continuation of the new service for at least a year from October 1995. The last two of these requirements were necessary in order to justify the effort which both DANTE and the research networks would have to put into an early transition from EMPB.

The final choice would also be affected by working capital requirements, which would be very different if research networks made all payments via DANTE instead of paying the contractor directly as they did with EMPB.

An investigation by DANTE, assisted by its Technical Advisory Group (a set of knowledgeable engineers from the research networks), concluded that the best option was to invite tenders for a new service. It was accepted that there might be difficulties due to the PNO environment at the time. Liberalization of EU telecommunications, due to take place on January 1 1998, was already having an effect, as individual PNOs were preparing for the competition they would face two years after the start of the new service. They had little incentive to cooperate, for example through the efficient delivery and management of half-circuits for use in a competitor's new developments, especially since such cooperation might reveal their own liberalization strategies.

Therefore, how effective an open tender would be was in doubt. In the event, DANTE received eight expressions of interest of which seven conformed with pre-tender requirements, followed by three tenders, two of which (from BT, British Telecommunications, Worldwide and Unisource Business Networks) satisfied the minimum technical requirements. After further negotiation and clarification of the tenders, the BT proposal was accepted.

As the major PNO in the United Kingdom, BT (through its Belgium-based subsidiary) was already planning and creating a transmission infrastructure covering the larger European countries on which it would be able to mount a range of international voice and data services. The contract with DANTE for the provision of the EMPB replacement enabled BT to implement its plan and to gain more experience in operating an international IP network sooner than had been anticipated. Under the terms of the tender and subsequent contract, BT provided a native IP service operating in parallel with an X.25 service, in which X.25 packets were transported on top of the IP service. The initial configuration of the BT network (named IBDNS, international backbone data network service) was based on 2 Mbps circuits with frame relay being used to provide connectivity to two research networks which could not justify a 2 Mbps access. Although BT was contracted to provide an IP service which had defined limits for performance and reliability and the same infrastructure could be used by BT to provide services to other customers, the initial network design was governed exclusively by DANTE's requirements. Access ports were available in capacities from 64 kbps to 8 Mbps for the IP service and 64 or 128 kbps for X.25. Ports with capacity greater than 2 Mbps were supported by multiplexing 2 Mbps circuits since no higher speed circuits were available at affordable prices. (In theory, 8 Mbps was another standard PNO circuit speed but very little equipment had been designed to operate at this speed and such equipment was expensive).

Timely delivery before the October 1 1995 deadline was going to be a challenge for any supplier and several steps were taken to make sure that it could be met. BT's commitment to providing service by this date and at the tendered price was conditional on DANTE ordering at least 170 units of access capacity before June 30 1995. (In its tender, BT had proposed a pricing scheme according to which the annual charge for an access port was related to a port with a set of multipliers, one for each possible value of access capacity, which was very similar to the set already in use for EMPB. With a 64 kbps access counting as one unit and a 2 Mbps access counting as 11.4 units, the BT condition would be met if sixteen or more 2 Mbps accesses were ordered.)

There were guarantees in the contract that provided for compensation if BT failed to deliver service at any of the committed access ports on time. BT also made arrangements to use its own and other PNOs' ISDN services in case of delays in the delivery of international circuits.

Getting commitments from the research networks to back up this order was essential as DANTE still did not have enough working capital to proceed without them. But it was difficult. In addition to the natural reluctance of any organization to make commitments before it needs to, some of the research networks were not confident that DANTE would succeed in managing the complete process of procurement, installation and operation of a completely new network service in a dozen or so countries, especially given the tight timetable that had to be followed. Access charges posed a particular problem. The research networks were not prepared to place an order until they knew what the cost would be; DANTE could only work out a pricing scheme if it knew how much BT would charge; and the BT charge was dependent on the number of accesses. This vicious circle could only be broken by DANTE making its own judgment of the likely take-up of the services by the research networks and taking the commercial risk associated with getting its estimate wrong.

The charging scheme that was adopted was similar to that used for EMPB. The principle of setting access charges which varied according to access capacity but which were independent of geography was maintained. The charge for each of the available capacities was related to the cost of the basic 64 kbps access by a standard multiplier. The same multipliers as for EMPB were used for capacities up to 2 Mbps. At higher rates, the multipliers were proportional to the 2 Mbps rate or even slightly higher; this was necessary since BT's charges were based on the cost of supporting the higher bandwidths with 2 Mbps circuits, with no discount for quantity and with the added cost of multiplexing equipment. These access capacities could still be attractive to the research networks that could make savings on the cost of local loops and interfacing equipment

As a result of DANTE's exhortations by e-mail and by telephone, the 170 unit threshold was met in time but this was not the end of the research networks' lack of faith. In order to manage its cash flow and pay the BT invoice that would be presented on delivery of the network service, DANTE required the research networks to make advance payments for the service to which they had subscribed. Just one week before the October deadline, one research network informed DANTE that it did not believe the new service would be in place on time, so they would not make the payment which was due. DANTE's forceful response was "no payment, no service".

The concern felt by the research network involved was not entirely without foundation, since BT was having difficulties in completing the installation of a circuit between London and Geneva which would carry a lot of traffic. However, BT put its contingency plan into effect and connected these two locations by means of an ISDN link. In order to minimize costs, the link's speed was limited initially to 128 kbps. A trial to adjust the link speed dynamically according to the load failed and so BT had no alternative but to maintain the 2 Mbps capacity using ISDN links until the planned circuit became available. Since the ISDN link had to be paid for at standard PNO rates (to another BT subsidiary at one end, but to Swisscom at the other end), the cost to BT Worldwide was high and DANTE agreed to pay a share.

On the whole, the transition from EMPB to IBDNS went smoothly, and the EMPB service was switched off by Unisource on October 2 1995. In the course of the following months there were a number of recurring incidents which badly affected the service to SWITCH; these were eventually traced to a fault in the Swiss access router. A more serious problem was the poor performance of the Network Operations

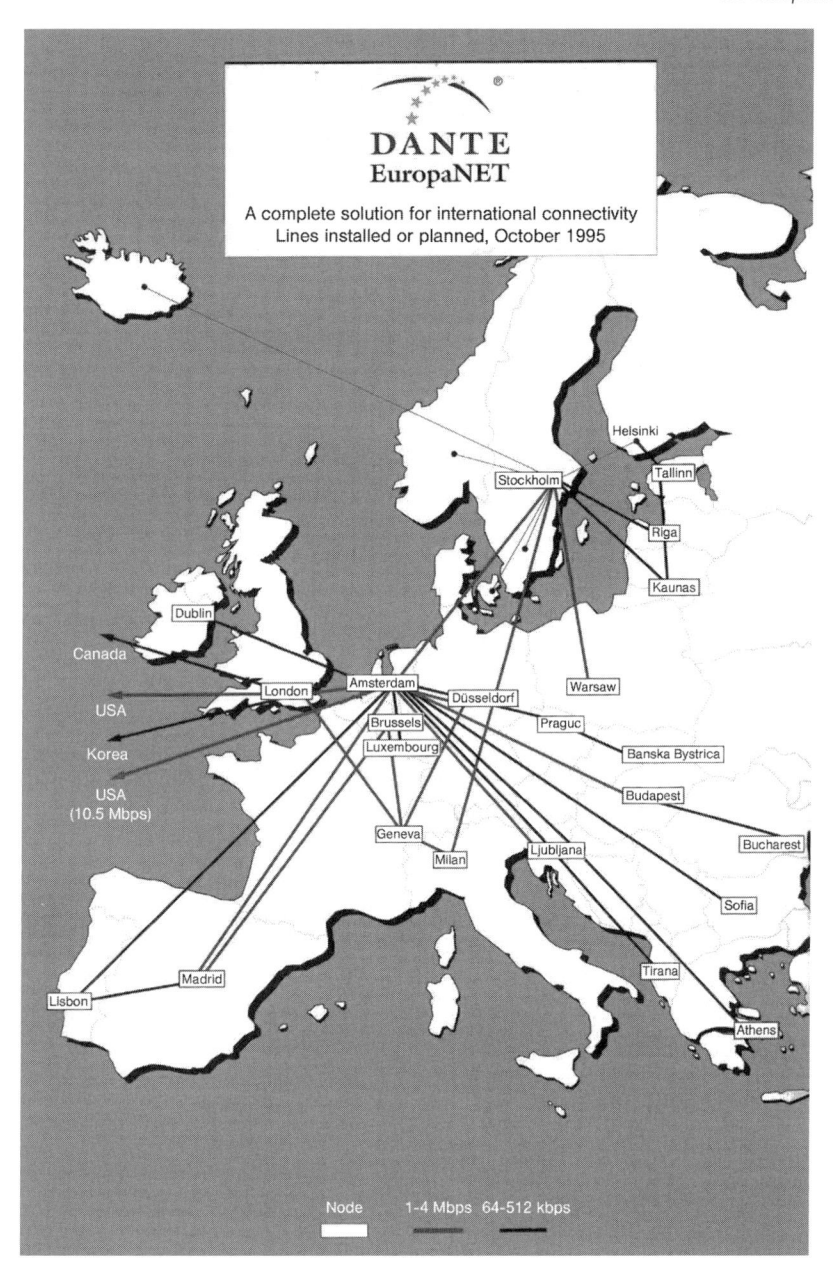

Figure 4.8 EuropaNET configuration. There is a color version of this figure in the set at the front of the book.

Centre that BT had established to operate IBDNS and it required intervention at a senior management level to remedy this. BT had set up a dynamic and capable project team to manage the installation of the new network, but had not been as careful in planning the operational phase. Managerial responsibility for IBDNS operations was held by a part of the BT organization which was technically very capable and which had a background in the IP development environment. Its relationship with other parts of the BT organization such as that which diagnosed line faults was not well-defined. As a result of DANTE pressure, responsibility for the IBDNS operation was transferred to a mainstream network operations group within BT. The result was a more rigorous operational approach, a reduction in the number of human failures, and a more systematic analysis and correction of equipment problems.

In 1994, BT had acquired a 20% shareholding in MCI, the major United States telecoms operator. One consequence of this was the extension by BT across Europe of MCI's well-established United States and transatlantic IP service. BT created a new infrastructure (named INCS, integrated network connection service) to support the extension, and in May 1996 proposed to move the EuropaNET (European multi-protocol backbone network) service from IBDNS to INCS. Although this meant yet another transition for the research networks, there were significant advantages in making the move. The new infrastructure was much bigger than that of IBDNS. This eliminated any remaining performance problems and access capacities could be increased quickly and easily. When the time came for the research networks to terminate their connections and move to the next generation service, there would be no pressure to make the termination by a fixed date. There were some concerns about IP routing for EuropaNET, in particular in relation to the sharing of transatlantic circuits with BT's commercial customers, but once BT had given assurances that DANTE would be kept fully informed of configuration changes, the transition was agreed. The EuropaNET IP service was moved from IBDNS to INCS between July 1996 and October 1996 and remained there until March 1998 when the last of the research networks had moved their traffic to the new TEN-34 network (Fig. 4.8).

The Protocol Wars

The protocol wars were undeclared and no peace treaty was ever signed, so it is hard to say when they started or ended. Wars in the plural: there were indeed several wars, with shifting alliances - proprietary solutions versus standards, Europe versus the United States, the PTTs versus the regulators, and pragmatists versus purists, plus other battlegrounds. The complete story would require a book of its own; here, the focus will be on how the research community in Europe saw the wars.

Even in the 1970s, and certainly by 1980, data-intensive research disciplines saw a clear need for international research networking. For example, in January 1982, the late Mervyn Hine sketched a map of the international backbone needed by the experiments planned at CERN's future LEP. Apart from bandwidth, it looks remarkably similar to the network needed a quarter century later by the experiments planned at the Large Hadron Collider (LHC). But in 1982 there was a big open question: which protocols should be used? The major computer vendors, notably IBM and DEC, vigorously promoted their proprietary protocols, SNA and DECnet respectively. Some segments of the research community had community standards of their own, notably the Coloured Books in the United Kingdom. The PTTs proposed X.25 services for the future, charged enormous sums for private modem links, and in many cases disallowed the re-transmission of any incoming packet, ie the customer's equipment should not act as a switch for traffic between third parties. People in Europe had heard of the ARPAnet, but it was not yet converted completely to TCP/IP.

There was rapid consensus in the research community that proprietary protocols could not be allowed to dominate in the long run. Moreover, the policy makers in most Western European countries and in Brussels reached the same conclusion as the EC struggled with the early stages of de-monopolisation of the PTTs. To allow any kind of competitive market, vendor-independent standards were agreed to be the only way forward. And for operational reasons, nobody wanted to see multiple network protocols running in parallel a moment longer than was necessary. The cost and inconvenience of obtaining global connectivity via multiprotocol gateways were prohibitive. Although DECnet in particular was to have a long and successful run in scientific networks, the war between proprietary and standard protocols had only one possible outcome. By 1985 the only question was: which standard?

In 1980, Hubert Zimmermann published an academic description of the OSI model for networking, developed as an ISO standardisation activity since 1978. By 1985, OSI was a reasonably full set of detailed technical standards, jointly developed by the ITU and ISO, with an apparently broad base of industrial support, notably including IBM and Digital, as well as the few remaining European computer firms and most of the PTTs. Furthermore, there was widespread official support for OSI as a preferred direction for government adoption and encouragement. Particularly noticeable were United States Federal requirements in the form of the GOSIP profile, and strong support from the United Kingdom Department of Trade and Industry and from the relevant Directorates of the EC. Obviously, OSI could not fail with this measure of official support, and it was technically attractive. One merely had to wait for the various vendors to release their OSI products, such as SNA/OSI and DECnet Phase V, and for the PTTs to provide the corresponding OSI network services.

Also in 1978, Vint Cerf and Bob Kahn had published a first version of TCP/IP, following nine years of experience with ARPAnet and fruitful interaction with European researchers such as Louis Pouzin and Peter Kirstein. By 1981, the basic TCP/IP RFCs (Request For Comments) were standardized. In January 1983, the whole ARPAnet, including all its applications and users, cut over to TCP/IP. Later the same year, Berkeley UNIX version BSD (Berkeley Software Distribution) 4.2 was released with TCP/IP included. The first widely available UNIX workstations with Ethernet connections (from Sun Microsystems) came to Europe that year with TCP/IP included for free. But of course, TCP/IP was not an official standard. RFCs were unofficial publications from a United States research project, and if you asked where to buy a copy, you were told to find it on the network and to print it yourself (to be fair, you could get a United States Department of Defense military standard for TCP/IP in book form, but it was not exactly the same text as the RFCs.) Obviously, "unofficial" TCP/IP was not a basis for building a global network.

It was in this context that many in the European research community had chosen OSI as their strategic direction by about 1985. RARE was created around the assumption of an OSI future; numerous emerging research networks decided to target OSI; CERN declared an OSI policy[2]; EARN announced an OSI plan; and of course the COSINE project was kicked off.

Four or five years later, strategies had generally switched dramatically, from OSI to TCP/IP[3]. Although the war continued for a while on both sides of the Atlantic, with the *coup de grâce* being administered to OSI by the release of the Web browser in 1993, it's clear that TCP/IP "won." To quote a famous phrase from Marshall Rose, OSI ended up as "roadkill on the information superhighway."

There are no doubt varying views on why this happened. Here we will mention two aspects: the fatal flaws in OSI, and the triumph of pragmatism. OSI had a very formal - almost mathematical - structure of seven layers and interfaces between those layers. A good design in itself, but with two major consequences. The first is that strict layering can lead to major inefficiency in implementations - seven layers make six interfaces, each of which adds overhead for message passing or procedure calls. The flatter and less formal TCP/IP model makes for more efficient implementation. Internet protocol designers today often debate whether a design feature is a "layer violation," i.e., one protocol layer interfering directly with another. This is formally impossible in OSI, but is sometimes a necessary engineering trade-off to improve performance.

The second consequence of OSI layering, and of the horse-trading that occurred in the ISO/ITU discussions, is that the Transport and Network layers (roughly corresponding to TCP and IP respectively) allowed several major non-interoperable options. At the network layer, the two options were "connection oriented" and "connectionless." We can summarise by saying that a connection oriented network (i.e., a virtual circuit network) matches the old PTT model of establishing paid connections between pairs of customers, whereas a connectionless model matches the concept pioneered in the ARPAnet, with anyone talking to anyone without advance notice, much better adapted to resilient routing and to flat-rate charging. At the transport level, there were also multiple options in OSI, but whereas the ARPAnet model offered only two transport options (TCP and UDP, User Datagram Protocol), OSI offered five, in a vain attempt to be all things to all men.

OSI could possibly have prospered with multiple transport protocols, but the diversity at the network layer was fatal. The US-GOSIP profile specified connectionless network service, but under strong pressure from PTTs struggling to maintain their monopolies, the profiles officially favoured in Europe mainly specified connection-oriented network service based on X.25. Obviously, the

---

2) Carpenter B.E., *Computer Communications at CERN*, Conf. *Computing in High Energy Physics*, Amsterdam, June 1985, proceedings ed. L.O.Hertzberger and W.Hoogland, North-Holland, 1986.

3) See footnote above.

international research community was highly resistant to a solution in which the networks in North America would be using a different basic protocol than those in Europe. This had its impact on COSINE, which included a pilot project for connectionless network service, but the transatlantic connection/connectionless battle remained, with the PTT alliance strongly pushing X.25.

At the same time, the use of TCP/IP was growing (some would say insidiously, and some would say inevitably) on practically every campus in Europe. As UNIX grew like wildfire with the proliferation of affordable RISC (Reduced Instruction Set Computer) workstations and servers, so did Ethernet and TCP/IP, and people discovered that TCP/IP was free, easy to use, and efficient. For example, Tim Berners-Lee discovered this at CERN before he wrote the initial proposal for the Web in 1989. Undoubtedly the availability of MIT's (Massachusetts Institute of Technology) X-Windows and Sun's Network File System (NFS) spurred this growth on campus. But unlike other campus solutions such as Appletalk or Novell Netware, TCP/IP was also quite easy to run over WAN links (even over X.25 links if that was all you could get). Even before the Web appeared in 1993, applications such as email, network news, and various information management systems to augment FTP were available on all types of computers used in the research community. So wide-area TCP/IP began to be used opportunistically in European research as the 1980s progressed. It was free, IP routers were reasonably priced, it worked well; whereas OSI software and hardware was either unavailable or very expensive. One can speculate that some vendors made OSI expensive to preserve a market for their proprietary solutions - if so, this was a fatal miscalculation. Researchers are nothing if not pragmatic, and they started asking their networking colleagues to provide TCP/IP support. Thus, TCP/IP appeared on IBM-compatible PCs, on Macintoshes, on Digital VAXes, and on mainframes, in addition to every UNIX box.

At the RARE Council of Administration meeting in Vienna in January 1990, RARE agreed to the fundamental argument of the pragmatists that TCP/IP should be recognized as a legitimate – though still interim - solution for the European research community. To quote from the decision:

"RARE, without putting into question its OSI policy, recognises the TCP/IP family of protocols as an open multi-vendor suite, well adapted to scientific and technical applications, which offers some facilities needed by part of the RARE user community that are not available with OSI today."

"RARE intends to ensure that coordination of TCP/IP in Europe is carried out as effectively as possible, by coming rapidly to a suitable arrangement with RIPE, the existing ad hoc TCP/IP coordination group, following the proposal by RIPE to RARE dated December 14 1989."

"The strategic implications of the above will be taken into account in RARE's programme of work."

Indeed, RARE forged a healthy relationship with RIPE in the course of 1990. In May of that year, at the first RARE/EARN Joint European Networking Conference in Killarney, a pragmatist's "birds of a feather" session was the first step to what soon became the Ebone. TCP/IP in the European research community had officially taken off, and OSI started to gather dust.

As a coda, we should not forget that the OSI reference model has served widely as a teaching tool in the academic community, and that some aspects of OSI have survived, for example in the highly successful Lightweight Directory Access Protocol (LDAP) which is directly based on OSI's X.500. The ASN.1 (Abstract Syntax Notation One) notation used in LDAP and in Simple Network Management Protocol (SNMP) data definitions is also part of the OSI endeavour. Although distinct from OSI, Standardised Generic Markup Language (SGML) was published as an ISO standard at about the same time as OSI, and today forms the basis for both HTML (HyperText Markup Language) and XML (eXtensible Markup Language). The great standardisation adventure of the 1970s and 1980s was not completely in vain.

5
The Interviews

This chapter presents a series of interviews with the heads of three European organizations heavily involved in organizing the pan-European research and education network. The different viewpoints highlight how all the European organizations collaborated, merged and competed, where that has eventually led to and what the future might hold.

5.1
Dai Davies

Dai Davies has been Joint General Manager of DANTE since its establishment in 1993. He previously worked for BT plc, initially as a development engineer and later in the international division of BT's business development and marketing group. He also spent two years with Deutsche Telekom and was Director of the COSINE Project Management Unit from 1991 to 1993.

What are the benefits and difficulties arising from the introduction of the network services?

The original interest in research networking in Europe in the 1980s was X.25. Europe was very much a leading region in terms of X.25 developments. The other factor about Europe in the late 1980s and through to 1996, was that the provision of telecom service across borders was a monopoly. It was very difficult to provide significant services in this monopoly environment. There were two reasons: One was a regulatory reason – only telecommunication operators could provide services. The other was a very practical reason – because it was a monopoly environment everything was very expensive. In a sense, network capacity, the arteries of the network, was rationed. It was very highly priced, and the operators wanted to make sure they kept it under their control.

What was interesting when I started with IXI is that there was a lot of acceptance of IP as being the way the networking technology was going to go. Another of the differences between X.25 and IP: the environment in research networking in the early 1990s was a war environment, a protocol war period. One group was interested

A History of International Research Networking. Edited by Howard Davies and Beatrice Bressan
Copyright © 2010 WILEY-VCH Verlag GmbH & Co. KGaA, Weinheim
ISBN: 978-3-527-32710-2

in IP, the other in X.25. The real objective which I saw in COSINE was to create a network that supported both approaches. EuropaNET, the main eventual outcome of the COSINE project, was a multi-protocol network. It supported access with X.25 and with IP. In a sense, it was a peace offering between these two warring camps. It was pretty successful.

In 1993, all of the major European research networks connected to EuropaNET at 2 Mbps, which in those days was quite fast. There were one or two countries that did not come in, the strangest exception was France, but everybody else, the United Kingdom, Germany, the Netherlands, the Nordic countries, all became part of this multi-protocol network.

When we set up DANTE, we took over the operational responsibility for EuropaNET. Since then we have built five further generations of research networks. We have done this in a relatively short period of time, replacing one network by another every three years on average. This haste has partly been driven by changes in technology, and most significantly by the liberalization of the telecoms markets in Europe. That has made an incredible difference to research networking on a European scale. Nationally, liberalization took place earlier, the big difference now, and this would have been true in 2001, you could get access to network capacity at a factor of 30 000 cheaper than was the case in 1991. It is an incredible change in the underlying cost of anything. That is why we have been able to build these huge GÉANT networks. GÉANT was a network which operated faster than the American equivalent, and with more capacity. Historically, the Americans had always led in research networking, as they had access to technology and a much more liberal market. In 2002, we had GÉANT in place, a 10 Gbps network with a much bigger footprint than the American equivalent. That was a major breakthrough.

Before that, we had gone through different stages of network building. We had gone from buying network service to building a network out of components. That was a gradual process. But by 1997, we were buying the transmission and the routing components, and building our own network. That process has got to the point now where we are acquiring fiber; we are equipping it with DWDM (dense wavelength division multiplexing) equipment. We are actually building a network from the most basic components. This has brought mainly positive benefits. It is more efficient, and more cost-effective for the most part. It also exposes some of the geography issues in Europe. Places at the edges of Europe do not have the same advantages as places in the center, simply because there is less traffic at the edges. Traffic from the edges goes to the center and traffic in the center stays in the center, it does not go to the edges. You always find more concentration in the center of a network. That means that center is cheaper, because you have more usage and economy of scale. This is one of the practical issues we are facing now: how do you have European cohesion when it costs you a lot of money to go to Spain, Portugal, Ireland, Greece, to all the places which are towards the edges? We still have to face this problem.

When we took over the network, the name EMPB did not sound very interesting, so we branded it EuropaNet. In the same way, we branded the most recent generations GÉANT, which is a very successful brand. DANTE's first result was EuropaNET, operating at 2 Mbps with some extension out toward Eastern Europe – Prague and Budapest got connected. We did not own any of the network equipment; we were still buying a service provided by, in this case, BT.

EuropaNET's successor, TEN-34, was a strange network. In 1996, you were starting to see liberalization, and slightly bigger capacity connections, but the situation in different countries was still very variable. We could only get 6 Mbps between Paris and the United Kingdom (provided by BT and France Télécom as a virtual circuit carried on a 34 Mbps line!) The fastest connection was a 34 Mbps circuit between Frankfurt and Geneva which we connected to our own equipment and which gave the network its name. Other parts of the network were bought as a service. This is very much the way the market started to develop

The major change came with TEN-155 (trans-European network at 155 Mbps), which started to be built in 1998 and provided the first real sign that prices were dropping and that capacity was becoming available. Part of it ran at 155 Mbps which was not a bad speed at the time. But there were also some connections at 10 Mbps and even lower speeds. The market was starting to liberalize and with TEN-155, based on ATM and IP technology, European research networking was starting to become world competitive. It was the first time we had a network where there was more or less enough capacity for the average user, so that users did not complain too much.

Then, we got on to GÉANT, the really huge breakthrough. In 2001, we had GÉANT, with some 10 Gbps connections. So you have gone from 155 Mbps connections as your basic building block to 10 Gbps, a factor of 60 increase. The new building blocks are not merely faster, they are also cheaper. You can see quite well developed connections to Poland, the Czech Republic, Hungary, becoming an integral part of the network, and also global connectivity to the States.

This is again an integral part of the network. This was another major breakthrough. You had a world-class high-capacity network in Europe. We leap-frogged the Americans at that point. We had a faster network. The GÉANT network is the breakthrough generation in networks as far as Europe is concerned. We covered more countries with faster connectivity. That developed for a three or four year period. Then, it was succeeded by GÉANT2 which has now been in place for about three years. One point about these networks is that there is a migration process which you have to take into account as well.

In what ways did each of the services above improve the facilities needed to support the work of end-users?

In the early 1990s, the users did not have anything. They had no connectivity. The first thing is that they started to experience real international connectivity within Europe and between Europe and North America in particular. It was inadequate, it was congested, but it was there, so that it was a major development as far as they were concerned. Then, what you saw was a gradual improvement in the performance, but not really sufficient capacity to do clever things. The network was always rather full. The first network where we started to do relatively interesting things for users was the TEN-155 network. This network was interesting because we could provide dedicated networks within this overall network. This meant that individual users could see what they felt was their own network. It gave them the advantage of having a relatively guaranteed performance in a congested environment. We built about 25 or 30 of these virtual private networks as part of TEN-155.

That made quite a difference precisely because users were guaranteed performance – users really could experience something which was not just a network connection, but a connection that performed for them. Therefore, we were providing some guarantees of quality in the days of TEN-155.

Then we moved on to GÉANT. GÉANT had so much capacity that nobody was worried about network performance. It was so big, the performance was guaranteed. What we started to do with GÉANT was to help users to take advantage of this very high capacity network. Networking is one of these things where you can plug the pieces together but it does not work. Networking is quite complicated. You have different end-systems with their operating systems, and you have different paths to the network. You can have all the pieces in place, you switch it on and it does not do what you expect. So, we started with GÉANT supporting users, particularly the high end users, who exploited the technology that was there in a way that made them achieve things they had not been able to achieve before.

The most interesting example was that of radio astronomy. The radio astronomers had been collecting data for years, recordings from radio telescopes across Europe. They had been putting it in on magnetic tape, and they then would fly all the tapes from the different centers to a central computer in the north of Holland. They would put the tapes on a computer there and they would run the tapes in parallel. So all the signals recorded from these radio telescopes were compared to one another. It took about 80 days to record the data and then you flew them to the Netherlands. It was quite a mechanical process. Straight away you realize that with a network like GÉANT, you can just carry that data. We put a lot of time and effort into helping the radio astronomy people exploit the network, because they had historically been getting data communications by flying magnetic tapes with a parcel courier. Now they had a network which enabled them, at least in principle, to put the data streams on the network and bring it to the Netherlands.

That was an interesting realization: with this very large high capacity performance network, you enabled users to do science in particular in new ways. But the practical aspects of it are quite complicated. As I said, if you just plug it all together, it does not always work. There is a lot of technical assistance and technical hand holding involved in supporting users of the new services on the GÉANT network.

GÉANT2 is different again. We do not just have an IP network in GÉANT, we have the ability to provide end-to-end paths at really quite high speeds – it can carry 1, 2.5, 10 Gbps. And you can do that for an individual user. The LHC activity really takes advantage of the fact that you can have almost dedicated high capacity links as well as an IP service. That means you can configure networks for people which they perceive as being their own network. And you have to manage that, you have to integrate all the pieces, and that gives a very powerful and flexible capability. That is what we are focusing on now in GÉANT2: supporting people to build their own virtual networks on our physical infrastructure.

That in itself raises problems in as much as you plug it all together and it does not quite work. So there is much more focus now, not just on providing people with connections, but looking at the way they perform, dealing with performance problems. Our emphasis is moving from simply providing users with high performance connections to helping them debug these connections to really make the performance available. Capacity used to be a problem in 1991, but not nowadays. Yet actually utilizing the capacity is still quite technically and operationally challenging. The next phase of user support is in terms of helping users to configure these quite complicated, quite large networks, and then really helping them to achieve the performance by looking at performance problems and by providing monitoring tools that look at the way the network is performing for individual users. That is where we are today in terms of user support.

How helpful and how important have the sources of funds been?

In terms of funding, without the European Union money, quite a lot of this would not have happened. The cheap parts of it might have happened anyway – the really cheap routes in Europe are between London, Paris, Frankfurt, and Amsterdam. That part is the most competitive set of routes in Europe. But once you go beyond that, it starts hurting – partly because the cost of links is geography dependent and the cost of a transmission system is very much related to the links. If you are going from Geneva to Madrid, you know it is going to be significantly more expensive than going from Geneva to Frankfurt. You can look at the distance and see Geneva-Madrid is four times the Geneva-Frankfurt distance. So the Geneva to Madrid route is going to be four times the price. There is little you can do about that.

The EU provides a degree of cohesion, so that the whole of Europe can benefit, not just the cheap parts. Cheaper parts might happen anyway. But without the EU money, you would not really build a pan-European network because the imbalance – partly geographic imbalance, partly cost imbalance – would be too big for the individual research networks to pay for themselves. EU money is getting close to 50% of the total funding of these networks. There have been networks, the second EuropaNET network, where there was no EU money. So it is certainly possible to build networks without EU money, but it is very much the glue that provides for bigger and better performing networks.

We do not actually see any national government money. We do see it indirectly because if we look at the total funding of the GÉANT network, some of it comes from the EU, but funding also comes from the connected R&E networks; and essentially they are normally using government money in one way or another to fund it. We see government funds indirectly, via the research network organizations in the different countries.

American money is interesting, because historically they did not really provide a lot of funding for transatlantic connections. If we go back to the early 1990s, the American government attitude was "we are the center of the Internet. Everybody should pay to come to us." And that is what happened. They gave a little bit of money to selected countries to show they were not prejudiced. Clearly speaking, Europe was paying the bill for the connection between North American researchers and European researchers. That has changed quite a bit in the past several years. Now the balance of networks is much more equal. The European network is as big, if not bigger and more powerful than the American network. The Americans are funding some of the transatlantic connections, and we are funding some of them as well. So from that point of view there is a balance, which is good.

As regards operators, our relationship is a relatively normal commercial transaction at arm's length. They compete with one another. From their point of view, they all learn quite a lot from what we are doing, because we are building advanced networks, and that is something that they need to do. However, we have straightforward commercial relationships with telecom operators. They may be very competitive, but at the end of the day, it is a contract. We pay money and we get either fiber or a service.

What are the strengths and the weaknesses of the organization and the management structure?

The strength is quite interesting in as much as we are consciously trying to be a European organization. So we have always heavily recruited from across Europe. It is not just a British company. If you talk to the engineers, you will find they are from Spain, from Romania, Poland, and so on. The nationality balance has changed over the years. When we started, we had quite a few Dutch people. I do not think we have anybody from the Netherlands any more. We had the last person working for us from the Netherlands about three years ago. Looking at the teams, you can see that young engineers have a strong interest in coming to work here. That is good: it means we have a sort of European culture and an understanding of some of the different national view points. That is a great strength.

The other strength we have is that we are good at financial management and we are good at negotiation. We are acting on behalf of a lot of people, and we get quite good deals. That is another major strength. Over the years, we have built up quite an impressive team of developers and operations people. Therefore, the quality of the staff and the commitment of the staff are high.

The weakness, I suppose, is that as a company we are owned by some but not all of the research networks. That means we work in a more complicated structure where we have a consortium which includes DANTE shareholders and non-shareholders and that mismatch is a practical issue. It does not stop things from happening but, for example, we own all the assets. As DANTE is a company, they ultimately belong to the shareholders. But, in fact, those assets should belong to everybody, to all the European research networks. Similarly, we built up our working capital over the years, and it amounts to some €8 M or €9 M now. That has come from everybody, but formally belongs to the shareholders. That sort of mismatch in terms of the ownership structure of DANTE and the organizational structure of the European research networking is a practical issue. That is the fundamental thing. If you ask "what would you change if you could?", that is what we are trying to change, the issue of ownership. DANTE should be owned by all of the organizations for whom it works, not a sub-set.

What were the pressures that led to the setting up of the main collaborative organizations?

There was no imposed requirement on the set up of DANTE. It was set up because a number of people thought it was necessary. It was the people that were involved who felt the need to establish DANTE. Not all of them actually took part, but most of them did. That was the position in 1993 when we were set up. There was a group of R&E networks who said: "we need this organization to work on our behalf. We need a European organization." And they established DANTE. The other structures that are there are quite different, in as much as there is a consortium of R&E networks, which are the people participating in GÉANT and in GÉANT2. We are part of that consortium. But that consortium only exists as long as it has a project to carry forward. It is project oriented. If we have another project, we can work that way.

Another organization is TERENA of course. TERENA is more of a trade association. It is a membership organization which people join. It offers certain benefits, but it does not, for example, have the funds or the commercial or technical organization to manage service. DANTE is an operational organization which does some R&D as well. But you can see the difference.

There are no links with governments as such. TERENA is mainly focused on the EU. To the extent that the EU supports pan-European research networking, it needs member states' acceptance of the budget item. The other point is that the member states have to provide roughly a little more than 50% of the total funding. They do not do that directly, but do so via the research networking organizations in their countries. We do not normally have any direct interaction with governments. We have it via their agencies.

What are the future directions?

Network generations last about four or five years, and in that period you set out what you intend to achieve at the beginning. And in the process of achieving that, you pretty well know what the challenges are going to be for the next four or five years. Initially, it was to provide a networking service, and then it was to provide more capacity. Then, it was to provide lots more capacity and some user support. Then, in terms of GÉANT2, it is a huge amount of capacity and increase in user support. But capacity is no longer a problem. The issues are performance: users have got the capacity but they cannot exploit it. Quality is increasingly becoming an issue. When they had nothing, just having a network was good. Now they are used to the network, but they want it to be performant and reliable. And achieving these things is no mean task. So what we are doing now is putting a lot more emphasis into monitoring and management of network performance, so that people get predictable and acceptable quality. That is certainly something to be developed further.

There are two other areas of importance. There are groups of users who are self-selecting. They know exactly what they want, they know how to ask for it, and you can interact with them in a relatively straightforward way. But there are other groups of users who really do not understand the technology. They are not interested in the technology. They know what they want to do, whether it is to study, whether it is science or weather forecasting or whatever; they need quite a lot of hand-holding to help them exploit the facilities that are there. They are not interested in the network technology. They do see the benefit. But simply plugging their machines in is not enough. So, looking ahead, providing more targeted user support to groups of people who are not really interested in networking is a major challenge.

We are starting to do that. It tends to be easier with the scientific disciplines, because they have some interest in it. But it is not just the scientific disciplines that can exploit this. The challenge looking ahead is really to make high performance networks more accessible for researchers in general. At the moment, if I look at the network usage, it is very much the scientific disciplines and those close to telecommunications that really exploit it. Making that more accessible more generally is the challenge which we need to concentrate more on. So it is more network performance and accessibility that I would see in the next five years.

There are some technical challenges as well, because historically, networks have been developed by making them faster. We went from 2 to 34, to 155 Mbps, to 10 Gbps, which is a pretty impressive increase in speed. But after 10 Gbps, we have actually increased the speed by adding more lanes to the motorway. What you had before were single pipe connections and you increased the speed of the pipe. In GÉANT, we have added parallel pipes as a way of increasing the network capacity. That makes economic and technological sense. But the next generation of technology, probably moving to 40 Gbps and to 100 Gbps, is on the horizon. The other thing we will be looking at is how useful that technology is, and if it works as well when deployed. So there is still a technology element, but I think there is a movement from just technology, which is what it used to be, to much more service and service support, which is a quite different sort of environment, but actually what is needed.

5.2
Kees Neggers and Boudewijn Nederkoorn

Boudewijn Nederkoorn (BN) retired in 2007 after working since 1988 as one of two Managing Directors responsible for SURFnet. He and Kees Neggers (KN), the second Managing Director, created the SURFnet network and the organization that supports it. Both were also very active on the international network level.

What has been your involvement in the RARE/TERENA area since the beginning?

KN: In the very beginning, I was heavily involved in the RARE/TERENA area and the COSINE project. I was one of the few people in Europe who were on both the EARN

Board of Directors and the Executive Committee of the RARE organization. I was also one of the driving forces of the merger of the two organizations because it did not make sense to continue with both of them. At that time, Boudewijn was active in the preparations of DANTE as an organization. In our view, we needed one organization to represent users, and another to provide services.

BN: We were involved at the very beginning of the IBM initiative that produced EARN. Later, I was involved in setting up DANTE, starting with the first meeting of the OU Task Force on June 28 1989. At that time DANTE was called the OU. On March 30 1993, DANTE was established in Cambridge and I served as a member of the DANTE Board of Directors from 1993 to 1997. Later I came back as a member of the Executive of the NREN Policy Committee of the GÉANT project.

What are the benefits and difficulties arising from the introduction of the network services?

KN: This can best be illustrated by looking at some examples. In the early 1980s, the only pan-European network was EUnet, set up by computer scientists. It was initially based on UUCP but moved to the Internet protocol suite, which was well supported by the UNIX operating system. In 1984, IBM introduced EARN, based on the proprietary IBM RSCS/NJE protocol suite. After tough negotiations with the European PTTs, who had a monopoly on data transport, IBM got permission to donate this network to the research community but only on the condition that EARN would move to OSI protocols and use the X.25 services of the PTTs as soon as possible. IBM donated a lot of equipment and lines to make that happen. Each country was given an IBM computer connected to each other with 9.6 kbps leased lines, including a connection to the already existing BITNET in the US. Based on proven technology the network worked instantly.

Obviously this triggered a reaction from the emerging national research networks trying to create networks based on OSI protocols. As a result, the RARE association was formed. The Netherlands offered to house an initial secretariat and pay for the start-up costs. Later the EC stepped in and gave additional support, all of which allowed RARE to incorporate as an association in June 1986 and take responsibility for the COSINE project. Peter Linington from the United Kingdom was the first president, Klaus Ullmann became vice-president and I became the treasurer. Both the United Kingdom and Germany already had a well-established research network organization at that time. In COSINE we were assumed to rely on the industry for products and on the PTTs for the network services. This really turned out to be an uphill battle.

BN: The COSINE specification phase was meant only to define the services that we needed on the OSI protocol stack. Industry and PTTs would do the rest. But the PTTs still being telephone companies at that time had no real data network. In their national environments they did provide some public data networking at very low speed based on X.25, more for transaction networking, not for general purpose networking. Internationally, almost nothing existed.

Therefore, in parallel to the COSINE specification phase, RARE declared pragmatically: "we cannot wait for this ultimate solution where the PTTs have all these nice public networks and all the computers support ISO-OSI protocols; we need a private international X.25 interconnect (IXI) network quickly". EUnet and EARN also supported this approach. COSINE people were also pragmatic and supported the idea. The EC was prepared to pay for an initial start of that backbone and IXI was created already in 1988, based on 64 kbps leased lines. Although much faster than the 9.6 kbps public data networks, this rapidly turned out to be not enough to cope with the growing demands.

KN: Campuses with UNIX computers started to use Internet protocols on their LAN. These LANs were high speed networks for that time and the support software arrived automatically when they bought a UNIX computer. LANs were actually able to carry big data streams while wide area networks could not.

BN: As a matter of fact, the Internet and EARN over IXI was a politically correct way of implementing services. Then the problems came. At the 64 kbps level, a little IP on top of that still worked but soon people started to need more capacity.

KN: IXI triggered research networks to implement private X.25 networks nationally as well in order to interconnect via IXI. We did that in the Netherlands in 1989, installing a 2 Mbps backbone network immediately. Then we discovered after a year that 2 Mbps interfaces on X.25 switches could only support about 350 kbps. Nobody had ever hit that wall in public networks because their use was limited to carrying transaction data. But we had much more traffic because of Internet on top of X.25. We had to do something. We took the 2 Mbps lines, E1s as they are called in Europe, and split them into a T1 which is 1.5 Mbps, the United States standard for leased lines, and 512 kbps which is what is left from 2 Mbps. We gave the 512 kbps portion to the X.25 switches, which was enough for them, and we used the T1 to directly interconnect Cisco routers. Suddenly the capacity limit was gone and the traffic grew rapidly. Needless to say that a 64 kbps IXI was no longer an adequate international interconnect.

BN: A document we wrote about our experiences had quite some impact because it proved that an upgrade to 2 Mbps of IXI would not solve the problem. Also OSI was not ready yet. We needed to do some native IP in the interim. This was around 1991. Many people had already moved to IP, but there were still groups who believed OSI over X.25 was the future, IP would die and a native IP interconnect as part of an upgraded "IXI" was not needed. We found we needed to go native in Europe as well. So we started the initiative to create Ebone outside of the COSINE process without any support of the EC. The first announcement of the Ebone proposal was at the RIPE meeting in CERN in 1991. We deliberately called it the Ebone92 proposal. In our view, Ebone services should have been taken over by DANTE as the ultimate NREN service provider. As soon as EuropaNET was there with the EMPB service, SURFnet switched its traffic from Ebone to EuropaNET but others decided not to do so. They stayed on Ebone much longer. It became a real split in Europe.

In what ways did each of the services above improve the facilities needed to support the work of end-users?

BN: With EARN, it was the time of email; there was a form of file transfer, and even of chatting. You could have a chat with somebody directly on a line by line basis. When we moved from EARN to IP services, some researchers were angry that we killed that chat function. We thought chatting was old-fashioned, not being aware of the role of chatting nowadays. Anyway, it was only supported on IBM mainframes. So most of the EARN users had no access to the chat.

Another important service at the beginning of EARN was the distribution list called "LISTSERV". That was one of the first cooperation-type services. It was, and still is, very popular. EARN built LISTSERV on basic original principles and it survives; I use LISTSERV every day. News was a service which originated on the EUnet networks and was later supported by TCP/IP. There was also the FTP. We had PAD service on X.25 which gave terminal access to a mainframe or minicomputer. X.25 as such was a service also, but only a carrier service.

KN: Talking about services, one of the surprises to everyone was the WWW.

BN: A number of navigation protocols appeared in that period. WWW was initially considered to be too complicated. Its slow response was assumed to be the result of complexity. The real reason was that when Tim Berners-Lee made his first demonstrations, it was not his protocol that was the problem; it was the capacity of the networks.

Do you remember GOPHER? It was heavily used for a while, and then in 1996 it was discarded. The WWW had taken over. WAIS (wide area information server) was another one. There were a number of emerging protocols, but WWW conquered everything.

KN: In 1993, AltaVista became available from Digital Equipment. It was the first search engine. The WWW and the search engines completely changed the whole landscape of services. It is interesting to note that most successful services originated from individuals and individual companies, not from standardization committees.

KN: Unfortunately, end-users have been a bit at a distance in the European environment. The whole networking scene is NRENs and some computer scientists, some protocol people.

I am sure that you made some improvement in the service to facilitate their work.

KN: That is an important point. You have two types of end-users, the advanced ones, and less advanced ones. This is true at the country level too by the way. How to serve them both well has always been a problem, because you cannot serve them with the same tools. The advanced users, like CERN, want the newest and fastest. The others cannot afford it and do not need it; they want something cheap, something proven; they do not want to take risks. There will always be tensions between these two groups. An obvious risk is that advanced users have to slow down. We have always been fighting that. In our view, by definition, the advanced research communities should have access to the best possible services. Otherwise, in a global economy, your research can no longer compete.

In the end, those buying your products are the other kind of users.

KN: In the end of course. So far, uptake has always been faster than anyone expected; soon the new advanced services were needed by everyone. But initially you have to find the funds to support the innovation needed by the advanced users. It is obvious that you cannot simply collect this from all users. In the Netherlands we solved this by having the Government subsidizing the innovation and the connected institutes financing the use. In Europe this is still a problem. The situation is more complicated by the lack of a well developed market for telecommunications in all places. There are 34 countries in GÉANT. In some it is technically impossible to provide the most advanced solutions, or even to have affordable prices for modest solutions. To find a single solution that fits all is impossible. Obviously developing areas need support, but Europe cannot afford to have this done at the expense of slowing down the advanced ones. It would rapidly lose its competitive edge in a global economy. But both goals could be served easily by taking a less monolithic approach and respecting the subsidiarity principle.

BN: Recently, everybody thought that the routed Internet was the solution for everything. Now we know this is not the case. That is why we started hybrid networking. Earlier on at the networking level, we pushed very hard for a private X.25 network which became IXI. Then we started Ebone, and, finally, we started this hybrid network. The technology was there, the need was there; it had to be done. Technology push is certainly something we use from time to time.

KN: And again this is a nice example of the difficulties in getting new services introduced on a European level. Hybrid networking was introduced in 2001 in the Netherlands. In the Netherlands we have the JIVE (Joint Institute for Very long baseline interferometry in Europe) correlator where they wanted high speed connections to telescopes. We also have active high-energy physicists groups that want high capacity connections to CERN. Both groups were very interested in experimenting with our point to point lightpath connections, recognizing the great potential of these new services for their research. We made lightpaths available for them: inside the Netherlands we connected JIVE with a dark fiber to NetherLight, and, also at our own expense, we installed dedicated 10 Gbps links outside of GÉANT from NetherLight to CERN to do the experiments. You know the results: the LHC network could not have been built on top of a routed network. It needs a dedicated lightpath network. It is because we pushed on that point that this technology was an ultimate solution. The LHC network is now an optical private network and so are the telescopes connections in the EXPReS (express production real-time e-VLBI - electronic transfer very-long-baseline interferometry - service) project, and both are using GÉANT2 lightpaths now after GÉANT also became a hybrid network.

How helpful and how important have the sources of funds been?

BN: In the start-up period of COSINE, some development work was wholly funded by the EU. But it was not yet the rule. For many years now, it is the rule that European networking is funded up to 50% by the EU and the remainder by the research networks. Research networks are funded totally differently in each country. Some years ago, in Germany, quite a lot of money came from the Government. Nowadays, almost all the money for operating the network and the development of the national German network comes from connected institutes. In the United Kingdom, almost all the money comes from the Government. In the Netherlands, the money used to operate the network comes from institutions; development and innovation costs are covered by the Government. Every country has a different funding system.

But at the European level, there is some type of cost sharing. As a result of the differences in local telecommunications regulations, the costs in the southern parts of Europe are usually much higher than in the center or the west. This means that these areas get the greatest benefit from Commission funding. Take for example the few connections from Greece to some neighboring countries: they are delivered by OTE (Hellenic Telecommunication Organization), the Greek provider; the total costs of these connections are higher than the total of dark fiber costs in the rest of Europe. In the economic heartland of Europe, circuit costs are lower and the research networks countries could acquire most of the capacity they need for about the same price as their net charge for accessing the overlay network after the EU contribution. All NRENs get the same percentage funding; it is the cost sharing procedure – agreed by the consortium – which results in access charges being only partially dependent on the cost of provision.

KN: With respect to the EC, it has been the main player during the whole development. Initially it had no money for networking. It only had money for research. COSINE was a EUREKA project and the EU and national Governments put up the money for the specification work: research, developing the protocols in more detail, and so on. Then it became more pragmatic and, for example, IXI was fully funded by the Commission, not just 50%. Nicolas Newman was the COSINE Project Officer. He was very pragmatic and very much interested in providing services where they were needed. He helped greatly to secure a budget for the IXI backbone. I remember presenting the IXI proposal to the CPG in Egham, just outside London, in 1988. The project was adopted there. Nicolas had already arranged for additional EU funding for it, on top of the specification phase funding. The only thing needed was the policy group support, which was given. EMPB was the next COSINE network service. Starting from EuropaNET, EU funding has always been close to 50%. But since it initially had to come out of the research budget it was a difficult fight. Researchers considered it their funds. Finally, we were successful in convincing the EC that they had to secure some money up front for pan-European networking infrastructure.

What about contributions from telecom operators?

KN: The first big donor was IBM with EARN. It was a huge amount of money. First they had to fight for the license, and then they had to pay enormous amounts of money for the lines – which they did. In addition, they provided the computers.

Then Digital Equipment came. They paid for the development of a special device called "Xbox", which was intended to provide an OSI migration path for EARN. At the same time they started to pay for the upgrades of the EARN network. Digital became the major sponsor of EARN in the early 1990s. Then, some PTTs got interested, in particular KPN in the Netherlands. KPN wanted to innovate and were interested in what we were doing. They were very helpful in providing international lines.

In the Netherlands, we discovered that if connected institutions pay for operation and the Government pays for innovation, and if both are ambitious, it becomes attractive for industry to join forces. SURFnet was quite successful in doing so. With SURFnet4 we were a launching customer of KPN's ATM service. SURFnet5 was based on a public call for tender, won by BT together with Cisco. They were not just providers but real industry partners. They spent a lot of money on our network. With SURFnet6, the first nationwide hybrid network, a Consortium led by Nortel was a major contributor. We are now trying to convince our Government that this is a win-win situation they should support on a structural basis.

What are the strengths and the weaknesses of the organization and the management structure?

BN: In 1984, the Dutch Government brought a document to the Parliament called "The informatics stimulation programme". There was a feeling that something had to be done about informatics, both in education and in research, in the market and industry. Those who wrote the document were quite nasty about developments within university computing centers. Kees and I were then in the Computing Centre at Nijmegen. The document said there was a need for motivation and innovation. It was also stated that there was no need to put any additional money into the universities, because it could be found easily just by modernizing university computing centers. These were considered to be dinosaurs. That was quite challenging. We started to put our heads together, all the university computing centers and also the universities' management people and board members. We decided to build a challenging plan. We obtained some funds for one year to build a plan to combine efforts, to make a cooperative organization, and to present something the Government could not refuse.

In 1985, this document was presented to the Dutch Government. It asked for just 1 billion guilders, about €450 000 000, for 5 years. This amount of money was not received very well. But there was a lot of pressure and the plans were challenging: not only should there be a national research network but also a national cooperation in collecting rights for licenses for software usage. We have a sister organization which is providing every university with the rights for every student to use Microsoft Office, and many other software and hardware facilities. This was already foreseen in that 1985 plan. It took one year before the Government decided to donate not €450 000 000 but one third of it for five years under the condition that universities and research institutes, and schools for higher education should cooperate in a Foundation. This Foundation would set up a national research network. So the SURF Foundation was set up in 1987, and on January 1 1988, Kees and I started to build SURFnet.

KN: There was also immediate money for interim networking facilities in 1985. That is where we also got the funds to do international things. We received a national node and an international link from IBM as part of the EARN donation. The interim money allowed us to extend the national node to all major universities with 9.6 kbps links, and install VAX/VMS systems to connect all universities directly to the backbone. The lines were expensive. We also got some money to support the set-up of RARE.

We always had an international dimension. We consider networking as valuable only if it is global. So, from the earliest days, we got additional money to do international networking and we still have that. In 2001 for instance, we installed the first 2.5 Gbps lightpath to Chicago, just to experiment with lightpaths. We also made that available for CERN users and others.

BN: We were keen to have a lean and mean flat organizational model at SURFnet and kept it like that for many years at a headcount level of less than 30. Then, the headcount exploded in a few years to the present level of 60. This is necessary because of the diversity of services we are involved in: end-user services, and so on. We are obliged to do it, but we are also eager to do it.

KN: We have always been active internationally. I was on the EARN Board, on the RARE Board, on the TERENA Board and was Chairman of the RIPE NCC for many years. I have been on the Internet Society Board for 10 years. I was closely involved in most of the initiatives for the network layer, IXI, Ebone, GLIF (global lambda integrated facility). Research networking is a global affair.

BN: And we had more people active internationally; Erik Huizer was one of the prominent members in IETF. The first IETF meeting outside the United States was in the Netherlands, organized by Erik. Erik-Jan Bos is active in GLIF and was one of the architects of the LHC OPN (optical private network). I was involved in DANTE as a Director and the first Company Secretary. The GÉANT project started with an Executive, and for the first three years, until my retirement, I was a member of the Executive. I was also involved in the set-up and management of the Dutch national top level domain registry, in the domain names. I was also the first Chairman of the Council of European top level domain registries, CENTR (Council of European national top level domains registries). I have been Chairman of the Amsterdam Internet exchange (AMS-IX) for the past four years. The AMS-IX, originating from SURFnet, is now the biggest Internet exchange in the world.

What are the future directions?

KN: In our view, development will go on for a while. There are still many things to do, like dealing with the IPv4 address depletion. Funding issues remain uncertain. Networking is becoming even more global. More countries are becoming a part of it. What we had in Europe when networks extended outside of Western Europe to all over Europe, we see this now on a worldwide scale. You have tensions between the advanced countries and the others, and we want to connect to everyone.

BN: At the same time, there is still a lot of work to do in the enhancement of the cooperation of NRENs in Europe. Not least at the level of organization and management structures. Almost all European countries are now united in TERENA as an association. All NRENs are also represented in the Policy Committee of the GÉANT projects. And there is DANTE, a company limited by shares. Only half of the NRENs own DANTE shares. Ownership, risk sharing and governance issues are difficult to improve as long as DANTE is not restructured in a way that is inclusive for all NRENs.

That is a challenge for the future. The other challenge is to keep track of user needs and technological development, and combine the two into something that works.

KN: Europe should be aware that it is not the center of the universe and it should accept that Russia, China and many others have internal arrangements different from European situations. Some in Europe believe that every country should have just one national research network. But China and Korea, for instance, have two well developed major networks. They are both important. In our view, worldwide connectivity is best served by creating a structure where each network can interconnect independently. Open exchanges are excellent vehicles for this. We usually accept the local habits and talk with everyone. The trick is to create synergies. For instance CERN also has a lot of good things to offer and our cooperation with them has been very fruitful from IXI, to Ebone, to GLIF. And the synergies are beneficial for many. With our investments in high speed connections and with the help of CERN expertise and CERN partners we developed an international infrastructure and exchange points that are not just beneficial for European networking but for global networking as well.

5.3
Klaus Ullmann

Klaus Ullmann is joint Managing Director of DFN. In addition to his responsibilities for the research network services in Germany, he has been heavily involved in research networking at the European level since the first days of cooperative activity. He was Vice-President of RARE when the organization was first established and later served two 2-year terms as President. He was Chairman of the DANTE Board of Directors from the company's creation in 1993 to 2002 and was re-elected to this post in 2005.

Could you please explain the COSINE project approach?

The COSINE approach was politically a bottom-up approach, starting from the countries. In nearly every country at that time there was some willingness to fund research networks. We created the DFN in 1984 for example. The Dutch were very close behind us. The Swiss network was created a bit later in 1986. At some point, politicians from the various countries' ministries said it was time for an initiative involving the EC to push forward research networking. As an administrative vehicle they used the EUREKA programme for a project which was created through the European Council of Ministers. The political impact of COSINE was very good, because the awareness at the political level of the need to fund both national and international research networking developed. The main impetus of the COSINE initiative was a political move both at the country and at European level to first create, and then maintain networking infrastructure for researchers. Since then – this was in 1988 to 1989 – the situation has been very stable.

The COSINE project produced the first manufacturer-independent network which was named IXI. It was the first X.25-based network. It was a private X.25 network which, for regulatory reasons, was a real advantage at that time. The market situation in Europe was completely fragmented into national markets. There was no real European market and the international links were extremely expensive due to the monopoly situation. Politicians were aware that there was a problem for Europe. By creating the European network operator, DANTE, we increased the awareness of politicians in Brussels that the monopoly situation could not create anything useful and had to disappear. They, then, did a very good job at de-regulating European markets.

The second effect of COSINE and the establishment of DANTE was the sustainability of the activity. It was clear that for some commercial reasons RARE was not the appropriate vehicle for running a big network at the European level. Then, Howard Davies and Dai Davies came in and there was a very fruitful cooperation between the research networks which is still very good today. This is my history of the European networking.

Of course nationally, I am one of the general managers of the DFN, our research network. We went through all the technology changes. The whole field is determined by technology changes which occur every three or four years. This is a very important boundary condition to all our activities. You can be sure that every three to four years, the whole technical scenario changes almost completely. Not only in terms of network performance or capacity, but from the technology point of view as well. We started with X.25 networks, then we went to SDH (synchronous digital hierarchy) networks; then there was an interim period when we used ATM. All these technologies, apart from some pieces of SDH, have completely disappeared. There is no X.25 any more. For technical reasons, there is no ATM any more. When ATM came up, people thought it was a long term future technology. But, this was not the case.

The most important technical difficulty is to determine at the right point in time that a technological change is taking place. One of the big achievements of David Williams was to have a very clear view on how networking should develop.

Six years ago, when he was president of TERENA, he said that the fiber network would be an appropriate solution for the research community. This was a bit of a vision in those days; apart from the technical risks attached to the fiber network, the market was not very well developed. But the market developed very well in most countries and today this is a reality. GÉANT is a fiber-based network, and several research networks, including ours, are also based on fiber. David was a sort of pioneer. People thought it might happen but they did not know. But David had a clear vision that this was the way to go, and that was correct. It was not very long ago, only five years.

What are the benefits and difficulties arising from the introduction of the network services?

There have been several network generations. Sometimes two generations have been used in parallel, sometimes one generation has been the technological successor of another. The direct technological successor of IXI was EMPB, funded by COSINE. IXI was based on 64 kbps circuits. EMPB was a big improvement as it had 2 Mbps circuits. In parallel with EMPB, there was an initiative started by Kees Neggers, Ebone. This had to do with the protocol wars taking place at that time. One camp said that TCP/IP was the future, and another camp, especially in the political arena, said that OSI was the technical future. EARN at that time was not dead, but there was no easy upgrade path for its facilities so its future prospects were not very good. But then Kees took the initiative to build up Ebone, which was a side track from the COSINE political environment. In terms of functionality, there was no major difference between EMPB and Ebone. Both networks were able to carry multi-protocol suites, they were able to carry the EARN traffic, the OSI traffic, the TCP/IP traffic, and also DECnet. They could be used for the different protocols available at that time. Even SNA applications were run on both networks. But, today, nobody speaks about SNA, or EARN, or OSI any more.

The TCP/IP suite was the successful one. This was the evolution for reasons which were not determined in Europe, one important aspect of the integration of the protocol state into the UNIX operating system. Without this development, maintenance of networking software would pose a huge problem. If it is embedded in the operating system supplied by the manufacturer, maintenance is his problem.

If you judge the EMPB versus Ebone, they were functionally the same. Within DANTE, however, we took the EMPB track. We decided not to use Ebone. We had gateways between the two networks in order to provide connectivity to the researchers, and make this problem invisible to users. Users are not interested in specific network technology, they want to have functionality. This worked very well. After a while Ebone was commercialized. It was transformed into a company which was later bought by KPN/Qwest. But then KPN/Qwest went bankrupt. EuropaNET succeeded EMPB. In time sequence, there was IXI, EMPB, EuropaNET, TEN-34, TEN-155, GÉANT, and GÉANT2.

The benefit of TEN-34 was capacity. TEN-34 was a trans-European network with an access speed of 34 Mbps. This was a big jump, reflected in the cost; the amount which we had to collect from the research networks increased sharply. The main benefit for the users was a big leap in the capacity provided. The next step was TEN-155 with 155 Mbps capability, and then GÉANT started with Gbps speeds. GÉANT2 is an implementation of David Williams' idea of a fiber platform. In GÉANT2, we have an optical platform and an IP service on top of it. But for specific services, we can build so-called virtual private networks (VPNs), which give you the option of filtering out user traffic which has specific characteristics. For example, we are finishing building an LHC optical private network which is taken from the GÉANT optical platform – it does not interfere with the IP service, it is a separate service. The Tier-1 centers of the LHC distribution system are always connected with 10 Gbps with CERN, so the data are pushed to every Tier-1 center worldwide, and from there the distribution to Tier-2 and Tier-3 centers is done on a regional basis. The Tier-1 network is the LHC European network. It uses the GÉANT platform on a broad basis. This would not have been possible without GÉANT. The new optical technology gives big additional options. In terms of traffic volume the growth of the IP service on the networks at the European and national levels used to be a factor of 2 to 3 per year. It was exponential growth. This has now flattened out. One of the reasons is that big consumers are going to use their own VPNs, but these private networks are built on top of the NREN GÉANT2 infrastructure.

In what ways did each of the services above improve the facilities needed to support the work of end-users?

Normally an end-user does not see any international research network, especially not the European part. Anyway, it is clear today that most scientific communities can no longer live without networking. It is very clear in physics. If you install something like the LHC, you must provide a 10 Gbps network to give data to physicists worldwide. Without a network, no data evaluation will take place. The computing power is not in CERN, it is distributed worldwide. There are other science groups working in the same way: biology is one example – genome database evaluations use a lot of network capacity. If you look specifically at university faculty members, most of them cannot live without good network connectivity: they must be able to reach everybody with whom they collaborate worldwide, and, today, the capacity for reaching them should be 10 Gbps in order to access bulky, huge datasets. That was one of the reasons. If you do visualization, do computing on a remote machine and visualize the results, you need a lot of memory. Today networking is a normal tool for most people. Even if they do not realize it, they are using the network.

To give you some numbers, for network infrastructure, the bigger European countries have roughly the same budget. We at DFN have a budget of €30–40 M per year. It is the same with GÉANT, so DANTE has the same budget. It is not a cheap tool that most scientists are using. COSINE was a big pusher for that, because it made politicians aware of the problems, specifically the financial problems. So in most European countries, ministries give money to their research networks. We are an exception. We have to earn our money directly from the universities. But in most cases, ministries are involved. So the main achievement of COSINE may not be technical, but political. It gave a stable political environment to networking, especially for funding purposes.

How helpful and how important have the sources of funds been?

Equipment suppliers and telecom operators do not play any significant role in funding. Here and there, some equipment suppliers help networks, especially the new ones, to come up, but that is more a marketing activity for them rather than a long-term involvement. The most important source of money for most research networks is the national ministry; and for the network at the European level, it is the EU. The effect of the COSINE project was not only that awareness was built at the national level, but it was also built at the European level. It was a very wise decision to have the CPG. The Chairman of the CPG was Peter Tindemans, and all the funding went through the EC. He found a way of convincing high level people in the EC that they should administer the project and that they should look at it not in a hostile way, but try to include the ideas behind the project into their future plans. This worked very well.

Today, the infrastructure funding at the European level, which is always designed as a sort of complementary activity to the national ones, is working very well. For GÉANT2 (the formal name for the collaboration between about 30 NRENs), funding is coming through the Sixth Framework Programme, and the Seventh Framework Programme for GÉANT3. There is no doubt that this will continue for the Seventh Framework Programme. This is a very good development. It gives a very stable financial environment.

There is a long history with North America. It started with a situation where the North Americans were very far ahead of Europe. Then in the 1980s, we started to speak about transatlantic links. The Americans said they would allow us to connect to their network. This was not appealing because we had to pay for all the transatlantic links. There were several political initiatives from national ministers and from the EC to overcome this situation and to share the costs of the links but for a long time they did not work. The United States had an excellent network at the time, the NSF network, which was really advanced. Then something really strange happened. They gave up their NSF network. They closed it. They said "the market will provide". That was a big mistake, the market did not provide anything and it was a mess. Then the American research institutes did something very similar to what we developed in Europe and in DFN. DFN is a private association supported by all the universities and research laboratories in Germany. It is a not-for-profit organization, and it is private. There is no ministry involvement. Of course, we get some funding here and there for projects. But, today, not even the operations are funded by the Ministry. We have to get the money from the universities. So the United States people did the same. They said: "the market does not provide and we want to organize our networking." They did not say: "as the Europeans did", because they are too proud for that, but basically they copied our organizational model. This initiative was launched in the 1990s; it is called "Internet2" today. It is an initiative with almost all important United States universities. They are now establishing a network which is very similar to the GÉANT network. So they are no longer ahead in technological development; if you compare them with research networks in European countries or at European level I think they are equal.

We have now found a good arrangement for cost sharing. When there is a new transatlantic link, it is not co-funded, because, for administrative reasons, that was difficult. But if we put a 10 Gbps link there, they put another 10 Gbps link at their cost and we adapt the technical concept. There is a very good collaboration between GÉANT2 and both ESnet which is an Energy Science network and Internet2. In the US, they have a different approach in the universities, they have Internet2, and some agencies have their own research network. NASA has two or three networks; the Department of Energy has a big network because it is responsible for LHC cooperation. There is a very good collaboration, both on the development path and operationally, especially in GÉANT2 in which we now collaborate closely on performance measurement tools. There is a good complementarity between the United States and Europe. On the economic side, all the problems we had at the beginning, not co-funding the links, are completely gone. On a yearly basis, we have four to five technical workshops on specific topics on which we collaborate very closely.

What are the strengths and the weaknesses of the organization and the management structure?

DFN has been built as a private association. If you look around in Europe, you find a similar structure in Switzerland. The organization in Switzerland is not an association, but a foundation I think. But there is a big distance between the federal ministry and Bern. That is the same situation we have in Germany. The political problem in Germany is that the Federal Government has no mandate to fund networks for universities. Universities are funded by the Bundesländer level. At the Federal Ministry, they could even get into trouble if they did anything. At the beginning of DFN, it was clear that, if we had to organize a finance scheme from the Bundesländer, it would not work, because with twelve people around the table, all politicians, it does not work. So we went to the BMBF (Bundesministerium für Bildung und Forschung), at that time the BMFT. They said we had to follow two paths. They had no mandate to provide infrastructure for universities. But we could get the ederal research laboratories into the activity. That was not a problem because I came from the Hahn-Meitner Institute which was 90% funded by the Federal Government and only 10% by Berlin. Max Planck Institutes are in a similar situation. They are 90% funded by the Federal Government and only 10% by the Lander. The second path was through technology. They have a mandate for developing new technologies. They gave us a lot of money, €10 M per year, to develop this area. This worked very well for 20 years and around 2000 they stopped this program. But, by then, we had a very good financing structure, because finance-wise we always separated development from operations. We took care that the financing stream for operations came from the users, the universities. Individual users do not pay, but universities do. This has been very stable. With this system we have a yearly budget of roughly €40 M. This income comes from the universities. There is a very similar financing structure in Switzerland. Holland is a bit different: SURFnet is owned by the SURFnet Foundation which has a political mandate to finance research with public money in Holland. But that is the only difference. In the higher spheres of SURFnet B.V. (Besloten Vennootschap), you do not find ministerial people.

In Germany, influence from the Federal ministries is zero. Twice a year, we hold a membership meeting. One to two hundred representatives from universities come together. In the winter we have it in Bonn and in the summer in Berlin. The Board is elected every three years, and they have to explain what they have done and what they are going to do in the future. You can be re-elected twice to the Board. So there is enough stability at the Board level. At first, I thought this would be very difficult and would not work but, especially after the ministry gave up financing development work, the solidarity among research laboratories rose to a surprisingly high level. So we have no problem with financing the network. This was a big surprise for me when the Ministry faded out from co-funding the activity. I am an employee of DFN. In Berlin we are 30 people. We have another group of 15 people in Stuttgart in charge of operations.

What were the pressures that led to the setting up of the main collaborative organizations?

The pressure or the impetus for doing this at the European level was simply the idea that if there is a national group doing research and it wants to have networking, it needs to organize their work. Most of these people belong to international collaborations and need to communicate at the European level with colleagues in other countries. Then, you have the big science, like particle physics, or nuclear reactor physics in Grenoble, for example. People go there with their equipment, measure things, go home, evaluate their data, and they want to keep in contact with their colleagues in Grenoble. This is a very natural development and we have to support it. This was a driving force to get these things together.

I am now in my second period as elected Chairman of the Board of DANTE. There is no difference from the first period; the motivation is the same. The question is only whether we need an organization like DANTE or not. What you have to analyze is how to organize these things. For networking, it is very useful to have a European complementary network. DANTE is very specific. It is not directly comparable to the NRENs because, as customers, DANTE has only NRENs – there is the little exception of CERN. One of the basic decisions we made when we created DANTE was that DANTE should not go directly to end-users or to universities or research laboratories, and do business with them – to give them access to the European network. There were two reasons: DANTE is organized like DFN. They have to look after themselves. We make no assumption in DANTE that the EU will pay for ever. The EU may stop funding and we still have to survive. Therefore, we had to create a situation where there is no competition between an NREN, which is a shareholder of DANTE and which funds DANTE, and DANTE itself. You can understand that if you start from the assumption that every country has its own NREN, and DANTE works for these NRENs. This is the basic idea. Secondly, if you go to their financial sources, it is very risky, from a financial point of view. What do you do if an institution does not pay? So we decided to leave that to the NRENs. They can solve these problems politically. If we bring these problems to the European level, it would be extremely difficult and costly. You would have to do everything that commercial ISPs do. A normal ISP has to deal with that. If we competed with ISPs, the situation would be completely different. We would be in competition with the normal ISP market.

What are the future directions?

What are the future directions of DANTE, and at the European level? Technologically, the problems are very similar at the European level to those at the national level. We have to develop further the use of the optical platform. The inherent problem is not as easy to solve as in the IP case. Informatics people say it is a multi-domain network. The domain is defined by the NRENs and GÉANT. GÉANT does not own the domain. Domain labels say who is responsible for the operations. For example in the case of GÉANT2, DANTE is using Alcatel equipment. The Dutch are using Nortel equipment. We are using Huawei equipment from China. So, technically, you find solutions which are different in detail. What we have to ensure is that we have a common multi-domain solution for users. The LHC network is a typical example: we plug together solutions that are different in their technical detail to get a big solution which works for users. There are lots of technical problems on the operational management level which we have to solve: common database; distributed database where we get the operational data from the domains, put them together on a new logical layer. This is a future direction for, for example, Seventh Framework Programme on the European level, and for us with DFN here as well.

Fortunately, we are now in a collaborative situation. Of course we are struggling from time to time, but I would say the mainstream is constructive. So you find people here and there, and in the academic environment, so that we always have contacts with people who see where the future is taking us. It is a big synergy effect which is organized through these collaborations. I cannot say specifically what the next technology will be because, if we look back, we cannot imagine that about six years ago we had only the facilities of TEN-155. This was a network which you cannot compare in any detail with the capacity, functionality, or reach of today's network. Everything has improved dramatically. So it is very difficult to make a prognosis more than 2 or 3 years ahead. What the future brings is very difficult to say. The only thing which we can be sure of is that things will again change completely. That is challenging and exciting as well.

> **Radicals and Conservatives**
> It is generally believed that the root of the very evident divisions that have been observed within the research networking community was the religious war between proponents of TCP/IP and OSI protocols in the early years of network

development. In reality, this is not the case. The TCP/IP versus OSI dispute was just a battle which formed a part, albeit an important part, of a longer-lasting conflict between two groups which persists today: rebels versus the establishment, radicals versus conservatives. If the OSI war had never taken place, the two groups would have found some other vehicle for carrying on their conflict.

The radicals believe in opportunism, making use of whatever short term means are available for promoting their cause, minimizing or even eliminating management overheads and bureaucracy, and being quick to adapt to a changing technological world. For the radicals, personal glory is there to be won, at least amongst one's peer-group. Failure is tolerated as long as the objective was sound. The conservatives are more concerned with long-term stability and making careful preparations to minimize the risk of problems. The people concerned may be ambitious but, in most cases, get satisfaction from working as members of a team with defined positions in a hierarchy.

In the particular context of research networking, and despite declaring that they have the same objectives, the two sides have different technical interests. For the radicals, for example, a system failure provides an opportunity to explore the technology at a detailed level and to demonstrate their competence by quickly finding and correcting the source of the problem. Conservatives, in contrast, prefer to avoid having failures in the first place, in other words, to create an environment in which failures never happen, and which, in consequence, is very tedious for the technical staff involved.

The objective of research networking, that is the provision of services which are in advance of what is commercially available and which the end-users can rely on day-in, day-out, to support their own work, involves, by its very nature, treading a very fine line between reproducing the services of the larger and more advanced ISPs on the one hand and suffering the consequences of supposedly reliable but incompletely tested equipment from manufacturers on the other.

The radicals are generally prepared to take a higher risk than the conservatives and, as long as the gamble pays off, they are perceived to be more successful.

Fortunately, in each of the stages in the development of research network services in Europe after the establishment of the Ebone and IXI services, the two sides have managed to make compromises on their own ideals so that, in the end, a unified service has been provided to all participating research networks in Europe. Compromise between two parties often leaves both of them equally unhappy but, taking a positive view, the stimulation of each party by the demands of the other has led, in the case of research networking, to success in meeting the community's objectives of providing high-quality network services to a very large community of students, teachers and researchers.

6
The Bandwidth Breakthrough

A research and education network has different objectives and requirements from a commercial organisation's network. However, this gives opportunities for national telecom operators and equipment manufacturers if they are willing to embrace them. This chapter looks at these differences and how the national telecom operators and equipment manufacturers, more aligned perhaps to commercial and their own requirements, have been persuaded to provide the required services.

6.1
TEN-34

The TEN-34 (trans-European network at 34 Mbps) project which supported the implementation and operation of the TEN-34 network was unsatisfactory for almost everyone involved. Nevertheless, it represented a step forward in two ways. First, it brought all the research networks together again, providing a common service, albeit one made up of disparate components. Secondly, the research networks did get access to international 34 or 45 Mbps circuits despite the unwillingness of PNOs to make them available. This created the first crack in the wall that the PNOs had built in an attempt to maintain the privileges of their monopoly position (which included the freedom to ignore customer demand when planning the development of their services). The crack would later be progressively widened, and eventually the whole structure crumbled

The research networks' requirements had been fully discussed and specified in the EuroCAIRN project. EuroCAIRN also reviewed the technology available to meet these requirements, and put forward a draft implementation plan for the services that were needed.

In a separate initiative, David Hartley (who was at the time Chief Executive of UKERNA, United Kingdom Education and Research Networking Association, the research network organization in the United Kingdom) called a meeting of all research networks to establish a group which could oversee the planning and implementation of a unified service covering the whole community. This included those research networks which connected to Ebone for their international service, as well as those which used EuropaNET. With some difficulties along the way,

A History of International Research Networking. Edited by Howard Davies and Beatrice Bressan
Copyright © 2010 WILEY-VCH Verlag GmbH & Co. KGaA, Weinheim
ISBN: 978-3-527-32710-2

a Steering Group was set up with one representative per research network and with DANTE providing a secretariat. The first task of the Steering Group was to promote a project that was provisionally labelled TEN-34.

The main items TEN-34 would need were:

- access to 34 Mbps circuits in order to increase the bandwidth available internationally
- equipment needed to support a general IP service able to make use of much or all of this capacity
- a test network, also composed of high speed circuits, to support the study and testing of ATM facilities.

The 34 Mbps circuit cost should be no higher than four times the cost of 2 Mbps circuits between the same end points. (The factor 4 had been recommended in a report to the EC on the future of research networking by Dondoux[1] and Oakley[2]. The way in which the IP service might be implemented was deliberately left open. Some research networks were already pressing for an IP service running directly on 34 Mbps leased circuits but the use of other technologies was not ruled out. In fact, there was widespread interest in the possibilities offered by ATM, which include the splitting of a single physical circuit into multiple virtual circuits which might be permanent (PVC, permanent virtual circuit), that is their existence continues indefinitely, or switched (SVC, switched virtual connection) that is, they are set up and closed down dynamically under the control of a management system which might, in principle, respond directly to end-user requests. The bandwidth on a virtual circuit can be fixed (and guaranteed) or may vary between minimum and maximum values, allowing the possibility of one application using the total line speed when no higher priority application is active. Constant bit rate (CBR) services can support video and audio applications which require their input data to be delivered at regular intervals. Variable bit rate (VBR) services are suitable for applications such as the transmission of IP packets which routinely cope with the irregular arrival rates of packets; they also enable high percentage utilization of circuit capacity to be maintained under conditions of heavy load. ATM was seen by the PNOs as the basic technology they would use to support a new generation of telephony-related services once the R&D process had been completed with a set of validation and demonstration activities.

The position towards the end of 1994 was that ATM switches were starting to become available on the market; the transmission of IP packets between two routers interconnected by an ATM virtual circuit had been successfully demonstrated. On the other hand, different suppliers had given different priorities to the development and implementation of sub-sets of the complete ATM specification. Because of this,

---

1) Jacques Dondoux had previously been Directeur Général des Télécommunications in France, that is, responsible for the government department which, when it was re-structured as a limited liability company, became France Télécom.

2) Brian Oakley, Chairman of Logica (a large United Kingdom software house) and previously Secretary of the United Kingdom's Science Research Council.

in combination with conflicting interpretations of detailed specifications, interworking between equipment from different suppliers was unreliable or even impossible. Management facilities were rudimentary.

During 1995, an ATM pilot in which all western European PNOs were participants was already in operation. Other organizations could apply to make use of the pilot network for the purpose of testing applications which made use of ATM services, but they had no means of accessing the PNOs' ATM equipment other than via an interface which offered the equivalent of a leased circuit of variable capacity.

Although EuroCAIRN had concluded that ATM implementations were not yet mature enough to be used in operational services, ATM clearly offered scope for developing quality of service (QoS) features that could be applied to TCP/IP services. While TCP/IP offered, and continues to offer, a sound basis for the continued enhancement of the data transmission infrastructure required by applications, it does have its limitations. In particular, it provides no guarantee of quality of service and, by itself, has only limited mechanisms for managing conflicting demands for bandwidth. The research networks were all willing to participate in the testing and development of ATM-based facilities with a view to introducing them into service at a later date.

At the beginning of 1995, the research networks had a requirements specification, an implementation plan and a project organization in place; the EC was committed to supporting the provision of high-capacity networks for research; the PNOs had 34 Mbps circuits in place, and price guidelines had been issued by two senior and respected leaders in the telecommunications industry. Progress towards the introduction of high speed service should then have been straightforward. But it was not.

There were clearly differences of opinion inside the EC as to the best way of providing support for research networking. In January 1995, the news arrived that DG III (ESPRIT/Information Technologies) and DG XIIIC (Telematics) would pool their resources and work together to select and manage projects in research networking under the headings of their respective Work Plans, while DG XIIIB (ACTS - Advanced Communications Technologies and Services/Communications Technologies) would act independently.

The ESPRIT and Telematics Applications Programs of the Fourth Framework Program subsequently included "Interconnection of European University and research networks at 34–155 Mbps" in the December 1994 Call for Proposals. The EC budgeted ECU30 M over two years for this activity.

The corresponding ACTS Work Plan included the "Interconnection of National Hosts" item. "National Hosts" had been set up by the earlier RACE programme. They consisted of groups of service providers and system developers. Details of their structure and activities varied between countries, but all National Hosts had the common objective of promoting the use of ATM facilities to support advanced telecommunications services. In some countries, the national research network was part of the National Host, but not in others. Since interconnection of National Hosts would involve the setting up of a high-speed international infrastructure similar to that being proposed by the national research networks, there was a strong possibility of duplication. In order to minimize the risk of this happening, the TEN-34

Steering Group decided to submit identical proposals to the EC via both the ESPRIT/Telematics and the ACTS routes.

A serious problem in preparing any comprehensive proposal was that the PNOs did not want to make their high speed circuits available at any price. They feared that an organization which acquired such a circuit might use its capacity to mount an alternative service for international telephone calls, undercutting the PNOs' charges which generated very healthy profits. They also claimed that they could not give special prices to the research networks because of the open network provision (ONP) regulations in force at the time. These required that the charge made for any service must be the same for all customers.

DANTE had submitted an outline project proposal to the EC before the January 31 1995 deadline and the new Steering Group worked hard during February and March to put together a full proposal based on the EuroCAIRN conclusions. Each research network approached its national PNO with an invitation to join the project as an Associated Partner, providing one or more half circuits that could be used to construct a suitable network configuration, and participating in work items covering the development and testing of ATM services. The benefits to the PNOs of joining the project were pointed out to them and an attempt was made to reassure them concerning the non-commercial character of the project by promising that there would be no voice re-sale activity and that an AUP forbidding the transport of commercial traffic would be applied.

The full TEN-34 project proposal had to be submitted to the EC before March 31 1995, and only a few positive responses were received from PNOs in time to be incorporated in it. In addition, there were some research networks which were not prepared to commit to participation in the project until the cost of doing so was clearer. In order to deal with these two difficulties, the proposal which was submitted provided for an initial phase in which the seeking of commitments necessary to supply an adequate number of 34 Mbps circuits and the costs of this provision would be refined. It would be open to additional PNOs and research networks to join the project at the end of this initial phase.

The result of the ACTS evaluation of the TEN-34 proposal was "not retained", that is, rejected and the evaluators chose a project called NICE (National Host interconnection experiments) for the interconnection of National Hosts. NICE would be supported by another project which had been shortlisted, namely JAMES (joint ATM experiment on European services), essentially a continuation of the earlier ATM pilot operated by the PNOs, although there were few details describing precisely what was being offered. Some research networks were already participants in NICE, and in the negotiations to define a contract for the project, DANTE was included as an additional partner representing those research networks which were not themselves partners. There was better news from Telematics, whose evaluators shortlisted the TEN-34 proposal with the obvious reservation that commitments to provide the necessary circuit capacity must be obtained from PNOs before the project could be approved. The JAMES consortium had also "hedged its bets" by submitting its proposal to Telematics as well as ACTS and was seen by the Telematics evaluators to complement TEN-34 very well. Therefore the EC recommended that the two groups combine their proposals and report to it within a few weeks on the feasibility of doing so.

The first meetings between representatives of the two groups were concerned mainly with each side giving the other more information about its intentions and priorities. The tone of these meetings was generally positive but, inevitably, some mismatches were uncovered; for example, JAMES was aimed at providing services to end-user organizations which would have no visibility of the ATM facilities used within the PNOs' network while TEN-34 would provide services to research networks with the aim of integrating TEN-34, research network and end-user organizations' equipment to support end-to-end services which exploited the possibilities offered by ATM. The lack of detail in the original JAMES proposal and the subsequent failure of JAMES' representatives to provide information which would allow this mismatch to be resolved, led the TEN-34 Steering Group to inform the EC in May 1995 that there was no basis on which a joint project could be built although the possibilities of PNO participation in TEN-34 work items concerning ATM trials and of the research networks using JAMES as the test network required by TEN-34 were left open.

At this point, there might have been complete deadlock if Unisource Carrier Services had not broken ranks and made the first crack in the PNO wall by offering to provide an IP service based on 34 Mbps circuits between the countries of its parent organizations (the Netherlands, Spain, Sweden and Switzerland) and half-circuits from these locations to other countries. In combination with similar (but as yet unwritten) offers from the PNOs in Italy, Portugal and Greece, and confirmation by CERN that it was willing to connect a French national circuit, terminating on the French part of its site, to equipment in Switzerland, this meant that plans for a viable, though incomplete, European network at 34 Mbps could now be progressed.

With the precedent now set, there followed a long and complex process of refinement of the TEN-34 proposal in which the research networks, the EC and PNO representatives were all involved. By the end of October 1995, agreement in principle had been reached between the research networks and BT, Deutsche Telekom, France Télécom and Telecom Italia for the provision of a managed data transmission service between their four home countries the FUDI countries (France – FR, United Kingdom – UK, Germany – DE, and Italy – IT) based on ATM virtual paths. Together with a modified proposal from Unisource for an equivalent service elsewhere in Europe and an agreement with the JAMES set of PNOs for the use of the JAMES facilities for validating new ATM-based services, all the components were in place for a project which fully met both the EC's and the research network's requirements.

The EC set a deadline of December 4 1995 for the submission of a final version of the TEN-34 proposals and there were frequent consultations between research network and EC representatives during November 1995 to ensure that the detailed project specification being prepared was compliant with all EC requirements.

Discussions with the FUDI group of PNOs had resulted in a proposal according to which they would provide an ATM-based data transmission sub-network between the four countries involved. Access to this sub-network at 34 Mbps would be provided and supported at each access point by ATM virtual paths with an aggregate capacity of at least 34 Mbps. The service would be subject to an agreed acceptance test. A detailed proposal indicating the costs of providing access at 34 Mbps was due to be given by each PNO separately to its respective national research network on November 22 1995.

There were parallel discussions with Unisource with a view to the provision of a similar data transmission sub-network between the four Unisource home countries. No direct connection between these two sub-networks was foreseen at the ATM or leased line level, but they would be connected at the IP level. CERN was one obvious connection point, using a national 34 Mbps line to the French part of the CERN site. The second interconnection point would be located somewhere in Northern Europe: Amsterdam, London and Stockholm were the main candidates.

Research networks outside both the FUDI and the Unisource groups were expected to hold further discussions with their country's PNO and then to decide how best to connect (as spur countries) to the most convenient IP node in the FUDI/Unisource (core) configuration.

Formal detailed offers from the FUDI PNOs were received less than two weeks before the deadline for submitting the contract text to the EC. Because some research networks were obliged to follow lengthy contract approval procedures which could only start when a detailed contract specification was in place, not all the research networks participating in TEN-34 were able to commit to signing a contract with the EC before the deadline. However, a group of four research networks (those of Germany, Italy, Switzerland, and the United Kingdom) acting on behalf of the larger group, with DANTE as the Coordinating Partner, submitted a formal proposal by the EC's December 4 1995 deadline. The proposal provided for further research networks to be added to the Consortium during the first quarter of 1996 (Figure 6.1).

The EC shared the PNO view of ATM as the "technology of the future" and was actively promoting the development and use of ATM equipment and services as part of its policy for the support of European industry. Therefore, any proposal involving the research networks and the funding of TEN-34 would have to include development and testing of ATM services as part of its work plan in order to be successful in the Fourth Framework Program.

The eventual network configuration, determined by the limited availability of circuits, consisted of two sub-networks; a managed IP service linking six countries and managed by Unisource, and a set of ATM VP (virtual path) half-circuits or leased half-circuits used to build the rest of the network. The two sub-networks were linked and exchanged traffic at four locations.

After this configuration had been agreed, it was still necessary to negotiate contracts with suppliers. Although there was a single contract with Unisource for its sub-network, the remainder of the circuits were supplied as half-circuits by individual PNOs. As a result, a total of 16 supply contracts between research networks and their national PNO had to be managed and coordinated. This created both administrative and technical difficulties which took many months to resolve, the PNOs continuing to adopt their pre-liberalization approach compounded by the innovations introduced by the use of ATM. For example, in some cases it proved impossible to persuade the two PNOs at each end of a full circuit to carry out scheduled maintenance at the same time so that the planned down-time for the circuit was doubled. A surprisingly large amount of effort had to be devoted to ensuring that the two PNOs providing each half of a single ATM VP agreed on common parameter values (e.g., cell transmission rates) for the two ends of a single circuit.

Agreeing an acceptance test procedure with the PNOs was also difficult. The FUDI PNOs insisted that they were only providing an ATM service while the research networks' position was that any transmission service must adequately support the IP service which was required. After much debate, this issue was resolved by introducing the concepts of provisional acceptance, which would take place when a circuit had successfully completed ATM tests, followed by final acceptance after successful IP testing. Final acceptance followed provisional acceptance automatically after a specified number of days unless the research networks involved produced evidence of unsatisfactory IP performance. In such a case, the clock would stop while the PNO and the research networks investigated the cause of the failure together.

A limited call for tender was conducted within the TEN-34 consortium (open to the research networks and their PNO suppliers) to award a contract for the Network Operation Service. UKERNA was the successful bidder and the NOC (Network Operation Centre) was set up in London in the first quarter of 1997.

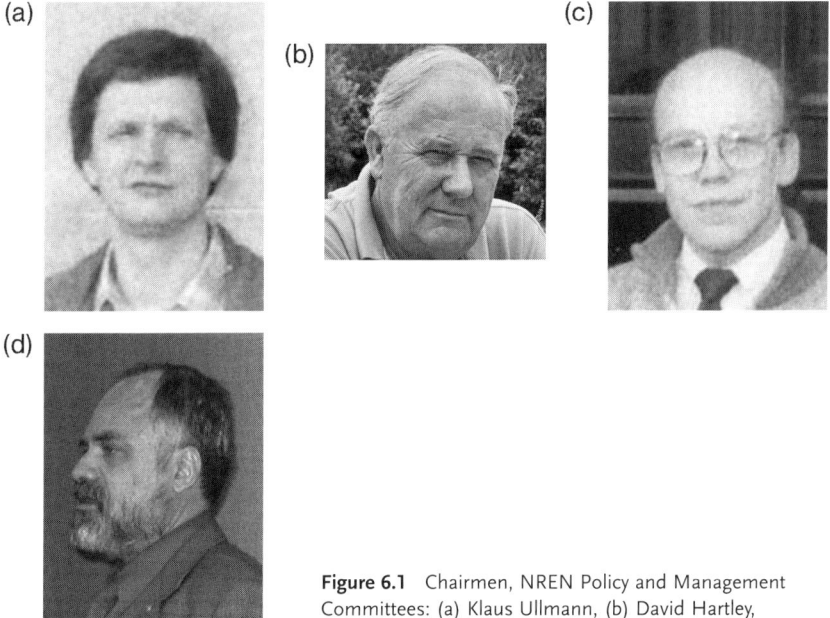

Figure 6.1 Chairmen, NREN Policy and Management Committees: (a) Klaus Ullmann, (b) David Hartley, (c) Fernando Liello, (d) Vasilis Maglaris.

TEN-34 topology
July 1998

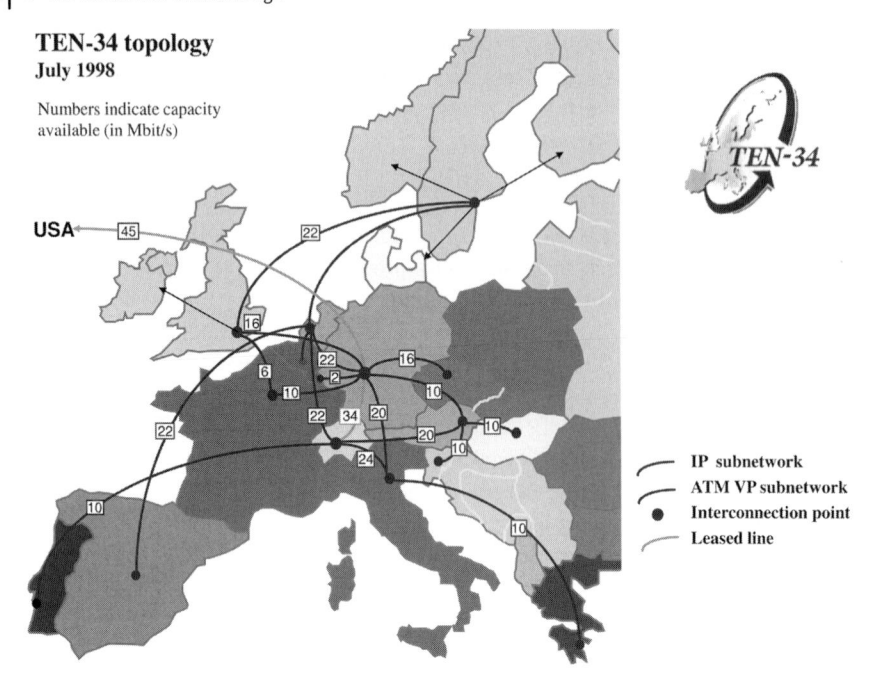

Numbers indicate capacity available (in Mbit/s)

Figure 6.2 TEN-34 topology, June 1998. There is a color version of this figure in the set at the front of the book.

The TEN-34 service started in March 1997, providing service to ten research networks. A further three research networks were connected in August 1997. The network configuration in July 1998 is shown in Figure 6.2. During the period of TEN-34 operation which lasted until the end of November 1998 the traffic carried by the network increased from 7000 to over 40 000 Gbyte per month.

6.2
TEN-155 and QUANTUM

"We have started to shed the dead weight of monopoly pricing of international bandwidth which has been holding back European research networking. We can now concentrate more on exploiting European imagination and ideas for delivering quality of service, QoS, to the research community."

(Howard Davies, General Manager of DANTE, on the launch of TEN-155.)

By the summer of 1998, the consistent growth of traffic in the TEN-34 network led to a gradual erosion of the previously good network performance. Additionally, more and more cooperative development activities in Europe were now based on the use of multi-media services. This required high QoS levels which could not be provided on a fully loaded "best efforts" IP network. The national research networks had responded by increasing their bandwidth capacities to 155 Mbps on a national scale. On a pan-European scale this sort of bandwidth was either not available or not affordable before January 1 1998. However, the liberalization of the European telecoms market caused the situation to shift.

Planning of a new project, QUANTUM (quality network technology for user-oriented multi-media), which would include the implementation and operation of yet another new network, TEN-155 (trans-European network at 155 Mbps), started even before TEN-34 was officially launched in May 1997. At the request of CSIC (Consejo Superior de Investigaciones Científicas), RedIRIS (Spain), DANTE (UK), DFN (Germany), GRNET (Greece), INFN (Italy), RENATER (France) and SWITCH (Switzerland) together with Telebit (Denmark) – a sub-set of the TEN-34 consortium – DANTE delivered a proposal to the EC on April 18 1997 in response to the Fifth Call under its Telematics Applications Program. Such a rapid introduction of new network generations involves a high management overhead but the partners in the new consortium believed that it was important to profit from the results of telecoms liberalization as soon as possible.

The broad objectives of the proposed QUANTUM project were to explore and subsequently to implement ways of providing improved QoS, particularly for multi-media applications, across a very high-speed (up to 155 Mbps) international inter-research network. Three phases were defined in the project proposal: experimentation/validation of alternative approaches using a test network in which Telebit would play a significant role, planning and procurement of a network service which would come into operation after the end of the TEN-34 project, followed by an operational service period. After this proposal received a positive evaluation by the EC the participants were invited to submit a detailed proposal with a deadline of December 25 1997.

In parallel with the EC's evaluation process, DANTE and the research networks had already been planning the successor service to TEN-34 with the working name of TEN-155. A specification of the service as seen by the research networks was agreed. In addition to a conventional IP-based service with access capacities of up to 155 Mbps, the specification provided for additional services with guaranteed QoS to be supported by a combination of ATM technology and new developments from the IP world. The possibility of creating multiple VPNs, with the use of the highest capacity VPN to support the IP service, was allowed for. It was felt that this time a unified and centralized procurement strategy for the successor service should be adopted, to improve the ability to negotiate a competitive supply price with a limited set of suppliers and to ensure a consistency of technical specification.[3]

Acting on behalf of the new consortium, DANTE issued a Request for Expressions of Interest on November 10 1997, and on December 23 1997 it issued an invitation to tender to organizations selected from those that had confirmed their interest. The deadline for responses was early February 1998. The intention was to start replacing components of TEN-34 as soon as possible after July 31 1998, when many of the

---

3) TEN-34 had involved contracts with 18 PNOs, leading to operational difficulties, network performance issues and higher costs.

TEN-34 contracts with PNOs terminated. It was expected that migration to the new service would take several months and that use of some of the TEN-34 circuits (e.g., those to countries where there would continue to be a PNO monopoly for international services) would be continued in TEN-155.

On February 13 1998, acting on behalf of the QUANTUM Consortium, DANTE received 16 responses to the invitation to tender issued on December 23 1997. The responses covered a range of offers from point-to-point connectivity to complete sub-networks. It had been expected that a much more cost-effective network could be built from these offers; however, the result was a rather mixed picture. It turned out that there were three distinct groups of countries in Europe when it came to progress in liberalization. One set of countries (Germany, Switzerland, the Netherlands, United Kingdom, the Nordic countries, France and Ireland) represented a reduction in cost of a factor of 10 when compared with 1997 prices, whereas for the second group of countries (Luxembourg, Belgium, Austria, Italy and Spain) the factor was 4; for Slovenia, the Czech Republic, Hungary and Greece the factor was 3.5. Portugal was the only country where the offers received for TEN-155 were actually more expensive than was the case for TEN-34. A further point was the availability of relatively high-capacity connectivity. Capacity of 155 Mbps was only available in the first group and in some of the countries in the second. There were still significant parts of Europe where infrastructure was both expensive and rationed.[4]

By April 1998 the QUANTUM proposal for EC support of the new network and related activities was approved by the EC's ESPRIT and Telematics committees. Altogether, €17 M was made available by the EC towards the building and maintenance of the new network until funding from the Fifth Framework Program could take over. On March 27, the QUANTUM Policy Committee agreed to DANTE's proposal to prepare three alternative costed proposals, based on the tenders received, for a further meeting at the end of May. There were many technical issues to be resolved with most of the potential suppliers. Delivery commitments, location of PoPs, provision of local access circuits (if necessary), and management of the managed bandwidth service (MBS) which aimed to provide guaranteed capacity and performance to particular groups of users were major topics which continued to require discussion and negotiation.

6.2.1
TEN-155 Takes Shape

At the end of May, the QUANTUM Policy Committee made decisions on several major issues concerning the network for QUANTUM. Next to a set pricing scheme, the committee members agreed on the principle that ATM would be used as

---

[4] The relatively homogeneous cost base of two years earlier gave place to a quite heterogeneous picture. Consequently, DANTE had to abandon the geographically independent pricing scale based purely on access capacity. Countries where international telecommunications were relatively expensive were disadvantaged compared to those where prices were relatively cheap. Thus liberalization had the divisive effect of making more capacity available but only in certain parts of Europe.

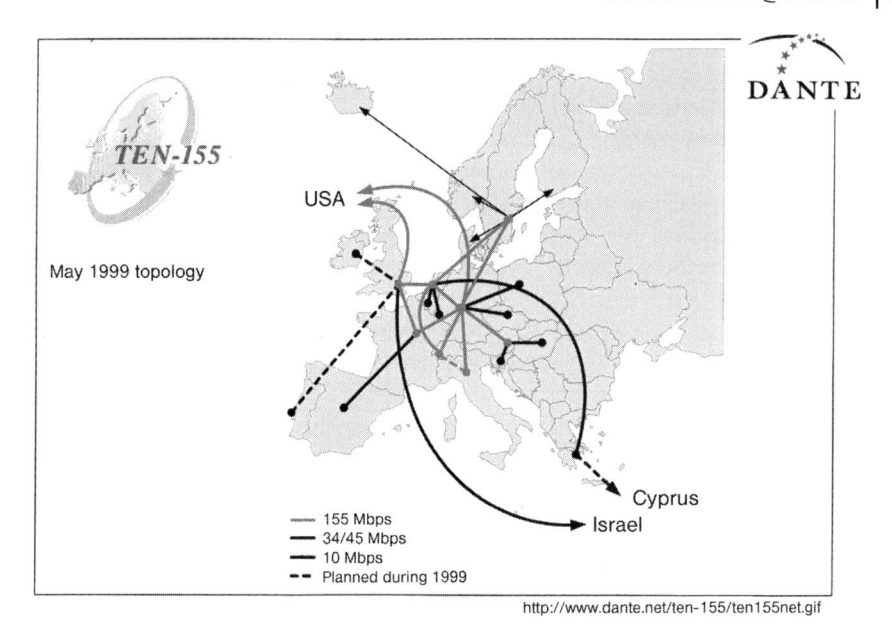

Figure 6.3 TEN-155 configuration, May 1999. There is a color version of this figure in the set at the front of the book.

a bandwidth management tool to optimize the use of the SDH circuits. The individual national research networks would have the choice between ATM or IP-over-SDH access to the network. QUANTUM would receive funding contributions from the EU's ESPRIT and Telematics for Applications programmes.[5]

Work on the TEN-155 network progressed well during the summer of 1998. The supply contract for the bulk of the capacity, awarded to Unisource Belgium, was signed at the end of August and was officially announced during an international press conference in Brussels on September 17 1998. Unisource Belgium would provide connectivity in Belgium, France, Germany, Italy, the Netherlands, Spain, Sweden, Switzerland and the United Kingdom. The contract was signed for a period of 3 years, with the roll-out of the network starting in December 1998. At the time, it was anticipated in the Unisource contract that the network would be upgraded to 622 Mbps by the year 2001.[6] The planned network configuration is shown in Figure 6.3.

On December 11 1998 the first production traffic flowed on TEN-155. The new network had access capacities of 155 Mbps in eight European countries and thus constituted the largest operational pan-European network. TEN-155 was officially

---

5) The QUANTUM Policy Committee also mandated DANTE to negotiate detailed arrangements with the EC ACTS program for the support of ACTS projects as well as with the Commission in general, to prepare the final EC contract for QUANTUM.

6) In fact, a new 622 Mbps central ring interconnecting Paris, Brussels, London, Amsterdam and Frankfurt was up and running by November 2000.

demonstrated during the launch activities of the EU's Fifth Framework Program at a two-day event in Essen in February 1999. A highlight was a visit to the TEN-155 stands by the German Federal Minister for R&E, Edelgard Bulmahn and Robert Verrue, Director General of DG XIII. Ms Bulmahn and Mr Verrue participated in a live video session between the partners of the MECCANO (multimedia education and conferencing collaboration over ATM network and others) project. The MECCANO project was the first user of the TEN-155 MBS. It was the first time a group of European researchers benefited from dedicated bandwidth made available in the TEN-155 network.

Altogether, 14 of the 20 TEN-155 circuits were carrying production traffic by the end of February 1999. In January, access port availability for seven of the (then) ten TEN-155-connected national research networks was 99.99% or higher.

Immediately after TEN-155 succeeded TEN-34, DANTE's network planning and engineering team carried out an analysis of the impact of providing more capacity to the European research community. The analysis compared international inter-research network traffic measurements on TEN-34 in November 1998 and on TEN-155 in January 1999. The measurements were derived from DANTE's international inter-research network statistics package. The analysis emphasized that international inter-research network traffic had increased by almost 50% during that period.

The roll-out of the TEN-155 network entered its final stage in March 1998. Except for Luxembourg, Portugal, Slovenia and Spain, all participating national research networks had completed their migration. Joining TEN-155 as a newcomer, the Polish research network POL-34 was connected with a 34 Mbps link to TEN-155 on March 10 1999.

In the meantime, TEN-155 became increasingly stable. High availability was recorded for the transit countries, which was related to the design of the network, especially to the rings and the dual links. In spite of a number of circuit problems, most transit countries had 100% ATM availability, with overall ATM availability calculated at 99.83% in March. IP access port availability for 11 of the 17 TEN-155-connected networks was higher than 99.94%.

RedIRIS (Red de Interconexión de Recursos Informáticos), the Spanish research network, migrated to TEN-155 on May 20 1999. The Israeli research network, IUCC (inter-university computation center), was successfully connected to the TEN-155 London PoP via a 34 Mbps link provided by the Israeli operator Golden Lines on May 21 1999. This connection was a result of the Q-MED (QUANTUM in the eastern Mediterranean region) project.

HEAnet, the Irish research network, connected to TEN-155 with an access capacity of 10 Mbps at the TEN-155 PoP in London on June 29 1999. The Portuguese Research network RCCN (Rede da Comunidade Científica Nacional) migrated to TEN-155 on June 30 1999. RESTENA, the Luxembourg research network, completed its migration on July 7 1999.

The overall access availability for July showed an improvement in comparison to the previous three months, although scheduled and emergency maintenance led to some service interruptions. Eight of the national research networks had 100%

access port availability in July, while average availability for the whole of TEN-155 was 99.52%.

A connection to Cyprus from Athens was established in September in the context of the Q-MED program. Within the network, the existing circuit connecting the TEN-155 PoPs in Brussels and Amsterdam was supplemented with a second 34 Mbps line between Brussels and Paris. The new link became operational on October 20. Similarly, an additional 155 Mbps line was delivered to connect the TEN-155 PoPs in Switzerland and Italy.

In October 1999, AUCS (AT&T Unisource Carrier Services) won a tender for the interconnection of TEN-155 and the European commercial which would be rolled-out over the following few months in four TEN-155 PoP locations across Europe.

In September, the average access port availability of TEN-155 had improved to 99.75%, with 9 of the 19 connected research networks enjoying 100% access port availability.

In November 1999, the figures for TEN-155 showed an average access port availability of 99.54%, with 10 of the 19 connected networks enjoying 100% availability. However, average access port availability in October reached only 99.10%, with 5 of the 19 networks enjoying 100% access port availability. The decline in the figures compared to the preceding month was linked to two major service interruptions in Belgium and France.

The interconnections between TEN-155 and the European commercial Internet via AUCS were gradually being rolled out: the interconnection in London became operational on November 8, only a couple of weeks after the set-up of the Geneva interconnection, while the existing AUCS connection in Amsterdam was upgraded. For December 1999, TEN-155 showed an average access port availability of 99.78%, with 6 of the 19 connected networks enjoying 100% availability.

In January 2000 an average access port availability of 98.28% was reached, with 13 of the networks enjoying 100% availability. The lower-than-usual average figure for January was mainly the result of two major interruptions in Poland and Portugal.

The last interconnection with AUCS/Infonet[7] in Stockholm was rolled out on January 5 2000, making the four contract-planned connections complete. Traffic congestion on the link led DANTE and AUCS to increase the bandwidth from 20 Mbps to 35 Mbps, and performance improved immediately afterwards.

In August 2000, DFN's access was upgraded to 310 Mbps. The migration to the new central ring connecting the United Kingdom, Belgium, France, Germany and the Netherlands was completed in September, with the re-homing of the PoPs. As a result, TEN-155 was running at speeds of up to 622 Mbps. The Infonet interconnection of TEN-155 to the commercial Internet was upgraded from 210 to 260 Mbps in October. The upgrade plan which had been formulated in April 2000 was then complete and the network configuration was as shown in Figure 6.4.

CARNet, the Croatian academic and research network, was connected to the TEN-155 by a 34 Mbps link to Austria on November 21 2000. CORDIS (Community

---

7) In 1999 Infonet gained management control of AUCS from its parent, Unisource NV.

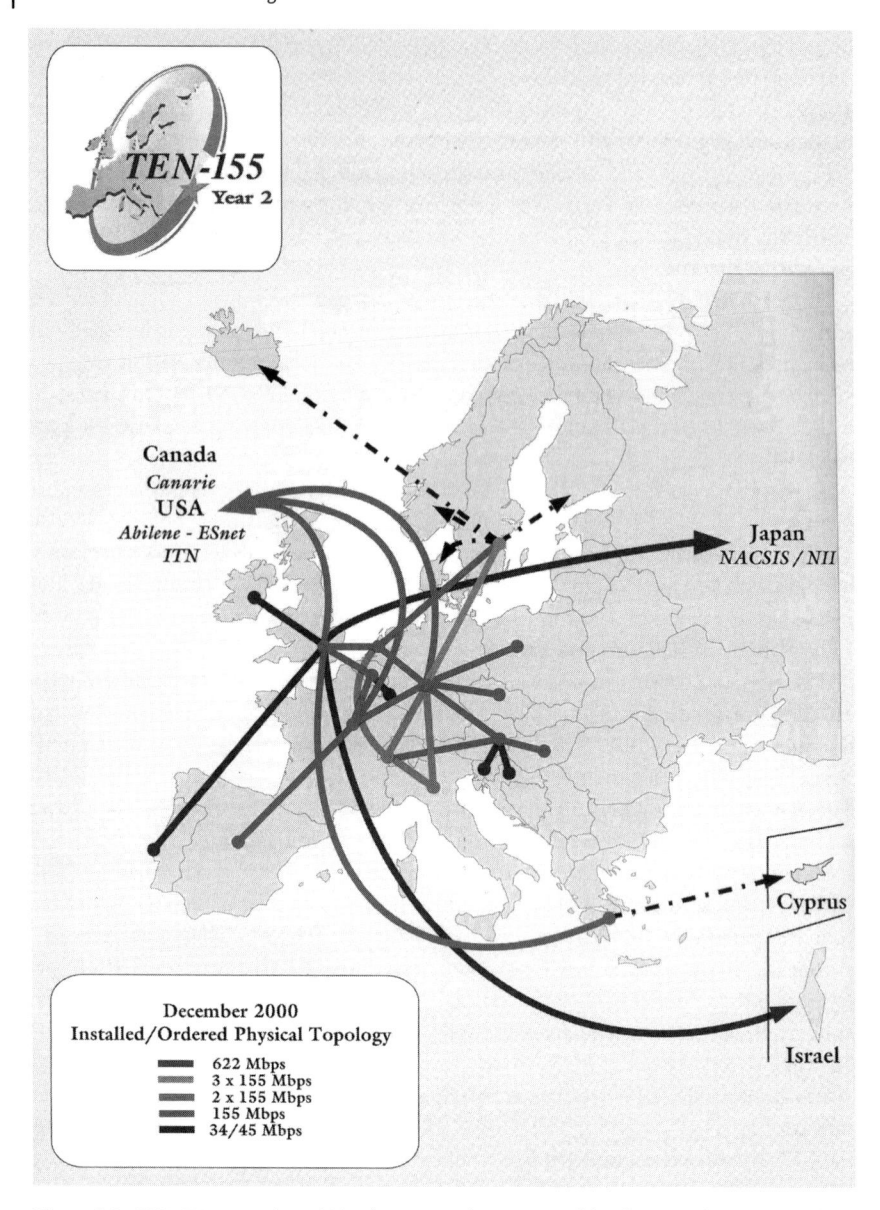

Figure 6.4 TEN-155 December 2000. There is a color version of this figure in the set at the front of the book.

Research and Development Information Service), the official European Union research and innovations information Internet service, connected to TEN-155 through RESTENA.

A 155 Mbps ATM link between France and Spain became operational on February 12 2001, half of which was dedicated to United States traffic under the DANTE World

Service. Two 155 Mbps POS (packet over SONET, synchronous optical network) circuits between Germany and Sweden became operational on February 19. The Infonet interconnection in London was upgraded to 155 Mbps on February 20, giving TEN-155 a 425 Mbps total interconnect with the commercial in Europe.

The backbone link of the TEN-155 network was upgraded between Austria and Slovenia on March 15 2001. Also on March 15, DFN upgraded its access to TEN-155 from 310 to 622 Mbps. The ongoing upgrade of the Infonet interconnection continued, with the new 80 Mbps capacity to Geneva giving TEN-155 a total interconnect of 445 Mbps with the commercial Internet in Europe.

The TEN-155 (155 Mbps) ATM STM-1 (synchronous transport module level-1) backbone capacity between Greece and the United Kingdom was doubled to $2 \times$ STM-1 on June 5 2001. A new POS STM-1 gateway to Infonet was added in Frankfurt am Main on July 3 2001, bringing the aggregate capacity of the interconnection of TEN-155 with the commercial to a total of 600 Mbps. The TEN-155 backbone was upgraded on August 14, when a POS STM-1 between the PoPs of Frankfurt and Vienna doubled the existing ATM STM-1 circuit.

In September, the interconnection in Amsterdam between TEN-155 and Infonet was upgraded to 622 Mbps overnight on the 9th. A new ATM STM-1 circuit between France and Switzerland was delivered at the end of that month.

Increasingly, cooperative development activities in Europe were based on the use of multi-media services, which rely on high QoS which cannot necessarily be provided in a "best effort" IP network. The TEN-155 MBS addressed this issue by allowing the definition of virtual private networks with committed bandwidth between national research networks.

As it was a new service, alpha and beta test phases were planned before the service became operational. The alpha test was carried out between the beginning of January and the end of March 1999, based on one pilot project and sites in a limited set of countries (France, Germany, and United Kingdom). The beta test phase lasted from the beginning of April to the end of June 1999 and involved eight projects/groups, with sites in most countries connected to TEN-155. The projects/groups were either involved in EC co-funded R&D activities (DYNACORE, dynamically configurable remote experiment monitoring & control; EDISON, European distributed and interactive simulation over network; SUSIE, and RCnet), research activities between Universities (ENCART, European network for cyberart), between research institutions (Czech physicists and CERN) or research activities within the QTP, QUANTUM test program (MPLS, multi-protocol label switching; and DiffServ, differentiated services).

During the alpha and beta phases, as well as in the subsequent period up to mid-September 1999, the TEN-155 MBS was successfully tested and used in 12 of the connected research networks, as well as in CERN. Overall, the alpha and beta test phases showed that the MBS was a useful service. A survey of the TEN-155 MBS was carried out in April 2000. The response to the questionnaire was good; 11 of the 18 groups which had used the MBS replied. The conclusion from the responses was that the service was performing well and was serving its purpose, but that some consideration still needed to be given to restructuring and simplifying the deployment process.

6.2.2
Intercontinental and External Connectivity

Within the context of migration to the TEN-155 network, DANTE's United States connectivity was upgraded from 45 to 155 Mbps by December 1998. Peering was arranged with ESnet while DANTE was investigating a connection to STARTAP (science, technology, and research transit access point), as well as looking into possible peering arrangements with the American academic and research networks vBNS (very high speed backbone network service) and Abilene.

On May 20 1999, capacity of the United States service at the DANTE Euro PoP in Telehouse, New York was doubled. In addition to the 155 Mbps link between Frankfurt and New York, a second 155 Mbps link was installed between London and New York.

Cooperative research between scientists in Europe and Japan received a boost when the interconnection between TEN-155 and NACSIS (National Centre for Science Information Systems), Japan was significantly upgraded on October 1 1999. The interconnection was based on a 10 Mbps IP service via the DANTE New York PoP to the TEN-155 PoP in Frankfurt and a 15 Mbps connection to the TEN-155 MBS at the TEN-155 PoP in London.

In addition, a 45 Mbps interconnection between those European national research networks using the DANTE United States connectivity and Abilene – one of the networks supporting the Internet 2 project in the United States – became operational in October 1999. This connectivity was further upgraded to 100 Mbps in February 2000, allowing better performance for research networks using this interconnection.

A new 155 Mbps line between Paris and New York became operational in October 2000. The connectivity to the Canadian research network CA*net was also upgraded from 10 to 15 Mbps. This connection was further upgraded to 30 Mbps (ATM) in January 2001. Multicast connectivity to the Canadian network was enabled the following month.

The interconnection with the American backbone network Abilene was upgraded by an extra 622 Mbps on an additional OC-12, optical carrier level 12 (POS) in December 2000. An agreement was reached with Abilene to provide the DANTE World Service customers with an international transit network (ITN) service, via which they had access to STARTAP and networks such as SingAREN, the Singapore advanced research and education network, APAN (Asia-Pacific advanced network), and so on. A new interconnection agreement with ESnet was also signed that month. The agreement was a milestone as it offered a shared-cost model for transatlantic connectivity for the first time. The lack of cost sharing in previous arrangements had been a major source of frustration.

In addition to the three existing circuits between New York and TEN-155, a fourth 155 Mbps line from Vienna came into service in February 2001.

In addition to the existing 622 Mbps POS line to Abilene from the DANTE New York PoP, an independent OC-3 (optical carrier level 3) was delivered on April 10 2001 for back-up and ATM-based projects. This freed capacity on the OC-3 formerly shared between Abilene and ESnet transit, allowing the line to be dedicated to ESnet.

During its lifetime, TEN-155 increased transatlantic connectivity from 155 Mbps in November 1998 to four times that amount by December 2001. In addition, high-speed interconnects with a number of important research networks in the United States, Canada and Asia were established.

6.2.3
The QUANTUM Test Program

The QUANTUM test program (QTP) was the technology-testing element of the QUANTUM project. Its goal was to evaluate emerging technologies with the aim of understanding how to implement operational services with them. Particular attention was paid to the provisioning of QoS, but also to multicast (IP and ATM), IPv6 and ATM signalling. Other efforts were devoted to understanding and developing techniques in support of these, such as QoS monitoring, flow-based monitoring, route monitoring and policy control.

The work was carried out by TF-TANT (task force testing of advanced networking technologies), a joint DANTE/TERENA task force. Activities started in November 1998 with a meeting in Cambridge, in which the areas of activity and the people responsible for them were identified. Subsequently, work was carried out to define in more detail the test proposal for each experiment, together with the finalization of the participants in each activity and the definition of a test plan.

Each activity was developed to a different level, having to do with prioritization within the task force: most of the members of TF-TANT took part in more than one activity; therefore there were simple time constraints on the possibility of performing all tasks at the same time. Other factors such as availability of test equipment influenced the development of the activities. An interim report on the results of the testing activity was produced in October 1999, while the final report was published in June 2000.

Work on IP multicast was very successful as in October 1999 a pilot IP multicast service based on PIM-SM (protocol independent multicast-sparse-mode), MBGP (multicast border gateway protocol) and MSDP (multicast source discovery protocol) started on TEN-155 and was transformed into an operational service in April 2000. The developments of the flow measurement and analysis activity of the task force were also partly deployed on the TEN-155 operational network and research network operational networks, especially in the area of traffic analysis and DoS detection.

The work on IP over ATM demonstrated that the use of ATM as implemented on TEN-155 was the most effective, whilst other mechanisms that might have been theoretically more efficient were either not developed yet or were not working properly.

All other activities produced many experimental results, but did not result in service specifications or in pilot services.

The QUANTUM project ended formally in October 2000. Preparation for its successor network GÉANT, the pan-European Gigabit research network, was well under way by then and in the summer of 2001 contracts were awarded for GÉANT.[8]

---

8) Planning had already started by September 1999.

The layout of the new network and migration from TEN-155 started at the end of the summer. Thanks to careful planning and plenty of overlap between the two networks, none of the European research networks, whether newly connected or TEN-155 partners, suffered any loss of connectivity when TEN-155 was shut down on December 1 2000.

The QUANTUM project had accomplished three important objectives: first and foremost, the successful deployment and operation of the TEN-155 network service. Besides the basic IP service, the MBS – offering guaranteed end to-end QoS – was made available to specific groups of users. In addition, significant testing was conducted under the QTP.

The TEN-155 era saw a breakthrough in both the cost and availability of bandwidth across Europe. After years of monopolistic prices in conjunction with limited available bandwidth capacities for pan-European connectivity, TEN-155 was the first pan-European network to close the gaps between bandwidth available and affordable nationally and internationally. Speeds within the network had now reached up to 622 Mbps, a substantial increase compared to its predecessor's 34 Mbps. The growing importance of the European Research was also reflected in the first cost-sharing arrangement reached for a transatlantic connection.

6.3
Relations with Telecom Operators

With a touch of commercial realism, DANTE profiled R&E networking as "network builders restricted by European politics". The internal view within the research network community might emphasise the differences between the various countries, yet the perceptions of the providers are that the research network representatives are all highly skilled, knowledgeable about latest network trends and commercially astute with a finger on the pulse of most aggressive network pricing.

From a provider perspective, it is not straightforward to place the R&E community and align it with common business models and market segmentation. Indeed, both national and international organizations can be put in different categories such as government (because of their funding source), SME (small or medium-sized enterprise – they have relatively few staff) or wholesale carrier (as a result of network size).

Besides the financial interest, there are other benefits to the operators in using a cooperative model when dealing with the R&E networks. Most of them deploy technology that is still the subject of R&D or in the early stages of deployment. The products that are needed to meet the R&E networks' demands are often not yet ready for full-scale deployment, and are hence not entirely suitable as the basis of a response to more conventional commercial demands or for immediate operational deployment. On the other hand, the learning experience from early deployment with a knowledgeable customer can influence which technology and services should be promoted on development roadmaps. Early deployment can be key to strategic success for carriers, as it can generate the new skills necessary to launch and support new products. The value of this learning is difficult to quantify or even to identify, as it is spread between product development, pre-sales, post-sales and operations which are separate units within large carriers.

In practice, the fit for European R&E networks does not sit comfortably with the existing alignment of carrier sales. European network carriers fall broadly into two categories, those with a strong national presence and larger Europe-wide (often global) operators. The national operators tend to deal with national R&E networks directly while the European network operators see more interesting opportunities within major European projects. European carriers will try to maximize revenue by offering the largest product footprint and portfolio. European R&E network strategies have led in the opposite direction as they have been trying to commoditize services and to select providers on the basis of their strongest footprint/region. The service portfolio has been reduced from fully-managed services to highly-commoditized products such as dark fiber and co-location space (PoP housing). The early R&E networks such as EuropaNET were fully managed, the supplier being responsible for the provision of all equipment and services, including configuration control and technology development. In subsequent network generations, the requirement for outsourced management has been reduced and carriers have been driven down the technology stack: first they lost IP routing, then ATM switching and wavelength services. Now, the lowest layer has been reached and they only provide fiber infrastructure and co-location, with a small amount of service management to provide on-site support and access to equipment. This means that the carriers that benefit most in this scenario are the ones with a fiber-rich footprint with ample quantities of fiber. Consequently, where carriers have their "built" footprint becomes more relevant, as fiber wealth is more important than network reach. The carrier industry has seen a series of developments. The extensions of international circuits to customer PoPs (tail circuits) were initially built on leased SDH capacity and/or half-circuit arrangements; this changed later to leased wavelength services where higher capacities were required. One real example which is now widely deployed is that the GÉANT network did not require active tail circuits and utilizes fiber as passive tails; this eliminates the requirement for expensive metro optoelectronics at the marginal cost of reduced management control.

One area of difficulty (or bone of contention) is inherent to early deployment which would normally be accompanied by a low service level. The research community can calculate or derive the anticipated values of service level parameters using industry standards or specific statistics provided by carriers or manufacturers, but these values are outside the limits that carriers are willing to commit to, for example, low bit error rates, aggressive guaranteed time to repair. On the one hand the R&E networks require the flexibility to perform and develop new network tests that can be intrusive or even destructive, while on the other hand it runs operational services on which the research community relies for its day-to-day operations. To manage the European network opportunities of non-productized service requests successfully, carriers need a combination of effective leadership and key account management supported by excellent technical and operational skills – something that is not easy to achieve.

6.4
Relations with Equipment Suppliers

The relationship between the R&E community and equipment manufacturers can take many forms: it can be about selling/buying a product or a complete technical solution, providing consultancy on architecture or services, sponsoring activities or projects, collaborating on R&D activities, and so on. All are different forms of business relationships which depend on mutual benefits.

This section describes the interest and opportunities for industrial companies in getting involved with the R&E community, and is concentrated on present situations.

6.4.1
Research and Education Networks as a Market

Manufacturers in the telecommunication industry should realize that R&E communities represent a distinct and entire market opportunity. People who have not approached this community directly have often made wrong assumptions; one of these is about market awareness.

The key is to understand that the R&E community represents a complete and distinct infrastructure from end to end, parallel to the commercial and public network operators. They may share resources at the very lowest level (optical fibers), but even at this level there is a tendency towards total separation. In other words, they represent a whole market opportunity.

The R&E acronym can be confused with R&D. R&D is a vertical activity in many business areas that focuses on discovering new knowledge about fundamental sciences, products, processes, and services; whereas R&E is a complete vertical segment in enterprise and service provider markets, as it is constituted by a complete chain of different stakeholders: campuses, research laboratories, computing centers, metropolitan and regional networks, research networks, and other global R&E backbones. "R&D" and "R&E" obviously have different meanings in terms of addressable market and business opportunities, although R&E supports and contains many R&D activities.

Market analysts are not much help in clarifying the situation, as they focus more on the end-user community rather than the infrastructure players: in most cases, the R&E community is positioned under one umbrella called "Education", often defined as "all institutions dedicated to academic and/or technical/vocational instruction, with the exception of certain training environments that are better treated as social services"[9]. That does not explicitly include all the network infrastructures that are necessary to connect all these institutions.

Apparently, many people still believe that university and research laboratory connectivity relies on public operators, or ISPs, which was the case in many countries just a few years ago. But deregulation has fundamentally changed the picture: the R&E infrastructure is made up of a myriad of purpose-built systems connected

---

9) IDC (International Data Corporation) Market Analysis, August 2005, IDC #33739, Volume 1.

together and managed by the community. Only a few are still built by commercial operators (for example, in some emerging countries).

R&E communities constitute an attractive market for equipment manufacturers, not only for those focusing on LAN technologies, but also for those focusing on infrastructure solutions (research networks, metropolitan area networks, i.e. MANs, and regional networks). The other wrong assumption is about business profitability. Some people may believe, for the reasons mentioned above, that R&E communities do not invest much in equipment and that they mainly rely on sponsorship and donations. In fact, a non-negligible portion of their budget is used for network and security equipment with the objective of maximizing the value they can get from vendor solutions. The reason is that vendors have to deal with production networks which combine state-of-the-art technologies and services without compromise on performance and reliability. In most places, this model cannot be deployed with donations and old technologies, although that does sometimes happen, in particular in areas where the digital divide persists.

Finally, an interesting lesson was learnt by industry when the Internet bubble burst in 2001. At the same time: (i) the Internet service providers who survived experienced a huge reduction in investment; (ii) the cost of network capacity decreased significantly (plenty of fibers and unsold SDH capacity), (iii) the research networks did not suffer proportionally from that crisis and actually almost maintained their budgets. The result made R&E communities a providential niche market for equipment manufacturers to counterbalance somewhat the drastic reduction of service providers' investment. The fact is that the R&E market, just like the public sector business in general, is stable and can reinforce any manufacturer's position in the long term.

6.4.2
The Research and Education Community as a Technology Incubator

The R&E communities differentiate themselves from commercial operators, not only because they have a different business model (they are non-profit organizations), but also because they have different end-users and applications. Of course, there is a significant proportion of users with only basic needs such as email, web browsing and file sharing, but many users require more advanced capabilities from the network, such as high capacity, guaranteed performance, multicast or IPv6 forwarding. These users would not get these services from commercial networks, at least not at an affordable price. The reason is that commercial operators focus on standard solutions that work for most customers and consumers, with data link capacities based on average usage (and not on traffic peaks of individual customers), from which they can expect maximum revenue and profit margin. Commercial operators can also fulfill any specific need with a customized offer, but in that case with a totally different economical equation. So that partially explains why R&E networks offer a very interesting arena for technology incubation.

From the equipment vendor's point of view, the R&E community deploys state-of-the-art technologies and services, and pushes them to the edges of new capabilities.

In many cases, these networks leverage technology building blocks offered by industry to create innovative services instead of simply deploying packaged services that do not fulfill their needs. At the same time, the R&E communities explore new paradigms that have yet to be considered by the commercial operators and that could forecast new developments in the telecommunication market.

By contributing to these activities, equipment manufacturers could reasonably expect some results from leveraging these R&E "long horizon" projects whose participants are the first people to have the chance of detecting new opportunities – which could assist manufacturers in moving ahead and keeping an edge on their competitors.

This multifaceted evolution of Internet technology can be represented by the three dimensions described in Figure 6.5. This representation does not match the academic network OSI model proposed by the ISO, although it still remains a reference when we address layer aspects.

In the vertical dimension, there are three distinct layers:

The forwarding and transport layer comprises both data and control planes in charge of transporting data from one point to another. This is the foundation of the infrastructure and contains all the capabilities required to perform this task (optical switching, IPv4 and IPv6 forwarding, etc.).

The management and policy and control layer embeds all systems and technology that control the network devices (network management systems, policy management, etc.).

The service and business layer is a relatively new concept that has started to be investigated and deployed in the R&E community but not yet in commercial networks. It contains all mechanisms and middleware required to coordinate network

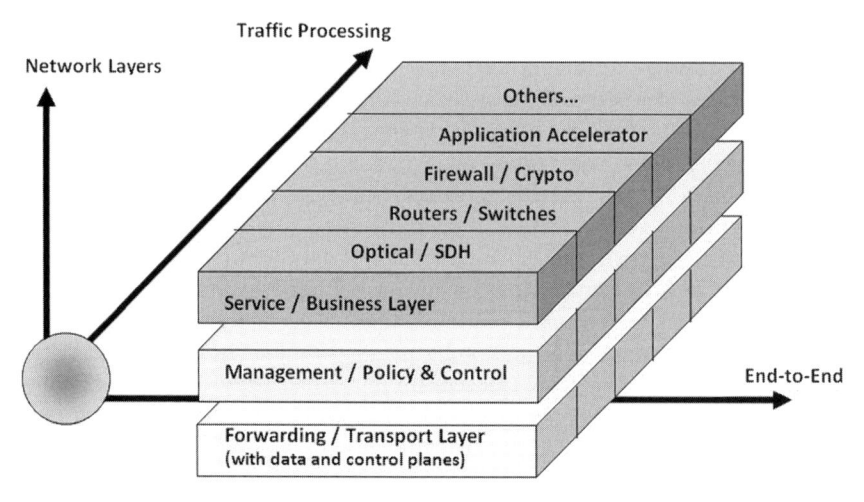

Figure 6.5 Representation of the three dimensions of convergence and interplay.

resources and capabilities from different stakeholders, in order to automate the activation of a service requested by an end-user or application (SOA – service oriented architecture – and web services). This layer is also the focus of standardization bodies and forums, in particular the IPsphere Forum (IPSF), now part of the Telemanagement Forum (TMF), an industry association focused on improving business effectiveness for service providers and their suppliers.

In the horizontal dimension, we have the spatial dimension, with E2E paradigm, very important in the R&E space because end-users and the applications they wish to use are rarely connected to the same network but interact via a chain of independent network domains, such as campus networks, MANs, regional networks, national research and education networks and other global R&E backbones such as GÉANT2. This requires a lot of interplay between the domains, both at the transport layer and the service layer.

In the depth dimension, there are all the types of traffic processing capabilities that are used in the chain of network elements. There is nowadays more focus on this dimension than in the past. One reason is that the emergence of optical layers leads the R&E community to study better integration and interaction with the IP layer. Another reason is the growing recognition of the role played by campus networks in the E2E paradigm. Adding these two parameters to the development mix increases the number of traffic processing technologies that have to be taken into account in an end-to-end circuit. Firewalls, intrusion detection systems, access control and application acceleration, could all be critical bottlenecks in a network for advanced services offered by the transit backbones.

A significant amount of work is conducted by R&E communities on technology convergence and interplays. Essentially, the telecommunication world is being transformed:

- The difference between enterprise and service provider networks is becoming indistinct.
- Routing and security technologies are progressively merging because it is becoming impossible to separate network security from other network functions.
- The new network technologies tend to simplify the number of transport layers, to reduce the cost of infrastructure and its operation.
- The convergence of multiple technologies and services (voice, data, and video) over a common infrastructure is mainly justified by its cost optimization and simplification. However, at the same time the infrastructure tends to serve multiple communities with different needs. That leads the R&E community to explore new paradigms such as virtualization.

Who else better than the R&E community knows that Multicast or IPv6 service are useless if a firewall in the campus does not support appropriate features? How much coordination effort is required between research networks to set-up an E2E Layer 2 circuit? How many grid applications sometimes suffer from very poor performance due to one single bottleneck? How does a huge data transfer impact other applications in the network if no prevention techniques are used?

The R&E community is already in the midst of this transformation and participation can bring a huge value to equipment manufacturers who want to plan longer term. Examples of R&E initiatives that already deal with some aspects of this issue include some of the E2E services, on-demand service activation, roaming and authorization, grid and IP/optical convergence.

Equipment suppliers can still greatly benefit; on condition, of course, that they take action in order to focus on the right initiatives to get maximum results for their future developments.

6.4.3
Research and Education Networks Need for Interoperability

The interoperability challenge can be considered from at least two angles. One is the interoperability of technology; the other is the interoperability of business processes. As far as technology is concerned, many standardization bodies and forums deal with this issue in order to allow customers to build complex networks in a multi-vendor environment. This work is obviously not only technically driven but also has political aspects. For example, a vendor that is very dominant in a market may not be very keen to develop interoperable protocols that would ease the introduction of new players into current customer networks. Conversely, the non-dominant players may push very hard for interoperable solutions, though not if they address new niche areas where they expect to be dominant. Likewise, a vendor may push one standard against another, not necessarily because it is better designed, but because it fits better with its own product portfolio. From the R&E community point of view, there is a need for interoperability between vendors because the model only works if services are available E2E across multiple independent networks. However, the possible result of depending wholly on vendor interoperability is to deploy an infrastructure that has the lowest common denominator characteristics, which is contradictory to the principle of pushing the technology to the edges.

Therefore, the deployment of vendor-specific solutions is difficult to avoid, but it can be done in a controlled way. The key is the divide and conquer approach: if the global network can be separated into independent pieces with clean and interoperable interfaces, then within the separate pieces, we can afford to deploy non-interoperable solutions that are fully controlled by one entity. For example, one piece could be one research network, or one autonomous system.

In theory, as long as its external interfaces are interoperable, the way in which a system is implemented within a domain does not matter much. The organization managing the domain is free to make its own choices without affecting others in the end-to-end chain, in particular by not imposing a choice of vendor on the others. Note that there are two different categories of vendor-specific solution: they can be vendor-proprietary solutions or something that has been introduced into a standardization process but implemented by only one vendor. Using items from the first category is very risky as there is a very limited chance of achieving any straightforward interoperability with this approach.

From a general point of view, interoperability is very important for all manufacturers as the network is becoming more global, with enriched interfaces between network domains, and more convergence with the application and the different data layers. This global convergence puts pressure on all vendors to follow the principle of standardization, even those who would prefer to maintain specific solutions in targeted areas for a certain period.

The second aspect of interoperability applies to business processes. This is as important as technology interoperability and sometimes the two get confused. A business process can be defined as a collection of related, structured activities – a chain of events – that produces a specific service or product for a particular customer or customers. The R&E community now realizes just how important it is for end-to-end activities and much emphasis has been applied to this in several projects in the last few years. A typical example of service that requires a good business process is the IP Premium service, as all stakeholders must agree how they will use the technology standard, how the service is defined and architectured, how it is implemented, provisioned and monitored. This is particularly complex, as the scope of a service is intended to be global. Since there are often parallel initiatives in different R&E communities worldwide, they have to agree on a minimum set of commonalities. Today, although the technology aspect is still omnipresent, the service and business layer where the technology is viewed at a higher level of abstraction has been given more attention.

A good balance between the two aspects is fundamental because there are interactions between them. For example, the use of a vendor-specific solution in one domain can be counter-balanced by an efficient and interoperable business process. In such a case, well handled coordination efforts combined with reliance on simple and widely-deployed interfaces is enough to build effective E2E services.

Chairing the TEN-34 Management Committee

David Hartley was Chief Executive of UKERNA, the organization responsible for the United Kingdom's national research network – JANET– for three and a half years from 1994. In this role, he had ultimate responsibility for ensuring that the United Kingdom academic community had good access to European and other international services, but he could have chosen to have one of his staff deal with this aspect of UKERNA's activities. Not long after his appointment, he had remarked that "European research networking was something that had, over a period of time, developed alliances, factions and schisms", the principal source of friction at the time being the different approaches adopted by three research networks (those of Austria, France and Ireland) which relied on Ebone to carry all their international traffic, and those which used EuropaNET.

David's previous experience of working at a European level was limited. As part of his previous job as Director of the University of Cambridge Computing Service, he had been involved in SHARE Europe (a club of IBM mainframe users), and then later, as a Vice-President of the British Computer Society, he chaired the first meeting that led to the creation of the Council of European Professional Informatics Societies (CEPIS). But even this limited experience had already taught him one lesson, namely that "at the European level, one has to proceed slowly and resolutely to achieve and maintain consensus". Despite this limitation, several of his European counterparts who tended to be friendly to the United Kingdom urged him to make use of his status as a "new kid on the block" to take some action to resolve the European tensions.

David subsequently invited the heads of all the research networks to a meeting to explore the possibilities for formulating a project in which everyone would participate. This led to the creation of TEN-34 and the appointment of David as the Chairman of its Steering Group.

Describing some of the incidents and issues that he had to deal with, he says:
"I knew very little about networking at the European level before 1995, and was only a little more knowledgeable in 1997. Having said that, I have no doubt that I am substantially the wiser for the experience. In the early days, the main problem seemed to be to persuade France to join in with what was going on in the rest of Europe. Austria and Ireland were also outside the fold, the three being involved with the Ebone Association whose clients were part research and part commercial. To my simple mind, all we had to do was to get France in and the other two would follow."

With one member appointed by each project partner, meetings of the Steering Group involved nearly 30 people. Various attempts were made at cutting the numbers down to a manageable size without causing diplomatic incidents. On the whole, they did not succeed. Almost everyone agreed that some form of executive committee would be much more effective, especially to handle social and day-to-day matters, but they would only agree to any delegation of authority to a sub-group if they were a member of it. David once commented that he only had to be seen talking to the representatives of two or more countries, then a representative of another would complain loudly.

A distressing characteristic of some organizations in the research networking community is a lack of commitment to things they have agreed to. David says: "I was invited to give a speech at the 1995 NORDUnet Annual Conference in Copenhagen and I gave this talk; TEN-34 had just reached an important milestone and I had prepared an up-beat presentation. But, immediately before me in the same session, someone from Telia (a Swedish PNO) gave a talk, and announced that they were going to provide a great network for NORDUnet. The Telia network was advanced. It was a good thing. It was ready, whereas the TEN-34 plan was still a bit scrappy at the time. I was completely upstaged. The message from the two talks was that the Nordic countries were getting a marvellous deal from one of the PNOs, and in the rest of Europe we were going to lag behind". David was very cross about that because he felt that he had been upstaged deliberately. NORDUnet people have always considered themselves more advanced than the rest of Europe – with justification. They were connected to the Internet before the rest of Europe and are very proud of it. It would have helped to maintain good relations, however, if there had been some recognition of the difficulties that research networks in other parts of Europe had to face. David was subsequently invited to the 1997 NORDUnet Conference where he was able to describe TEN-34 in some detail because by then TEN-34 was successful.

David can point to other lessons from his period of office. He says: In order to manage a project like TEN-34, it is absolutely essential to have a voting mechanism in place so that everyone can see that the process of taking formal decisions is transparent and democratic. But you must never actually take a vote. If you do so, those who voted against will play the I-never-agreed-to-that card endlessly. Instead, you must sit tight and find ways of moving towards consensus. If necessary, you can put on a deliberate loss of temper to speed things up when antagonists will not compromise: "OK, if we can't agree on this we had better pack up, go home and abandon the project!" – accompanied by a threatening shuffling of papers. Consensus sometimes involved choosing not the best, but the least bad alternative, meaning that everyone was unhappy about the result they had agreed on, but at least the unhappiness was fairly shared.

7
Support for Applications

Originally, networks provided an infrastructure over which data could flow between users and applications. Nowadays, the network infrastructure must also provide the services that the end users require to communicate. This chapter discusses a few of these new services, addressing how they developed and how they influenced the offerings we see today on the modern Internet. It also discusses some of the more hidden aspects such as security and responding quickly to issues.

7.1
Security and CERTs

With the ever-growing number of interconnections between networks managed by different service providers and users, the openness of the networks exposed the connected user organizations to a small but steady number (by today's standards) of attacks and incidents. The Internet worm in November 1988 and the DECnet worms of 1989 were early examples of "denial of service", that is, they created an overload of some essential system resource with the result that there was no capacity left to handle normal user operations). They generated an underlying feeling that the network was fragile faced with experienced attackers and showed that there was the potential for developing harmful ways of exploiting weaknesses and vulnerabilities. Therefore it is not surprising that already in 1990 during the 2nd CERT (Computer Emergency Response Team) Conference[1] Christopher C. Harvey spoke about "The Development of Response Teams in Europe". This early involvement is also visible in that the ESA's Space Physics Analysis Network (SPAN) became a founding member of FIRST (Forum of Incident Response and Security Teams), "the" international umbrella organization of security and incident response teams, in 1990.

At the same time, security needs were discussed from a totally different angle: the application users needed security functions to ensure confidentiality and authenticity

---

1) CERT was established by DARPA (Defence Advanced Research Projects Agency) in the aftermath of the internet worm in December 1988. Starting in 1989, it organized an annual conference. In 1993, this role was taken over by FIRST as the international umbrella organization of CERTs and security teams.

A History of International Research Networking. Edited by Howard Davies and Beatrice Bressan
Copyright © 2010 WILEY-VCH Verlag GmbH & Co. KGaA, Weinheim
ISBN: 978-3-527-32710-2

of email and other services. As the underlying protocols were recognized, at least in the case of TCP/IP, as being inherently insecure by more and more people, attention moved upwards in the protocol stack and focused increasingly on building security into applications.

Overall, it can be said that at some point in 1990 a critical mass in terms of experienced and curious experts was available in Europe; they decided it would be better to prepare beforehand and do something about the growing uncertainty regarding security – or rather lack of tools and procedures for providing it. So a RARE "Security" Working Group was established and, until 1992, it continued to discuss a broad range of related security issues. Since the participants were themselves members of the research network communities, they were able to trigger actions inside their networks and organizations; the working group members promoted the importance of security and many of today's results can be traced back to them.

While discussions had started earlier, it took some time to come up with a number of common notions and understandings. Therefore, the changes resulting from the group were not immediately obvious but by 1991 and 1992 more and more projects related to security were being kicked off. A typical example is the DFN project that developed a PEM-enabled (privacy enhanced mail) email client based on X.509 certificates and all the supporting tools, libraries and components needed to run the organizational infrastructure. (X.509 is one of the protocols in the X.500 set of OSI protocols which were designed to support directory services.)[2] Although the initiative built on earlier projects which made use of the X.400 set of OSI standards for e-mail and messaging, it confirmed the early insight that building security into applications was the only way of helping to protect end users.

Beside such application-focused projects, experts were concerned about how to handle the problems users and their organizations faced if one (or more) of their systems had problems. Even in these early years it was becoming obvious that many users were not knowledgeable enough to identify early signs of successful attacks. Much of the damage caused could have been avoided if the affected users had reacted more promptly after the security of their systems had been breached in some way.

Meanwhile, inside the RARE working group, consensus was established to look more closely at the question of whether Europe needed a CERT/CC (CERT coordination center). NORDUnet had established a security team back in 1991, and the first government agency to join the European "security club" was the CCTA (Central Computer and Telecommunications Agency) from the United Kingdom in that year. In 1992, SURFnet was the first national research network to establish a formally chartered CERT for its own constituency. The team, which was known for its first 10 years as CERT-NL and which later changed its name to SURFnet CERT, joined the global incident response community that same year. Also in 1992, DFN issued its call for tender that led to the establishment of DFN-CERT on January 2 1993.

---

2) While this work was used to gain considerable experience and to build many libraries with the basic functions, X.509 only gained widespread acceptance many years later. On the other hand, PGP (pretty good privacy) became popular and was the tool of the trade for all security experts for many years.

A few months later, June 1993 marked the beginning of a project called "RARE CERT Task Force" chartered by the RARE working group. Also based on a call for tender, the Woolwich Centre for Computer Crime Research (University of Exeter, United Kingdom) was selected to further analyze the options available in Europe to respond to the growing threat of incidents. Two interesting tasks in their work plan were a "Campaign to persuade all European networks to set up CERTs and to join FIRST either as full or liaison members "and" Coordinate the creation of an organizational structure within and between European networks so that security incidents can be dealt with quickly and effectively". Neither of these goals was fulfilled in the short 18-month project, but seeds were sown and would eventually develop into healthy plants.

7.1.1
Establishing a Regional Identity

During the 5th Workshop on Computer Security Incident Handling in the United States in August 1993, many European teams and experts involved in this topic actually met for the first time. SURFnet CERT invited all of them to a meeting that was held later in September that year in the RARE office, with the aim of facilitating the Woolwich Centre project. This was the beginning of the European CERT development which has been carried forward by volunteers and with strong support of the teams and TERENA ever since.

During the meeting, in which no commercial CERTs were represented yet, all agreed that efforts in each national research network would bring a real benefit for everyone. Attacks were becoming more widespread and automation was becoming an issue. (For example, a self-reproducing virus might be unleashed which would infect one target computer and then make use of an easily found address list to target many more. In addition, scanning and probing for vulnerable systems became common practice, resulting in a continuous level of something called "internet background noise", unauthorized and potentially dangerous packets addressed to all systems on the network.) Infections could spread very quickly and it was important to extend the incident coordination aspects to as many networks as possible. While you can take steps to secure your own networks and perimeter, your security is greatly improved if you can depend on others to do the same with theirs. It was expected that the European teams would cooperate, share information and also share some responsibilities for helping other research networks to develop their own teams. Again, such outreach was based solely on the work of volunteers and support by TERENA.

To summarize the consensus among the experts, here is an excerpt of the meeting:

- Use FIRST as an already established forum with similar interests.
- Support a European special interest group within FIRST.
- Integrate new European teams – including non-FIRST members – and help teams to gauge their operations, apply for FIRST membership and so on.
- Build up trusted relationships and support the cooperation with non-European teams.

- Enable the participation of other teams with a clear interest in the European situation.
- Communicate common problems and characteristics to other teams worldwide, emphasizing (if necessary) the specific European dimension.
- Research the need for improved European incident handling coordination.

As a result, in 1994 RENATER (France) as well as the German government team at the German Information Security Agency (BSI, Bundesamt für Sicherheit in der Informationstechnik) joined the small community; in 1995 SWITCH-CERT (Switzerland), CERT-IT (University of Milan, Italy) and JANET-CERT (United Kingdom) were added. By the middle of 1995, nine European teams were collaborating, seven of them responsible for research networks and two for governmental institutions. Seven more research network teams were in the process of formation and planned to join the growing community. Indeed the success of this development also brought the Annual CERT Conference to Europe when FIRST chose Karlsruhe, Germany, as the conference location in 1995, drawing much attention to the European teams.

So while this part of the RARE CERT task force was rather successful, the final report pointed out that some form of coordination between European IRTs (incident response teams) other than bilateral links should be organized, especially with respect to incident coordination. This point proved to be rather contentious and while some proposals were made, none was accepted. To reach consensus the TERENA task force "CERTs in Europe" was created in May 1995 to draw up a proposal for a way out of the deadlock. The task force's constitution provided for representatives from various national research networks and its final report was greeted warmly by the TERENA members at their General Assembly in Rome, October 1995: a project was to be started to further define the service specification and to pilot the service on the basis of the outlined concept.

The current *ad hoc* cooperation of existing teams was important and showed much potential, but at that time it was thought that a more fundamental approach should be taken to solve the underlying problems and to meet the scalability demand for a truly coordinated approach that would be crucial in the future. To summarize the ultimate tasks and advantages of a European IRT coordination center it was stated that the center should:

- build trust relationships between all European teams and act as a clearing house,
- care for the European part of the CERT world, while conveniently being in the same time zone,
- be aware of the specific details of the European situation and regional problems,
- provide know-how for other teams,
- introduce new teams to the FIRST community,
- build the European part of the global "picture".

To be able to address the need for such coordination efforts, various approaches could be taken, resulting in different levels of support and coordination. The TERENA "CERTs in Europe" task force considered several approaches, three of which were considered viable: incident response team support, basic incident coordination, and full incident coordination.

These approaches were initially developed as separate entities but it soon became obvious that they were actually three stages of the same model. This model offers a level of service which increases from incident response team support towards full incident coordination. At each step, services are added.

An abstracted treatment of this layered coordination model can be summarized as follows:

Incident response team support: Support functions are needed to enable cooperation and coordination. Examples of such functions are meetings, contact information, information services, secure communication, and promotion. The maintenance of this service can be handled inside business hours.

Basic incident coordination: In addition to the incident response team support services, this level focuses on the need for incident coordination to complement the incident handling which is mainly taken care of by the existing teams. Coordinating an incident implies channelling relevant information to the right teams and building the bigger picture to improve quality of service. The expertise, facts and background information gained from the coordination effort should be made available to all the teams. The basic incident coordination service should be available outside business hours as well as inside.

Full incident coordination: While all basic services necessary to coordinate incidents have been addressed in the previous level of service, extended and additional services are needed in the areas of security vulnerabilities, education and security technologies, in order to allow proper prevention measures and support for the technical know-how and work of the coordinated teams. In the longer run, this value-added approach will prove to be more effective than just coordinating a random distribution of expertise among teams. The full incident coordination service must be available 24 hours per day, 7 days per week.

Obviously the result of the task force's work was not a proposal for one or more individual solutions to the coordination problems of incident response teams in Europe and beyond. Instead, a coordinating model was proposed which offered a migration path from a simple support function to a professional infrastructure for computer security incident handling within Europe. National and network-oriented teams would provide incident handling capabilities to their constituencies. The coordination of their work and international issues would be addressed through incident handling coordination, which was to be supported at a European level.

The task force's recommendation to TERENA was to implement the basic incident coordination service right away. While important parts of the incident response team support service were already being provided through the voluntary work of single teams, the coordination issue could only be dealt with in a formalized and funded fashion because of the resources needed for this task. While the task force's report clearly stated that a larger number of teams would be necessary to justify the move away from bilateral agreements between teams towards a structural hierarchy, this carefully phrased statement was lost. Instead, many focused on setting up the infrastructure, while leaving the other – much more important functions – in the capable hands of volunteers. All this lead to a three-year period during which various projects were suggested, prepared, and drafted, to create something that was called a European coordination center.

Finally in 1997, this project was started and continued until 1999 as EuroCERT. There were various inherent problems, as some CSIRTs saw this team as a competition to their own activities. Indeed, the name EuroCERT did not resonate well with national CERTs which were concerned that this CERT would want to simply take over. Technically, the bilateral agreements in place together with the cooperative support inside the community were efficient enough not to need support from another level of hierarchy.

While some people pointed out that the discontinuation of EuroCERT proved the point that no coordination was really needed, it merely proved that running a CERT is something different from coordinating CERTs. The main criticism was that EuroCERT simply did not add very much value to the overall processes.

7.1.2
Today's Activities

When EuroCERT was discontinued in 1999, TERENA called all experts together to assess the overall needs once more, and to discuss what would have to be done about the loss of services that had been provided by EuroCERT, in particular the organization of the European meetings and infrastructure support to facilitate information sharing and exchange.

Interestingly enough, the meeting came to the conclusion that the lessons learned led to another operational model. As the services were indeed quite different from each other, they could be grouped in three categories:

- The services that need continuity and have specific requirements like trust management, especially:
  – contact database,
  – team and team member authentication,
  – accreditation and certification.

- The services that benefit from the support of volunteers and do not require continuous personal support:
  – regular meetings,
  – specific working groups.

- The services that had not been well-developed and that would need further study by all involved before they could be considered for further up-take:
  – coordination of multilateral incidents,
  – mandatory reporting.

The experts and volunteers – with strong support from TERENA – then produced a formal specification of the first category services. After its adoption, the whole process was put out to tender. In September 2000 the "Trusted Introducer" service started. Its main objective was – and still is – to introduce new CERTs into the established community.

In addition, volunteers have been instrumental in defining important cornerstones of the security infrastructure, for example the RIPE IRT object, which allows people to look up the designated CERT for a given IP address or domain via the RIPE web site[3] or the WHOIS client. Other activities were coordinated with IETF Working Groups, in particular GRIP (guidelines and recommendations for incident processing), producing RFC 2350 as a best current practice document, INCH (incident handling), defining exchange formats designed for CERTs and IDWG (intrusion detection working group), defining exchange formats and protocols for intrusion detection systems and related applications. And above all, the regular meetings were coordinated between the TERENA secretariat and CERTs that could provide meeting space and logistical support.

7.1.3
The Trusted Introducer Service

The trusted introducer service has been providing accreditation and infrastructure support services for the European CERT community since September 2000. The key idea is simple: to be part of the security infrastructure trust is needed among the players. But trust is not easily gained, rather earned and given by others. To help the CERTs develop and foster trusted relationships, information about both operational parameters and key policies is collected. Operational parameters include contact information, emergency numbers, service portfolio and identities of team members. Key policies deal with the way sensitive information is handled and protected, under what conditions it is provided and to whom, what code of practice the team supports, and so on.

Accreditation is a voluntary process. A team signs up and during an initial time period as candidate, all necessary information is requested, provided and checked. By accepting the accreditation, a team agrees to support the trusted introducer accreditation process, which also includes four-monthly updates of the team information. This is to ensure that the team database is up-to-date all the time and to guard the quality of the accreditation. But naturally, the accredited team agrees to be truthful and to adhere to the standards set by themselves during their accreditation – in regard to such various topics as their service window, their information management policies and their code of practice in general.

A team could actually provide false information during the candidate phase, but then all accredited teams have access to this information and review new candidates. Therefore if a team acted "strangely", this would be reported and followed up accordingly. All accredited teams support the service itself with a small annual fee, and gain access to more value-added services that will be described below in more detail. The governance of the trusted introducer is indirectly in the hands of the

---

[3] www.ripe.net.

accredited teams themselves – their team representatives elect a review board that oversees the service and they review all escalated problems that teams bring to their attention. In such a way, sanctions, like termination of an accreditation, can be handled in a balanced way, by ensuring that the quality and impartiality of the service can be guaranteed.

As the accredited teams share a common baseline set of code of practice, policies and information available, tailored services are provided to further facilitate their communication and coordination. Accredited teams get access to:

- a detailed database containing information about all registered teams and (in detail) accredited ones,
- subscriptions to secure (encrypted and authenticated) mailing lists,
- a secure repository for further information and documents,
- an out-of-band alerting mechanism based on voice mails and SMS (short message service),[4]
- registration and maintenance of RIPE IRT objects.

The future will require even stronger coordinated activities of all teams involved, as the changing landscape of common threats calls for shorter response cycles and coordinated mitigations. To support this, the information exchange between teams – on a bilateral or multilateral basis – needs to be improved. This requires new technologies which, for instance, allow the direct push and pull of required data.

Consequently, the demand for all teams to adhere to defined and agreed common standards is becoming more important, so there is a discussion of ideas that effectively build on the current accreditation levels, to add the concepts of verification, and certification. In fact, this natural development mirrors best practices which are being increasingly adopted by European industry and governments in and beyond the realm of information technology. As an example it can be noted that the ENRON case in the United States, which led to an increased demand for transparency of financial and accounting processes in companies, has been one of the enablers of a growing demand for transparent, accountable, verifiable and certifiable ICT and security processes. Essentially, the people holding the budgets want security to deliver Euros – and want to be able to certify that.

Therefore, the trusted introducer's independent and objective accreditation system is an excellent starting point to add on certification in due course.

7.2
COSINE Sub-Projects

It happened once upon a time....

The email in Figure 7.1 is 20 years old. Its bits have lived on many different storage media since it was sent, but it still sits inside "1988" e-mail archive, just a

---

[4] As the internet itself might become unusable due to a widespread virus outbreak or servers of the CERT community might be jammed with high loads of traffic rendering the systems unusable, other means of communication not depending on the internet itself must be available.

```
Received: from SEKTH.BITNET by SEARN.BITNET (Mailer X1.24) with BSMTP id 4059; Mon, 12
 Sep 88 13:12:03 GMT
Received: from kth.se by KTH-BITNET-GATEWAY ; 12 Sep 88 10:57:23 GMT
Received: from rtr59b.kth.se by kth.se (5.57+IDA+KTH/3.0) id AA00173; Mon, 12 Sep 88 12:57:00
 +0200
Message-Id: <8809121057.AA00173@kth.se>
Received: from GEMINI.#DECnet by rtr59b.kth.se; Mon, 12 Sep 88 12:51 MED
Date: Mon, 12 Sep 88 12:56 +0200
From: Torgny Hallenmark LDC <th@seldc52.BITNET>
Subject: RE: e-mail contact
To: ALLOCCHIO@SYNCTS.INFNET

Hello,
My EARN/BITNET address is TH@SELDC52
If you want to use Internet style addressing also following address should work:
TH@LDC.LU.SE
Regards from Lund in Sweden,
Torgny Hallenmark
EARN/BITNET: TH@SELDC52
Internet: TH@LDC.LU.SE
VAXPSI: PSI%24020031020720::TH
```

Figure 7.1 An early e-mail massage.

few clicks away from the spam message which was deleted just seconds after its annoying delivery.

If you have a closer look at this piece of electronic antiquity, you will easily notice a number of strange features in it; just look at the e-mail addresses. A glimpse at the e-mail headers and the addresses proposed in the correspondent's signature give a picture of a very different networking world. The Internet was just "not there yet". If you wanted to use Internet style addressing, "it should work", but the Internet is mentioned as the second choice, after EARN/BITNET and just before a proprietary implementation of X.25 real-time mail. And, indeed, the message arrived on another proprietary messaging system, the self-named. INFNet (INFN network)

At that time, networking had challenges to face which nobody even knows about nowadays. The first was that there was not a single network. Different networks, using different network protocols were living side-by-side, often on the same campus, not talking to each other. Succeeding in sending an e-mail message like the one above, crossing many different networks, was something only very few people could achieve, and e-mail was one of the few (maybe the only) application that could cross boundaries.

In the above scenario, the few network users quickly realised that this situation was not going to be sustainable for long; something had to be done to unify solutions. But of course everybody believed that their own solution was the best one, and the others should just migrate to it. Moreover, the few colleagues across the Atlantic who were playing with IP networks were obviously computer science people playing games, and they were not to be taken so seriously – that was the main opinion among "real" users.

Systems and applications must talk to each other! And of course, at least on paper, there was a full set of specifications with a self-explanatory name: OSI specifications, which were developed by ISO and also issued by CCITT as its X. series of recommendations. They even provided the ability to carry multimedia parts inside e-mail messages, they were talking about directory services and certificates, and they were the future.

At least this was what the decision-making bodies were convinced of, and given the fact that the "real users" needed to make at least e-mail interwork more easily, at the time of that e-mail, RARE set up its first set of Working Groups and of course WG1 was the one to work on e-mail. This was the first attempt to pull together people who were working on application services and it was a great idea. When they first met, most of them only knew on paper what OSI was but they had a clear mission: make it live, make it work, and deploy a set of services to users.

Between 1988 and 1991 there was a lot of work being done and the EC buzzword for computer networking was OSI. Very few people, including those in the computer industry, really used and tested OSI specifications in real life deployment but members of the RARE WGs were pioneers. For e-mail, the people in WG1 quickly became experts in the full X.400 specification (which, just to make things more complex, was updated meanwhile to a new version by CCITT), while the X.500 series was the daily breakfast for WG3 participants. Some people started to implement code matching those specifications themselves, others joined efforts with the OSI development teams of the major vendors of that time to integrate their products – and indeed make them really interwork with other implementations. Yet others started to create bridges (or "gateways") between OSI implementations and the application systems used daily which were around (proprietary or just covering a different set of the options allowed within the standard). Setting up effective communications between OSI applications and their equivalents in the TCP/IP world was just one activity amongst many.

Implementation of the OSI specifications required a human network to be set up first. There was a clear need for interactions between people, not only because of the technical requirements – setting up the application communication parameters, for example – but mainly because, for the first time, it was necessary to enable interworking between different implementations of the same application in different operating systems and environments. Just to make things more complex, even if X.25 was the background network layer for everyone, existing networks were all using different protocols internally (DECnet, SNA, TCP/IP, United Kingdom Coloured Books, etc.) and of course, people wished to use the other capabilities of these infrastructures as well as transport for their applications. Given the technical difficulties in making the bits interwork correctly, WG1 members quickly became a very efficient and integrated network of human experts. It was the beginning of successful European and worldwide collaborations.

At the beginning of the 1990s, the RARE MHS experimental project was almost a production reality and a number of gateways to other messaging systems were in place, allowing global messaging in a quasi-transparent way, provided that the users typed in a not-so-friendly X.400 e-mail address which looks like, for example:

$G = $ Claudio; $S = $ Allocchio; $P = $ garr; $A = $ garr; $C = $ it;

At the same time, our North American colleagues had also joined WG1, but of course they preferred TCP/IP as the transport mechanism for OSI rather than X.25, and in 1991 WG1 people decided it was time not only to standardize what they were doing at the CCITT, but also to integrate their work into the TCP/IP world. WG1 sent a couple of scouts to explore the IETF world in what was subsequently dubbed "the St. Louis meeting". They did a good job and established the basis for the newborn IETF WG X.400-operations. When they came back, WG1 decided to mount an "educational expedition" to explain to the TCP/IP natives how to use OSI and make it work. The expedition landed at the following IETF meeting, in hot, humid Atlanta in mid-August, and after some initial quarrels with the locals, having survived the serious health hazards due to the 18 °C air-conditioning systems, everybody started to work happily together. The bridge between OSI and TCP/IP applications was built and in the following years it produced a successful series of IETF standards, from e-mail gateways to Directory Services. It was also the inspiration which brought multimedia alive in Internet mail (MIME, multipurpose Internet mail extensions), ignited LDAP specifications and led to the only OSI specification which really proved successful in the long term and is still happily alive: the X.509 certificates.

It was time to move from experimental services to a common coordinated effort, and the various proposals which were written under COSINE started to become operational only in 1991/92. At network layer, IXI was replaced by EuropaNET, which also supported IP, and COSINE sub-projects S2.1 MHS service, and S2.2 MHS gateway service came alive.

In 1992 it became clear that some of the OSI applications would never fly, in particular FTAM, but others like X.400 and X.500 were well on their way. At the same time, in a little corner of the Innsbruck Conference Centre at the 1992 European Joint Networking Conference an unknown expert named Tim Berners-Lee was presenting his ideas about HTML/HTTP (hypertext markup language/hypertext transfer protocol) and the World Wide Web: "interesting, but what is it useful for, apart from reading online documentation more easily?" was Claudio Allocchio's comment and that of WG3 too, "The biggest mistake we ever made" was a much later statement by Erik Huizer, WG3 chair at that time.

The COSINE MHS service quickly turned the RARE MHS experiment into a production level service. A full mesh of message transfer agents (MTAs) was established across Europe and North America and X.400 multimedia message traffic was flowing across it daily. The deployment of the service was so successful that a number of commercial X.400 providers (at that time most of them were tied to the national telecommunications monopolies) also decided to peer with COSINE MHS. A number of participants in COSINE MHS even obtained recognition from national regulatory bodies as an ADMD (administrative management domain) – X.400. Now, e-mail communication with non-R&D partners was made possible. An explicit peering with another EU project, Y-net, which had the commercial environment as its target, was also working successfully.

COSINE MHS could also exchange messages efficiently with all the other existing messaging systems being used by the R&D community. The COSINE sub-project was providing the MHS gateway services, mainly to the rapidly growing TCP/IP world using SMTP (simple mail transfer protocol), but also to everything else that existed, and more notably, between everything else that existed. EARN/BITNET mail, DECnet Mail-11, SMTP, United Kingdom Grey book messaging could all talk to each other, not only to the X.400 service. A global messaging system was established for the first time.

In the following years, mainly when MIME became more robust and IP networks were deployed reliably in Europe, the COSINE MHS service continued to be the main messaging service in the R&D world, while it transparently migrated from X.25 to IP transport. For a long time, it remained the only exchange point to non-R&D messaging systems, before the Internet as we know it now was created. But it also became clear that a messaging system based on a concept too closely tied to the hierarchical human organization behind it (in the style of just one, or a few central operators per country) was not going to scale to larger traffic numbers. And the "S" – simple – in SMTP or ESMTP (extended simple mail transfer protocol) eventually turned out to be a winning factor. Nevertheless, the COSINE gateway service was there, providing a transparent connection service between different systems and standards. This was yet another successful result of COSINE sub-projects, enabling a smooth migration to the "winner" in messaging: ESMTP with MIME support, a migration which lasted many years. An interesting detail: the COSINE S2.2 gateway service ran much longer than the COSINE project itself. The service was eventually shutdown in 2004, 12 years after its inauguration, and when it was turned off there was a complaint from the United Kingdom National Health Service: they said they were not able to send messages with X.400 to a correspondent hospital in France, which was of course located on the Internet. Somebody, maybe once a month, was still using it.

In the end, the history of COSINE sub-projects and of OSI applications deployment and subsequent migration to IP applications is a success story. People learned how to collaborate and work together in a very complex and challenging scenario. They succeeded in making complex different implementations interwork for the first time, despite the fact that in some of the standard specifications, some pages had the astonishing sentence "this part of the protocol is for further study" (and, probably, it was never studied afterwards). People also learned features of the OSI specifications which were later introduced into IP equivalent protocols/applications, like the X.509 standard, or the concept of peer authentication among messaging clients, or the concept of the LDAP suite. There was a forum for exchanging information freely and openly, in all those meetings of the RARE WGs, meetings which could be held anywhere around Europe provided the name of the city was "Brussels/Bruxelles", at least during COSINE project deployment. The COSINE project also had another great success story: it made many European experts go and actively participate in the development of the IETF and of IP itself, which at that time was still a very United States-centred activity. This participation started with messaging and directory services, but quickly spread all over the other activity fields of the IETF. Twenty years later it still deserves credit for what it did. It also cost someone what was a fortune at the time: there was an agreement among the Europeans and their American colleagues that the first European to publish an RFC would pay for the drinks at the following WG1 meeting dinner. RFC 1405, published in January 1993 was the winner, and the next WG1 meeting was in Switzerland: wine was very expensive in that country at that time, and messaging people were not exactly abstainers.

7.3 Grids

The idea of the grid came to Europe from the United States at the end of the 1990s and provoked great interest in the HEP community that was always desperate for large and affordable computing power. Georges Metakides, head of the EU's ESPRIT program at the time, came to CERN early in 2000 and met with the committee of the particle physics laboratories responsible for developing a strategy to address the enormous problems of collecting, managing and processing several petabytes of data to be produced by the new Large Hadron Collider a few years from then. Following a recent Computing in High Energy Conference, most of the members of this committee were convinced that something like the new computing model presented by United States computer scientists Ian Foster and Carl Kesselman would be the best performing and most convenient approach to merging the large number of distributed resources which physics laboratories had around the world. The system had to be seamless and would have to provide all of the several thousand physicists involved in the LHC enterprise with easy access to a virtually infinitely powerful virtual computer center.

The synergy and dependence on an extended and powerful research network infrastructure was immediately obvious and this is why, following Mr. Metakides's visit to CERN, the first exploratory discussions for EU specific funding of some grid prototype projects were redirected to an imminent call for network research infrastructures. It must be said that Mr. Metakides, contrary to the general tendency of the EC bureaucracy never to take risks, understood the potential of this innovative technology and "invented" a considerable budget (€10 M) to start EU-DataGrid, the first EU grid flagship project.

This was the beginning of the adventure with the EU on grid projects in early 2000. Some of the first phone discussions with EC officials were not easy. From the grid users' perspective, it was necessary to move fast and maybe bypass some EU rules, whereas the EC officials needed to make sure that the most important project of its kind in the EU program was also correct from a legal and administrative point of view. The beginning of the relationship was somewhat bumpy, but turned out to be the start of a long and solid friendship which is still ongoing today.

Indeed, this is not the only episode in which the major enabling role of the EU and some considerable risk taking on its part must be acknowledged. Another example of the EC going a long way to support the international scientific community was when it was decided that grid computing needed to go further than Europe and start to expand and reach scientific communities in China, Latin America, the North African countries and so on. It was not easy to do this within the strict rules of the EU, but they took the risk, made it possible to aggregate the right collection of scientists and grid developers and their efforts were successful: activities and collaboration with all those continents continue to this day. Unfortunately, it is highly probable that many of these projects (EUMedGrid, EUChinaGrid, EUIndiaGrid, OMII - Open Middleware Infrastructure Institute - Europe, ICEAGE – international collaboration to extend and advance grid education) will no longer be supported: the era of pioneers and risk takers could be over.

Grid projects and research networks proceeded in close synergy and mutual "interaction" for the last years. Grids needed a highly reliable and affordable research network infrastructure to build on. For their part, the research networks needed grid applications to demonstrate the capabilities of widely available bandwidth, to prove the value of projects like GÉANT, and in so doing to justify the continued funding of EC research programs.

Now we are on the fringe of a new evolution in distributed computing and we see the grid concept moving towards cloud computing, elastic computing, Web2.0 and so on. All these new kinds of models are a natural evolution of the distribution model based on the grid, but they address more sophisticated issues of semantics, content management, ease of use and so on. It is clear that the experience of the grid technology has been very successful, but the cost of running large production grid operations is very high when compared to more conventional cluster and data centers. As in the case of the grid deployed by the physicists of the CERN LHC, that has become a major obstacle for a wider adoption of the grid and for an effective industrial takeover. EU and its partners in the research networks and in the grid community have another major opportunity to explore these new models of computing, while leveraging the precious experience of these last several years. In particular, recent network progress on dynamic lambda networks together with virtualization technology appears to offer an elegant and very safe way to implement large distributed grids which could also be secure enough for mission-critical industrial applications.

The World Wide Web
The development of high-capacity networks and of the World Wide Web (WWW) provides a striking demonstration of the unpredictability of the outcome of research projects and of the synergy that can sometimes lead to dramatic changes in areas far remote from the original research topics.

The initial concept of the WWW when Sir Tim Berners-Lee first embarked on its development was as a tool to assist in the analysis of data from high-energy physics experiments and in the presentation of the results of the analysis. Without high-speed network facilities to support the distribution of very large amounts of data to physicists distributed throughout the world and to enable millions of people to use it as a routine part of their daily activity, the WWW may have remained an interesting applications package used by a relatively small group of enthusiasts who were prepared to tolerate slow response times when they wished to interact with remote machines.

At the same time, the enormous increases in data transmission capacity resulting from the activities of the research networks over a period of 10 to 15 years might have remained largely unused except by a relatively small proportion of research workers who are capable of generating vast quantities of data and who could put up with awkward user interfaces which the average computer user would find difficult to understand and to exploit effectively.

In combination however, these two separate threads in the field of telecommunications research have transformed the way in which the nations of the world go about their business. In the most advanced countries, three quarters of households have broadband access to the Internet and the use of the WWW is a matter of routine – an outcome that no one foresaw in the 1980s when these developments got underway.

Besides being used for information access and exchange in education, government and commerce, the WWW has also had a social impact which was never predicted and which has been made possible through the use of web applications such as FaceBook and blogs. These social developments are continuing and their impact in the long term on language, culture and personal relationships remains to be seen.

The introduction of these technologies also has a dark side. Four fifths of the world population does not have access to the Internet (in Africa, only 5% have access)[5] and the resulting "digital divide" will be a source of friction for as long as it exists. High speed networks provide improved access to a host of valuable information sources and services. At the same time, they make it easier to access undesirable services such as on-line gambling and pornography. It has always been the case, however, that when one group of people makes an invention with the best of motives and in the hope of improving the state of the world, another group of people will seek ways of using the invention for purposes which are considered to be undesirable. New knowledge is almost impossible to hide once it has been published, officially or otherwise. Individual researchers cannot be held responsible for the ways in which other people exploit their work but members of the research community should always be aware of any dangers that might result from their efforts and should strive to prevent misuse of the new devices or systems that they create.

Overall, the WWW and the network services that support it are seen to be a force for good. They justify the resources and human effort devoted to the projects that have produced them. They provide strong support for the case for continued funding of advanced academic research which allows individuals to conceive and implement ideas which do not necessarily have an immediate application.

---

5) See http://www.internetworldstats.com/stats.htm.

8
Regional Perspectives

This chapter presents the networking advancements seen from the perspective of several different regions around the world. Western Europe, Eastern Europe, the Far East, Russia and South America and Central America are represented. It helps explain some of the different problems encountered during the setting up of the networks in these areas and how they were later connected to the European research and education network.

8.1
NORDUnet

NORDUnet (Nordicic university network) provides connectivity for the Nordic national R&E networks, but it also has another fundamental function: to serve as a platform for international collaboration. This has been an equally important task throughout the 25-year history of Nordic networking cooperation.

During the early 1980s when the NORDUnet community was forming, networkers in the Nordic countries learned to work together for a common goal. These early contacts became vital in the mid-1980s, when European collaborations began to take shape. Nordic networkers were very active in these early collaborations, and as a group they were a stronger force than a single participant from one country would have been.

In the 1980s, the first significant European collaborations in the networking field were EARN and RARE. NORDUnet and the Nordic research networks participated in both of these, but in the late 1980s the Nordic networking community decided to move in a direction based on views at odds with those of many other European networks. In building the NORDUnet network, the NORDUnet community was determined to make use of the TCP/IP protocol in the Nordic backbone. But the Internet protocol used in America was not accepted as a part of pan-European networking plans. The difference between the Nordic stance and that of other European organizations meant that NORDUnet was closer to its American collaborator, the NSF.

In the early 1990s, NORDUnet was a driving force in bringing the Internet protocol to Europe, and was one of the initiators of the first pan-European IP backbone, Ebone.

A History of International Research Networking. Edited by Howard Davies and Beatrice Bressan
Copyright © 2010 WILEY-VCH Verlag GmbH & Co. KGaA, Weinheim
ISBN: 978-3-527-32710-2

Nowadays, NORDUnet's major platform in European cooperation is DANTE, which manages the pan-European research network GÉANT.

Over the years, members of the NORDUnet and the later NORDUnet communities have participated in international working groups and in projects developing new networking technologies. NORDUnet has been involved in valuable collaboration with the Internet2 project in the United States since the end of the 1990s. In Europe, NORDUnet has participated in the large 6NET (large-scale international IPv6 pilot network) research project, testing IPv6. And most recently, NORDUnet has become an active member of GLIF, an organization dedicated to developing optical networking.

8.1.1
EARN, First Steps in European Collaboration

In the mid-1980s, the European research communities were energetic in setting up new collaborations to ensure networking development and standardization in Europe. The NORDUnet program began in 1985. EARN (European academic and research network) was initiated in the early 1980s by the computer manufacturer, IBM, which had already sponsored the BITNET network in the United States. In 1984, IBM began to donate hardware to European universities; meetings for computer scientists were organized to plan an academic research network in Europe. In February 1985, the EARN association was established and started its operations.

The Nordic countries took part in the EARN collaboration from the very beginning. Already in 1985, Denmark, Finland, Norway and Sweden were connected to EARN, and Iceland established its connection in 1986.

In its early years, the EARN network proved to be an important service. Although EUnet had already been built by UNIX users in Europe, for many academics it was EARN that gave them the first chance to send e-mail to other researchers and network with them. Peter Villemoes, the General Manager of NORDUnet, recalls that at this early stage, EARN was the major backbone in Europe: "EARN was the basic service for universities in Europe, without any doubt."

However, the EARN network used provider-specific technology, the NJE protocol and RSCS, created by IBM. The European research networks could not have their future activities on proprietary technology, so they had to consider other alternatives.

EARN was supported by IBM for four years, but in 1988 the funding was to come to an end. Nordic networkers began to plan ways of using the EARN lines, and the X.EARN project was established. Soon the project evolved into a more ambitious model: a network that would carry multiple protocols to connect the Nordic research networks.

Frode Greisen, the former EARN President, believes that EARN helped the development of Nordic networking: "Nordic researchers benefited from having a service before the Internet developed internationally. To some extent, bandwidth provisioned for EARN was used to carry other protocols too, which probably facilitated Internet development in the Nordic countries. It was easier to get bandwidth for

EARN, since it was providing a real e-mail and file transport service for the established community of mainframe users, easier than for development for the initially smaller numbers of Internet users."

For Nordic networkers, the EARN service was a vital stepping-stone in the development of their own Nordic infrastructure, the NORDUnet network.

8.1.2
RARE, Harmonizing European Development

The EARN project gave European computer scientists a chance to collaborate but, at the same time, plans were made to establish a new cooperative organization. EARN had been dependent on the products and standards of a single company. For the European academic community, that could not be a solution for the future. European researchers therefore considered ways of harmonizing the development of networking protocol standards to ensure the interconnection of the research networks. With this purpose in mind, European networkers established a new association, RARE (Réseaux Associés pour la Recherche Européenne).

Peter Villemoes points out that RARE was clearly established as a reaction to EARN: "RARE was to some extent set up to make sure that we got a non-provider-specific technology for European backbone networking – that is still the goal we have today. We set up RARE because we couldn't just rely on one provider to decide the future."

RARE has its roots in Germany, where computer scientists were trying to organize the development of networking protocols in the early 1980s. In May 1985, a workshop, hosted by the EC and attended by representatives from the European academic community, was called in Luxembourg to consider future collaboration.

In the Luxembourg meeting it was decided that a unified network infrastructure should be set up to support research and academic collaboration. It was also proposed that an association should be established to foster European research networking. The Dutch Ministry of Education and Science provided an interim secretariat for the association, and RARE was formally founded in June 1986 under Dutch law. The RARE secretariat was opened a year later in Amsterdam.

The NORDUnet Community was a main contributor in setting up RARE. However, towards the end of the 1980s the Nordic position in RARE was weakening because of the difference in views on protocol standards. In 1987 a number of European countries together with the EU established the COSINE initiative. As its name indicates, the purpose of COSINE was to build a pan-European network based on OSI protocols. RARE became the contractor for the work and promoted OSI in Europe.

In the meantime, Nordic networkers could not wait for OSI standardization. Instead, the Nordic research network, NORDUnet, would include several protocols – including the American TCP/IP which was not accepted by other Europeans.

Peter Villemoes says that Nordic collaboration in RARE progressed smoothly while the NORDUnet program was officially committed to the OSI model, but the situation changed when NORDUnet clearly moved to TCP/IP and "RARE maintained their purpose of setting up OSI networking in Europe. So, when we diverted from that path, we had some kind of opposition with the RARE Management."

The COSINE project eventually managed to build the IXI network which connected 18 countries together. Yet the need for IP services was already understood in most countries, and IXI was succeeded in 1992 by EuropaNET, which supported both X.25 and IP protocols.

EuropaNET was the real outcome of RARE and COSINE, but it was not the only one. Within RARE and COSINE collaboration it was realized that Europe needed an OU to provide a European backbone, and the national R&E networks established a new organization for that: DANTE, founded in 1993.

After setting up DANTE, the mission of RARE was fulfilled and it had to look for another role. In 1994, RARE and EARN were merged to form TERENA, which basically took over the tasks that previously belonged to RARE: it carries out technical activities and provides a platform for discussion to develop research networks. The Nordic countries continue to participate actively in the work of TERENA.

8.1.3
Ebone, the First Pan-European IP Backbone

At the beginning of the 1990s, the protocol war was still going on in Europe. The Nordic national R&E networks had chosen to include the TCP/IP protocol of the Internet in their Nordic backbone NORDUnet, but in many European countries belief in the OSI model was still strong.

NORDUnet was the most developed IP network in Europe in the early 1990s, connecting the five Nordic countries to the Internet in the United States and to the European networks. In other parts of the continent there were some isolated IP networks, but they were not interconnected and the traffic between them had to go via the United States.

To get the European IP networks connected, an idea for a pan-European IP backbone, Ebone, emerged. The reason for Ebone was simply the inability of the pan-European backbone services based on the X.25 protocol to cope with the volume of research traffic demands for IP. A native IP backbone was needed. The plan was initiated by SURFnet in the Netherlands, and by the members of the NORDUnet community, especially networking experts in Sweden.

The Ebone92 proposal was sent out in September 1991 and Ebone was set up during 1992. It connected Stockholm-Amsterdam-Geneva-Paris-London-Stockholm, Bonn-Stockholm, Bonn-Geneva and London-Montpellier, thus making IP connections between many European countries possible. Peter Villemoes, the General Manager of NORDUnet, says that Ebone "meant a lot to our ability to provide services to our users. To begin with, it solved our problem of getting good IP connectivity to other countries in Europe – also to some extent to the United States, but mainly to Europe. So we benefited a lot from Ebone."

According to Kees Neggers, the Managing Director of SURFnet, Ebone also served as an example for future European backbones: "Ebone really showed that native IP networking on a European scale was possible and needed. Within a year the CPG agreed to officially allow native IP next to OSI networking as part of the COSINE project. This finally released a lot of money for pan-European IP backbone networking and for the creation of EuropaNET."

The Ebone initiative also brought NORDUnet and SURFnet closer together and strengthened cooperative ties, a relationship that continues today. Both NORDUnet and SURFnet are driven to translate new technologies into better services for the research networks. In this approach most notable is the introduction of new and better transport backbone services, both intra-Europe and to the United States. But also on the middleware and application level there were and still are several good collaborations.

8.1.4
NSF, the American Connection

The NSF (National Science Foundation) is an independent agency of the United States government that has played a pivotal role in the history of the Internet. The agency was originally established in 1950 to promote the progress of science, health and welfare and to secure the defense of the country. In the 1980s, NSF took on the task of financing new computer networks to provide better networking services for computer scientists.

The ARPAnet network was financed by ARPA, later DARPA (Defense Advanced Research Projects Agency), but the universities that had no defense research were not included in ARPAnet. In the early 1980s, these universities without DARPA support turned to NSF to get funding for a new network. The plan was looked upon positively by NSF and it sponsored the building of the CSNET in 1981. In the mid-1980s, NSF decided to establish a new network to link the supercomputer centers in the United States. The NSFnet came online in 1986.

Towards the end of the 1980s, other institutions and networks, like the CSNET, began to connect to the NSFnet, turning it into the major networking player of the United States academic community. Eventually, the NSFnet became the main governmental network and the backbone of the Internet. The ARPAnet was dissolved in 1990 and the responsibility for the Internet passed on to NSF.

Nordic collaboration with NSF began at the end of the 1980s. As the first international R&E network outside the United States, NORDUnet was connected to the NSFnet at the end of 1988. Since then, NORDUnet has had a special relationship with NSF.

Steven Goldstein, formerly NSF Program Officer for international inter-research networking, was the primary NSF contact for NORDUnet for many years. In his view, in the early 1990s NORDUnet was clearly set apart from other European networks: "The rest of Europe at the time was mired in complex network protocol politics over the OSI suite, PTT monopolistic intransigence, and hierarchic government sponsor control. I can recall one NORDUnet meeting where one of the speakers kept referring to "NORDUnet and Europe" as if they were very separate and distinct entities."

NSF established an ICM (international connections management) program to take care of international Internet connections and NORDUnet also participated in the program from 1991 to 1997. NSF contributed funds for the NORDUnet connection, in the mid 1990s paying a bigger share of the interconnection cost than for any other international partner. According to Steven Goldstein, NSF was willing to co-fund the connection because NORDUnet was a real partner. NSF managed the Internet in the early 1990s during its phenomenal growth. However, by the mid-1990s the privatization of the Internet had become evident and the role of the NSF changed. NSF stopped funding the NSFnet and the backbone was decommissioned in 1995. Instead, NSF would fund the universities directly to enable them to buy services from commercial providers.

The ICM program also ended in 1997. At the time of its ending, Peter Villemoes and Steven Goldstein exchanged e-mails thanking each other for the long collaboration. In his message to Villemoes on September 30 1997, Goldstein wrote: "This is a "bittersweet" day for me. ICM, which has been so much a part of my life, sees its last light today. ICM provided us unprecedented leverage to build a global foundation for the Internet. I don't think that we shall ever have as much opportunity again. But the Internet world has matured around us, and it is indeed time for the ICM star to fade. I, too, look forward to continued collaboration with you, personally, and between NSF and NORDUnet in the NGI (next generation Internet) and Internet2 arenas. Long-time partnerships, proven through the years, are to be honored and preserved."

The collaboration did continue. When ICM ended, NSF was already preparing a follow-on program focused on advanced networking. The NSF program for high performance international Internet services (HPIIS) ran from 1999 to 2003 and NORDUnet was one of the few European research networks accepted as a participant.

The HPIIS program was created to provide a basis for the development of the next generation of networking applications. An integral part of the program involved organizing a connection to STARTAP in Chicago in order to exchange traffic with the American research networks, vBNS and Internet2.

Today, both NORDUnet and NSF participate in international GLIF collaboration, continuing the development of network technologies. The long history of collaboration with NSF and American networking organizations has made NORDUnet a wanted partner in international cooperations and NORDUnet is well recognized among the networkers in the United States.

8.1.5
DANTE, Coordinating European Networking

Today, DANTE (Delivery of Advanced Network Technology to Europe) is the major organization coordinating pan-European research networking. It was established as a non-profit limited company in 1993 in Cambridge (United Kingdom) and it is owned by the European research networks. DANTE works in collaboration with the EC which grants funding for DANTE projects. The mission of DANTE is to plan, build and operate pan-European research networks and to provide the infrastructure for networking research projects. DANTE and TERENA are the principal collaborating bodies in European research networking and they both have their origins in RARE.

The idea of DANTE emerged in the context of RARE's COSINE project. In the early 1990s, COSINE was building a pan-European research network based on OSI principles. This was the time the research networks in Europe began to realize the need for a new organization. The research networks proposed a European OU which would provide a European backbone; and the OU became DANTE. DANTE started taking over what COSINE had produced and slowly made that into an IP network in Europe.

The outcome of COSINE, the IXI network, was further developed in 1992 to include IP services and was renamed EMPB. When DANTE was established in 1993, it chose the name EuropaNET for its backbone services which were based upon EMPB.

At that time, NORDUnet had the Ebone service for IP connections to Europe, so there was no immediate need to migrate to EuropaNET which did not have enough capacity. However, by the autumn of 1993 it had become clear that EMPB's IP service was functioning and several countries decided to leave Ebone to move to EuropaNET. For example, JANET of Britain and SURFnet of the Netherlands decided to use DANTE network services and migrated from Ebone in 1994. NORDUnet also considered the move and connected to EuropaNET later in 1994.

The real turning point in European networking came when the EC began to support the creation of a 34 Mbps network in Europe. The planning of TEN-34 began in 1995 and the network became operational in 1997. In less than two years, it was replaced by a new network, TEN-155, which was launched at the end of 1998 followed by GÉANT, which began operations in 2001 with 10 Gbps links between the larger countries. Its successor was GÉANT2 in 2005.

Peter Villemoes admits that during the first years of DANTE there was a period of suspicion, but DANTE is nowadays the major cooperation platform that NORDUnet shares with other European research networks.

8.1.6
Internet2, towards New Applications

NORDUnet and Nordic networkers have had collaboration programs with American networking institutions for a long time, so it was natural that NORDUnet was also interested in establishing collaboration with Internet2, and its backbone network Abilene, when they were initiated in the late 1990s.

Internet2 is an American consortium set up in 1996 to develop advanced network applications and technologies. It is led by over 200 universities which work together with governmental and industrial partners to ensure the transfer of new applications to the global Internet. Internet2 is therefore not a replacement of the general Internet but provides testing facilities for new technologies. For this purpose, the Internet2 community has created Abilene, the high-performance backbone. The Abilene network began operating in February 1999, and its deployment was completed by the end of the same year. An upgrade to 10 Gbps was accomplished in 2003.

NORDUnet was the very first research network outside the United States to begin negotiations with Internet2 over a connection to Abilene, even before Abilene was put into operation. At the last minute, NORDUnet was "beaten" by the SURF Foundation of the Netherlands, which signed the contract first. Thus, when it signed the MoU with Internet2 in September 1998, NORDUnet was the second European research network to do so.

The Abilene connection was implemented in 1999 as a 155 Mbps ATM link between a NORDUnet router and an Abilene router in the Teleglobe building in New York. The link was dynamically shared with SURFnet.

According to Heather Boyles, the Director of International Relations for Internet2, the partnership has focused on working collaboratively in several areas: NORDUnet and Internet2 have first of all provided interconnection for advanced higher education and research networks, supported collaboration between faculty, researchers and students, and developed new technologies and services.

In the summer of 1999, the interconnectivity of NORDUnet and Abilene was tested with high-quality audio and video conferencing. New technology was employed to have Internet2's President and Chief Executive Officer, Douglas Van Houwelling, speak at the NORDUnet conference in Lund, Sweden, from his office in Michigan. Boyles points out that "the network engineering that it took at that time to make such a high-quality, high-bandwidth video-conference over our respective networks possible was significant, and the NORDUnet and Internet2 network engineers and applications developers learned quite a lot together."

NORDUnet's direct connection to research networks in the United States was terminated in 2003, after which NORDUnet began to use the European GÉANT for United States research traffic. But even though NORDUnet traffic now goes via GÉANT, the research collaboration with the Americans is still organized directly.

Inspired by Internet2, NORDUnet also proposed a Nordic NORDUnet2 program in 1998. The networking projects within the program ran until the end of 2002. NorduGrid was one of the most significant achievements of NORDUnet2 project. Peter Villemoes said that it was essentially the only functional grid in the world. Another program, NORDUnet3, was initiated in 2003. It was approved by research councils in all the Nordic countries in November 2004.

8.1.7
The 6NET Project, Testing IPv6

The largest European Internet research project of recent years has been 6NET (large-scale international IPv6 pilot network). The project was initiated in 2001 by networking company Cisco Systems, Inc., DANTE and a number of national R&E networks. The goal of the project was to operate an international IPv6 network to gain more knowledge of IPv6 by testing new applications and services.

IPv6 has been created to replace the current Internet protocol IPv4. The ever-growing popularity of the Internet has led to a shortage of IP addresses and the main purpose of IPv6 is to find a solution to this problem. The 6NET project was aimed at testing how IPv6 would work in realistic conditions when used in a large-scale international inter-research network.

The 6NET project started at the beginning of 2002 and continued until July 2005. During these years, the project built an IPv6-based network connecting 16 countries.

Over 30 partners, both institutions and organizations from the research sector and private companies have taken part in the project. The total investment in the project has been €18 M of which €11 M has been support allocated by the EC.

NORDUnet and the Nordic member networks have been active participants in IPv6-related development projects, including 6NET. NORDUnet has been one of the main contractors of the project and has provided the Nordic part of the 6NET network. During the project, NORDUnet has also organized workshops and conferences, thus disseminating the experiences gained from 6NET. The 6NET backbone network was set up in the central Nordic countries in 2002 with 155 Mbps links from Stockholm to Frankfurt and London, and links from Stockholm to Copenhagen, Helsinki and Oslo. In summer 2004, NORDUnet upgraded the Nordic 6NET links to 1 Gbps.

During its lifetime, the 6NET project provided a learning experience for European networkers. Jari Miettinen, the 6NET project coordinator for NORDUnet, believes that the 6NET project has hastened the deployment of IPv6 in the Nordic countries. "It offered a large-scale international test-bed which could be used to construct a realistic routed network and test the network's behavior in the field. In this way, the personnel of the Nordic network operations centers gained experience and the router hardware and software matured."

Although this European research project on IPv6 has ended and coexistence with IPv4 will continue for decades, the gradual deployment of the new protocol and the exhaustion of the IPv4 address space will extend the use of IPv6. The next step will be the conversion of network services to run over IPv6.

8.1.8
GLIF and Lambda Networking, the New Light

The most recent network development activity of NORDUnet is the test-bed for lambda networking, NorthernLight. The test-bed has a star topology from Stockholm to Copenhagen, Helsinki, and Oslo. A link to Amsterdam connects NothernLight to other lambda structures in Europe and in the United States.

NorthernLight is a part of the GLIF (global lambda integrated facility) collaboration, a worldwide virtual organization supporting R&D in the field of lambda grids. Lambdas are considered by many to be the next major phase in the Internet evolution, leading the way towards optical networking. The idea in lambda networking is to use different wavelengths of light, "lambdas", in optical fibers for separate connections. Each user community has its own individual set of lambdas, and because it is possible to send multiple wavelengths on one fiber, the potential capacity of the network is increased.

As in the early days of the Internet, experimental work and the development of new innovations is fostered by research networks. The history of global lambda collaboration began in 2001, when SURFnet, the network for higher education and research in the Netherlands, and TERENA organized the first LambdaGrid meeting in Amsterdam. The first research-only lambda was set up between the Dutch NetherLight and the American StarLight in Chicago.

SURFnet's Managing Director Kees Neggers has been the initiator both in Ebone and now in GLIF. The European IP backbone Ebone was established in the early 1990s because it was realized that OSI and X.25 would not be a solution – GLIF was established in the early 2000s because "routed IP was no longer enough to serve the needs of the R&E community. Direct lambda or light path connections may be a better way forward to serve the most demanding users."

NORDUnet is now an active participant in GLIF collaboration, but it took some time to join in. NORDUnet was at first skeptical about lambda development. In Europe, the first collaborations to work with SURFnet were CESNET (Czech educational and scientific network) of the Czech Republic and UKERNA of the United Kingdom. NORDUnet stepped in as the fourth European partner.

In 2002, Tom DeFanti of the University of Illinois at Chicago suggested that NORDUnet consider having a lambda connection to SURFnet's StarLight link and consider taking part in the collaboration. At this point NORDUnet was not yet ready to use lambda because of potential problems in scalability. When General Manager Peter Villemoes suggested in March 2003 that NORDUnet should join in the lambda experimentation and set up a link between Stockholm and Amsterdam, the proposal was accepted.

A 2.5 Gbps link between Amsterdam and KTH NOC in Stockholm became operational in August 2003, connecting NORDUnet to the Dutch NetherLight. Amsterdam in turn connected to CERN in Geneva, CzechLight in Prague, StarLight in Chicago (with 10 Gbps links), and later also to UKLight in London.

NORDUnet was ready to extend lambda connectivity to other Nordic countries and thus create the NorthernLight. The links for a 2.5 Gbps system from Stockholm to Copenhagen, Helsinki and Oslo were installed in December 2004, but because of the new technology involved, it took a few months to get the network up and running.

Nowadays NORDUnet is fully part of GLIF and one of the European driving forces. In fact, the GLIF organization was formally established in a meeting hosted by NORDUnet. In August 2003, the Global LambdaGrid Workshop was arranged as a part of the NORDUnet conference in Reykjavik, Iceland. In that conference, GLIF was formed.

The members of GLIF are national R&E networks, countries or institutions that have enough bandwidth for production traffic and have extra capacity for scientific testing purposes. Because bandwidth is not as expensive as it used to be, many R&E networks now have enough capacity and can make it available for computer scientists studying lambda networking.

GLIF collaboration seems to grow every year: in 2004 the GLIF meeting in Nottingham, England, was arranged by invitation only. Sixty people were invited, networking managers from major research networks from all over the world. From Europe, the participation was restricted to SURFnet, UKERNA, CESNET and NORDUnet. The interest in future collaboration was great, and TERENA began to prepare secretariat support for GLIF.

As a consequence of the lambda collaboration, the GÉANT2 network in Europe is, for instance, now implementing lambdas in its design – and Abilene is working hard on that too.

8.2
CEEC

Although the first network activity in the CEEC (Central and Eastern European countries) started during the Soviet period, the environment at the time was rather complex. According to the economic strategy of the former Eastern bloc, each country was responsible for different ICT tasks. Mainframes, minicomputers, microcomputers, controllers, operating systems – development and production of each of them were associated with a specific COMECON (council for mutual economic assistance) country.

Universities and research institutes belonging to the national academies of sciences were the first users of new equipment and software, and it was their role to make it work. It took considerable effort and time to integrate the computers with communication systems and the communications possibilities were very limited, even nationally. Even in the more developed COMECON countries there were just a few links between universities and research institutes in the largest cities. In the late 1980s there were experiments with networking on a national scale but, because hardware and software quality was poor, to make things work engineers had to dig deeply into technical details, so people working in the field became highly skilled.

There was very little international computer networking cooperation in the former CEEC because the technology was not ready, and of course communication with Western countries and organizations was not encouraged. However, it was possible for individual researchers to visit other countries. Thanks to the personal contacts of the related researchers, in the late 1980s some CEEC got themselves connected to EARN/BITNET by 9.6 kbps lines. On the other hand, Internet connectivity was not possible because of the COCOM regulations which prohibited the export of the necessary equipment to the COMECON countries. So cooperation with Western countries was very limited, and joining international groups was very difficult. But everything changed after the political upheavals of 1989.

8.2.1
External Support

After 1989, rapid evolution of research networks, the acquisition of international connectivity and services, as well as international cooperation all became possible throughout the region, the Czech Republic, Hungary, and Poland, in particular, taking advantage of the new openings. Progress nationally was closely related to the joining of the European research networking associations (EARN and RARE) as well as to direct external support by some devoted research networks (especially ACOnet which had the Austrian government and the University of Vienna behind it, and also GARR, with the Italian INFN in the background). The Austrian government initiated a program of paying half of the costs of international links to the CEEC. That was very important because although the links were very slow they were expensive at the time and it would have been very difficult for the CEEC to pay the full line cost. Austrian initiatives contributed significantly to the creation of CEENet, the Central and Eastern European network. Austria was one of the founding members even though the association was meant to benefit Eastern European countries; "Eastern" was given a flexible interpretation. The main activity of the organization was to exchange information and know-how.

A very welcome move by NATO (North Atlantic Treaty Organization) was to support a series of training workshops organized by TERENA and CEENet (Central and Eastern European network association). Copies of the proceedings were sent to each country so that the information they contained could be disseminated widely. The workshops that took place in different locations were very important for engineers. Because of COCOM, the Eastern countries had not had access to the latest technologies. The workshops provided unique opportunities for engineers to learn about advanced equipment and to get hands-on experience of configuring it. This was crucial for know-how transfer and for increasing people's skills in the CEENet region.

8.2.2
The EC's PHARE Program

The EC's PHARE (Poland and Hungary: assistance for restructuring their economies) program, which in 1994 covered Albania, Bulgaria, the Czech Republic, Estonia, Hungary, Latvia, Lithuania, Poland, Romania, Slovakia and Slovenia, was very important in helping to provide international links to the Eastern region. Within the EC, DG I was responsible for relations with states outside the EU and set up the PHARE program with the general objective of helping the beneficiary countries of Central Europe to advance their economies to the level of those in Western Europe.

Having solicited proposals from other Directorates within the EC for activities that would contribute to achieving this objective, DG I established a project to connect the research networks of the CEEC to the European backbone that was already being supported in the West by DG XIII. In countries which had no research network, the benefits of creating such an entity were promoted (but each country was left to decide for itself how such an organization should be structured; the only external condition that was applied in each country was that there should be a single access to the pan-European network. Two or more national organizations sharing a common access was not recommended but was accepted; two national organizations which could only intercommunicate by sending traffic into the international network was not.)

At first, DG I officials tried to manage this activity themselves but they were not successful; they had little or no appropriate technical knowledge and no appreciation of the speed with which technology was changing. As a result, their well-meaning actions did little to satisfy the intended beneficiaries who were interested in using only the most up-to-date equipment and techniques. To correct this problem, the EC issued a Call for Tender for the management of the activity; the result was the award of a management contract to DANTE.

DANTE staff, supplemented by other specialists who DANTE engaged for the purpose, had experience of procurement and other EC procedures which was lacking in the CEEC. They visited nearly all of the PHARE countries and talked, not only to the engineers, but also to university managers and government officials, explaining why computer networking was important for research communities. The PHARE project played a major role, especially as PHARE contributions came early and were well-timed. The coordination from DANTE was very significant. The topology of the network had structure and was designed to optimize the flow of traffic.

CEENet, having operated as a complementary organization to TERENA, also played an important role in activity coordination because its members talked both to PHARE people and to NATO, and tried to use available resources more effectively. Each of these organizations was very experienced and contributed greatly to the development of the region. Support was provided at a time when help was really necessary, very soon after the political changes. It helped the evolution of university networking in the region, which developed very quickly, and showed how experience and expertise could be shared between countries.

8.2.3
National Infrastructures

From the very early years, there were differences in telecommunications infrastructures from country to country. Some countries were better developed than others. For example, in Czechoslovakia, Hungary, or Poland, telecommunications systems for implementing networking services were better than in, for example, Ukraine, Bulgaria, or Romania. Until about the mid-1980s, all telecommunications infrastructures were for phone services only. Data services were just being introduced and used infrastructure originally designed to support phone services. The luckier, more highly developed countries had better infrastructure for implementing the new services. There were cables everywhere; nearly every village had telephones and major cities had good cable connections. It was easy to build computer networks where there was good telephone infrastructure. In other, less developed, CEEC, there was practically no infrastructure at all, although in some cases the picture was already changing. For example in Romania, a comprehensive set of fiber-optical cables was laid between the major cities and was being brought into service during the period of the PHARE networking activity. However, there was no equipment to support data services, no immediate plans to purchase any, and the local copper-based infrastructure was in a very poor state. In Albania, fiber had been installed in parts of Tirana, the capital city, but nowhere else and it was not yet in use. The net effect was the same in both cases: there was no usable infrastructure. These are just typical examples of how difficult it was at that time to make significant progress in research networking. Economic conditions were different in each country and, obviously, networking possibilities were related to economic and communication developments.

Another very important element was how successful the researchers were in convincing their governments to fund the evolution of networking. In all these countries, the economy was in a relatively poor shape and there was strong competition for resources for research and education. To convince governments that building a research network was a priority and that they should provide significant funding was not easy. The network was something that did not already exist and bureaucracies were not good at striking out in new directions, however compelling a case might be from the point of view of its proposers. In the Czech Republic, CESNET managed to persuade the Minister of Education to provide significant funding for research networking infrastructure as early as 1992. The ministry provided 20M Crowns, which was a very large sum, to build a national infrastructure. It continued this funding for several years. Hungary also had a group of senior officials who took the trouble to understand how EC programs might be exploited most effectively and arranged for the complementary national funding to be included in the government's budget.

Research and education communities in other countries were not as successful, at least not immediately. Success was often related to the position of education, especially at university level, in the government's scale of priorities and to the status of the Academy of Sciences. (Note that, according to the conventions in place at the time, universities' activities were devoted largely to teaching; research was carried out under the umbrella of the Academies of Sciences.)

In some countries, there was strong competition and no cooperation between universities and the Academy of Sciences. In Romania, for example, the two groups could not agree on a common infrastructure, and today there are still two academic networks, one for universities and one for the Academy of Sciences. The Czechs were luckier there too: in 1992, the original project to establish the Internet was for universities only, but the following year, the Czech Academy of Sciences joined the project and decided to have one infrastructure, one funding, and so on. The Hungarian case was really advantageous: joint networking activities of the research and higher education communities started in the late 1980s. The other extreme is characterized for example by Russia and the Ukraine: more than two organizations in a single country have claimed to act as the research network. Azerbaijan is another country where two organizations responsible for networking have been set up, one for higher education, and another for the Academy of Sciences, so that two organizations have been competing for resources for many years. Obviously, convincing governments to fund two organizations is much more difficult and is not generally successful. Moreover, in accordance with their membership policy, international (European) organizations accept just one representative national organization per country. As a result of all these factors, separate research networking organizations in most countries have either joined or at least started to cooperate closely in order to fight together for optimum local and international conditions for their operation.

8.2.4
Pan-European Connectivity of the CEEC

By the mid-1990s, some of the more developed CEEC (Central and Eastern Europe Countries) had improved their internal research networks and their international connectivity so that the state of their research networking started to be commensurate with that of their Western counterparts. The first step was their taking part in the EuropaNET activities which were devoted to building a European network operating at Mbps speeds. Connecting to EuropaNET was an important milestone for the CEEC and, with a low speed connection in place CESNET was able to exploit the opportunity provided by the 1994 joint INET'94/JENC (Joint European Networking Conference) event of the Internet Society and RARE, a big conference which, in 1994, was held in Prague. A temporary high speed (512 kbps) EuropaNET access had been established by CESNET and DANTE, funded by a supplementary grant from the EC/PHARE together with very positive cooperation of PTT Telecom and Czech Telekom. The EC grant was sufficient to cover only the period of the conference and its associated workshop but the Czech Ministry of Education agreed to provide continued funding to keep the upgrade in place after the conference for the benefit of the research and education community.

Another milestone was the start of the TEN-34 project when, for example, HUNGARNET (Hungarian academic and research networking association) was in a difficult situation until the Ministry for Education approved finance for the Hungarian TEN-34 connectivity and the Hungarian telecommunications company agreed to cooperate in the TEN-34 activities.

These were major advances which set examples for other countries in the region. They showed how important it was to work within an international framework and helped to explain with concrete examples that countries of similar size in Western Europe had this kind of bandwidth.

8.2.5
European Projects

After the closing down of the EuropaNET service in 1996, there was a series of pan-European network generations, each generation providing increased capacity and more extensive geographical coverage than its predecessor. Each network generation has received funding support from the EC. DANTE, the "operational unit" of the European research networks, has been the coordinating partner in a consortium of the participating research networks and has had responsibility for implementation and operation of the network services; and a committee consisting of one representative per participating research network has had overall control of policy.

Of the research networks in the PHARE countries, ARNES (academic research network of Slovenia), which had taken over the Yugoslavian position in COSINE when the Federation broke up, and HUNGARNET were shareholders in DANTE from its beginning. They have also been partners in each of the consortia established for the successive projects TEN-34, TEN-155 (QUANTUM) and GÉANT.

This was an important achievement since the membership of ARNES and HUNGARNET in DANTE and in the TEN-34 consortium served as an example to be followed by the other CEE (Central and Eastern Europe) research networks. It also played the role of demonstrating acceptance by Western (mostly EU member) countries and of the EU as full and equal partners in European research networking activities.

Although in the case of TEN-34, it was not possible to provide a connection for all the interested CEE research networks from the same start-of-service date as the West Europe research networks because of the difficulty in acquiring the necessary circuits, practically all interested TEN-34 partners were connected to the TEN-34 network shortly afterwards. Later, all interested research networks were also able to join DANTE.

The situation with TEN-155 (within the QUANTUM project) was much easier and smoother for most of the CEE research networks which were interested in joining. However, until 2001 (the start of GÉANT) SANET, the Slovak academic network association, accessed the European backbone (TEN-155) only via Prague. In addition, Poland was not directly connected at that time to the European backbone but instead, together with the Baltic States, accessed both TEN-34 and TEN-155 indirectly via NORDUnet. In the case of Poland, a satellite link between Stockholm and Warsaw was used.

Some other research networks, like those in Romania and Bulgaria, were connected somewhat later. Two of the PHARE countries had serious difficulties. Bulgaria lost connectivity for several years when the national network organization was closed down, and in Albania, domestic unrest in Spring 1997 caused a planned connection to be abandoned because it was too dangerous for Western engineers to travel to Tirana to install the necessary equipment.

8.2.6
The Significance of GÉANT

The entry into service of the GÉANT network in December 2001 marked a major milestone for the research networks of the CEEC. Although some countries in the region were still struggling with organizational and technical difficulties, most of the research networks were now operating at the same level as those in Western European countries of a similar size. In particular, the Czech Republic, Hungary, Poland and Slovakia were all nodes in the core configuration of 10 Gbps circuits and their engineers were playing a full part in the development activities associated with the network. The research networks in these countries had now succeeded in catching up with their Western counterparts and were now full and equal partners in the continuing development of research networking for the benefit of Europe as a whole – a remarkable achievement in a little over 15 years after the first moves towards integration with the West.

8.3
Asia and Pacific

In the early 1980s, the first R&E networking between Europe and the Asia-Pacific region used UUCP over a dial-up connection between EUnet at CWI in Amsterdam and AsiaNet which connected Australia (ACSNET, academic computing services network), Japan (JUNET, Japan UNIX network) and Korea (SDN, system development network) among others. The initial connection was used mainly for e-mail and news. There were also dial-up connections to both the East and West Coasts of North America. The dial-up connections were typically made between once per day and once per hour. Typical bandwidth was either 1200 bps or 2400 bps in the early 1980s, increasing later to 19.2 kbps and then to 64 kbps. Large files such as news archives were shipped by air mail in order to save international telephone charges. In some cases, an X.25 connection was used instead of dial-up, giving greater reliability and 64 kbps bandwidth. CSNET with dial-up or X.25 was added in the mid-1980s, offering more Internet-compatible (then ARPAnet) services such as the PMDF (PASCAL-based memo distribution facility) e-mail package. An International Academic Net-Workshop (IANW) was held every summer (mostly in Europe after 1980). This series of workshops helped to develop the global research network community and is the place where the European research and education community met its counterpart in the Asia-Pacific region.

By the time that IP connections to NSFnet in the United States were opened in 1986, traffic had built up so much that dial-up connections were no longer viable and many European and Asia-Pacific research networks installed leased-line connections to the United States. Leased-line connections between Europe and Asia-Pacific followed naturally but for several years these leased lines were set up as a result of bilateral agreements between organizations at each end.

8.3.1
Leased Line Connections

The bandwidths of the initial leased line connections were typically in the range from 19.2 to 64 kbps. In the Asia-Pacific region, many people considered that their primary intercontinental link was to North America; their link to Europe was secondary. With some minor exceptions, Asia-Pacific research networks paid for the full-circuit cost to Europe as they did to North America.

SINET (science information network) in Japan led the European connection effort by having a 19.2 kbps link to JANET in the United Kingdom in 1989. The bandwidth was increased to 2 Mbps in 1996, 15 Mbps in 1999, and 150 Mbps in 2002. The connection was moved to GÉANT in 2003 with 2.5 Gbps, and was expected to be upgraded to 10 Gbps in 2008. Thus, there was a half-million-fold increase in capacity in less than 20 years.

The JANET-SINET link was changed from a direct connection between Japan and United Kingdom to a Japan-Europe circuit via the United States in order to take advantage of lower costs through North America. Taiwan took a similar approach by adding a US-UK extension – with smaller bandwidth – to the Taiwan-United States link.

Korea and China followed a pattern similar to SINET's. Korea had an initial link of 64 kbps to the United Kingdom in the 1990s. China established the China

(CERNET)-United Kingdom (JANET) link in the early 2000s. This became part of phase 2 of TEIN (trans-Eurasia information network) in 2005.

India offers another unique example. The Tata Institute of Fundamental Research (TIFR) established the first international research and education connection in India – to CERN in Geneva. It ran the DECnet protocol and was used to support HEP experiments in the 1980s. The TIFR link was eventually converted to the Internet protocol and became part of ERNET, the education and research network in India. Singapore set up its European link in the early 2000s, in addition to its North American link in the1990s. The European link eventually became part of TEIN.

TEIN was formed by combining it with the link between Korea and France and for the first time the communication link charge was shared by Europe; more details are given in the next section.

8.3.2
Trans-Eurasia Information Network

From one point of view, any bilateral agreement which increases the capacity of the connection between two world regions is to be welcomed but, in the history of connections between Europe and the Asia-Pacific region, a few of the bilateral initiatives that were proposed or implemented were ineffective because they were not compatible with other developments that were being planned. This was particularly the case when a government minister provided funds for a new connection which, naturally, had to terminate in his country and for which promotion of his own political reputation counted at least as much as prospective benefits to the research community. With time, mechanisms for coordination between the two regions have improved and the importance of bilateral arrangements has diminished.

A major step forward was approval of TEIN by the Asia-Europe meeting III (ASEM III, October 2000, Seoul, Korea). At ASEM III, the Republic of Korea, the EU and Singapore jointly proposed the TEIN project to interconnect research and education networks in Asia and Europe, in order to promote better information exchanges and research collaborations by providing faster and more powerful connections between Asia and Europe.

To materialize the initiative, the first phase of TEIN (TEIN1) was launched between Europe (RENATER) and Asia (KOREN: Korea advanced research network) in December 2001. The TEIN1 (Korea-France) was jointly managed by KISDI (Korea Information Society Development Institute), Korea and RENATER, France under the sponsorship of the Ministry of Information and Communication (MIC), Korea the Ministry of Research, France and the EU.

France (RENATER) and Korea (KISDI) established a Korea-France link of TEIN by directly connecting the KOREN in Korea and RENATER in France on December 5 2001. TEIN1 was first implemented using ATM technology with a bandwidth capacity of 2 Mbps SCR (sustained cell rate) and 4 Mbps PCR (peak cell rate). Network demand was high from the beginning. In response to the increasing demand from both Europe and Asia, the Korea-France link underwent three upgrades, to 10 Mbps, 34 Mbps and then to 155 Mbps between March 2002 and December 2004.

8.3.3
Trans-Siberia Link in the 2000s

Many telecommunications links between Europe and the Asia-Pacific region pass through southern Eurasia or through North America; in either case, they have a length of 20 000 km or more.

A direct link between Europe and the Asia-Pacific region through Siberia which, with a length of 10 000 km is the shortest route, was not put in place until the early 2000s when the GLORIAD (global ring network for advanced applications development) project was initiated. GLORIAD connects Europe to Asia through Russia and also provides routes between Asia and North America and between North America and Europe. The trans-Siberia route has the advantage for real-time traffic of cutting the round-trip time by half.

The GLORIAD project also created new network and science communities of Eurasia-Asia, Russia, and Europe – and opened up opportunities for collaboration among Northern Eurasia countries. GLORIAD links Europe with several cities in Russia (St Petersburg, Moscow, Novosibirsk, and Khabarovsk) as well as Asia (China, Korea) and North America (Canada, United States).

8.3.4
Network Development

TEIN has contributed to work on diverse applications between Europe and Asia, including Traffic Measurement, Physical Science, mobile IPv6 network, HD (High Definition) distribution and collaboration, e-learning and telemedicine.

The TEIN project also added the trans-Siberia link from Beijing in China to Europe to the network, operating at 2.5 Gbps. Figure 8.1 shows the TEIN network configuration.

There have been many collaborative IPv6 experiments in Europe and the Asia-Pacific region, involving, in particular, three leading Asian countries on IPv6; China, Japan, and Korea. Korea was the member of the 6NET Consortium in 2002–2005 which managed a large-scale international IPv6 project funded by the EU's Fifth Framework Program. The project built a native IPv6 network connecting 16 countries in order to gain experience of IPv6 deployment and the transition from IPv4 networks. TEIN was used extensively to support experiments through the use of a dual-stack (IPv4 and IPv6). Noteworthy applications included high-definition video streaming of cultural events.

Japan and China also carried out collaborative projects on IPv6 with Europe, for example the WIDE (widely integrated distributed environment) project. NTT (Nippon Telegraph and Telephone) participated in the 6NET project through its European office.

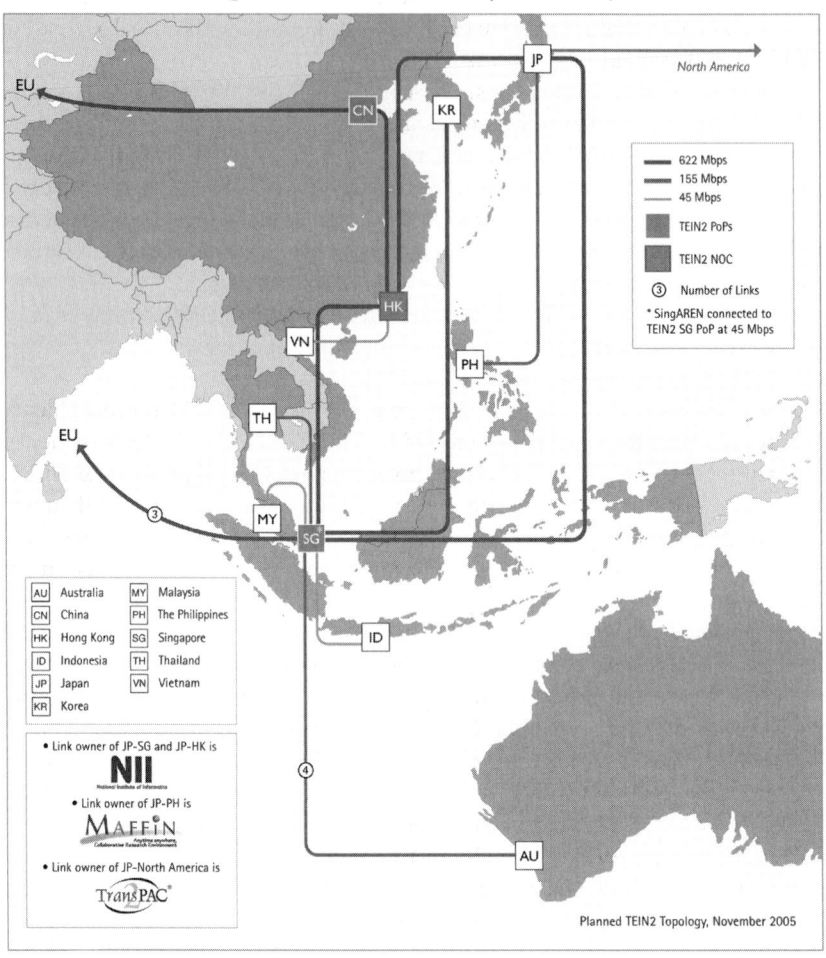

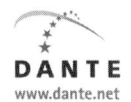

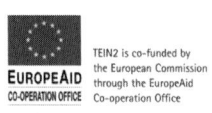

Figure 8.1 TEIN2 configuration. There is a color version of this figure in the set at the front of the book.

8.4
South East Europe and the Mediterranean

Connecting the countries of South East Europe to a pan-European network presents a number of special difficulties. These countries are a long way from the economic centre of gravity of Europe; this makes their links more expensive than the European average, even if the telecoms operators apply circuit charges which are related to cost (and not inflated by exploitation of a monopoly). In general, their economies are less developed than those in Western Europe which makes funding more difficult. And the political tensions in the region impede the establishment of cooperative projects. Despite these difficulties, the number of countries with a research network connected directly or indirectly to the pan-European backbone has steadily increased thanks to funding contributions from several different EU programs as well as patient, but persistent, diplomatic negotiation by many people. The same factors apply to the countries on the south and east coasts of the Mediterranean.

8.4.1
GRNET/Greece and SEEREN

Through its membership of the European Union, Greece has been able to take advantage of the possibilities offered by EUREKA and by the EU's sequence of Framework Programs. It was a participant in the COSINE project and an IXI connection to Athens was planned but not implemented because of difficulties in acquiring a 64 kbps circuit between Athens and Northern Europe, IXI had been transformed into EMPB by the time that the connection was put in place.

In 1998, staff of GRNET (Greek research and technology network) took the initiative, with the support of the Greek government, of trying to set up links with the research and education communities in neighboring countries and improving their access to the Internet. The first positive result was the connection of UNICOM-B (universal integrated communication-Bulgaria) to GRNET by means of a 128 kbps circuit provided by OTE at its normal price. At the same time, CyNet, the Cyprus national research and education network, was connected to GRNET at 2 Mbps. In February 2001, Yugoslavia was connected to GRNET at 2 Mbps with OTE again applying its normal charge. In July 2001, the link to UNICOM-B was upgraded to 6 Mbps. This time, OTE provided the connection in the form of a tunnel service through a 34 Mbps circuit which led to a large reduction in cost.

By 2003, more countries were ready to join in and SEEREN (South-East European research and education networking) was set up with funding support from the EU to interconnect the national research networks of the region, to provide them with access to the GÉANT network and its interconnections with other world regions, and thus to work towards a reduction in the "digital divide" between South East and Western European countries.

With GRNET taking responsibility for project management and with technical support from HUNGARNET and RoEduNet as well as DANTE and TERENA, the research networks to be connected were those of Albania, Bosnia Herzegovina, Bulgaria, the Former Yugoslav Republic of Macedonia, the Former Republic of Yugoslavia-Serbia and Montenegro. The budget was set at €1 M for a service duration of one year. As a result of a formal procurement, in August 2003 a contract for SEEREN was signed between GRNET and OTEGlobe. The connections to Athens were:

- Tirana 2 Mbps
- Sarajevo 2 Mbps
- Sofia 24 Mbps
- Skopje 4 Mbps
- Belgrade 34 Mbps

SEEREN became operational in January 2004. A poster showing the SEEREN configuration is shown in Figure 8.2.

A successor project, SEEREN2, with the same objectives as before but with more ambitious targets for capacity was prepared but could not start until October 1 2005 with a planned duration of 30 months. Since the SEEREN project officially ended on December 1 2004 and contracts with the telecoms suppliers were only funded until this date, a loss of connectivity for South Eastern Europe was threatened but was prevented when GÉANT agreed to take over the supplier contracts, subject to matching funds being made available from the SEEREN partners. The GÉANT move highlighted the cooperative approach to research networking in Europe and allowed regional research collaboration to continue.

An international tender calling for connectivity elements for the beneficiary countries was launched in November 2005 and the first SEEREN2 connections were established in January 2006, connecting the research networks of Serbia, Montenegro, Bulgaria and Former Yugoslav Republic of Macedonia, using circuits acquired as a result of the November 2005 procurement as follows: Athens-Belgrade: STM-1 (155 Mbps) with an add-drop multiplexor (a device which allows low bandwidth traffic to be added to or extracted from a high bandwidth traffic stream) in Sofia to serve the Serbian research network.

Athens-Skopje: $1 \times E1$ for the first year of operation, later upgraded to $2 \times E3$ (68 Mbps) to the Former Yugoslav Republic of Macedonia server.

Belgrade-Podgorica: $2 \times E1$ (4 Mbps) to serve the Montenegro research network.

Belgrade-Doboj: Gigabit Ethernet over a CWDM (coarse wavelength division multiplexing) link to serve the Bosnian research network.

Although a circuit supplier was selected, it was not possible to connect the Albanian community due to the lack of any contribution from the Albanian government towards the cost of international links, which is a contractual obligation for the beneficiary partners.

The network configuration allowed the four participating research networks which were already connected to GÉANT2 (Greece, Hungary, Romania and Bulgaria) to provide transit services to the others which, together with their user communities were consequently the main beneficiaries of SEEREN2.

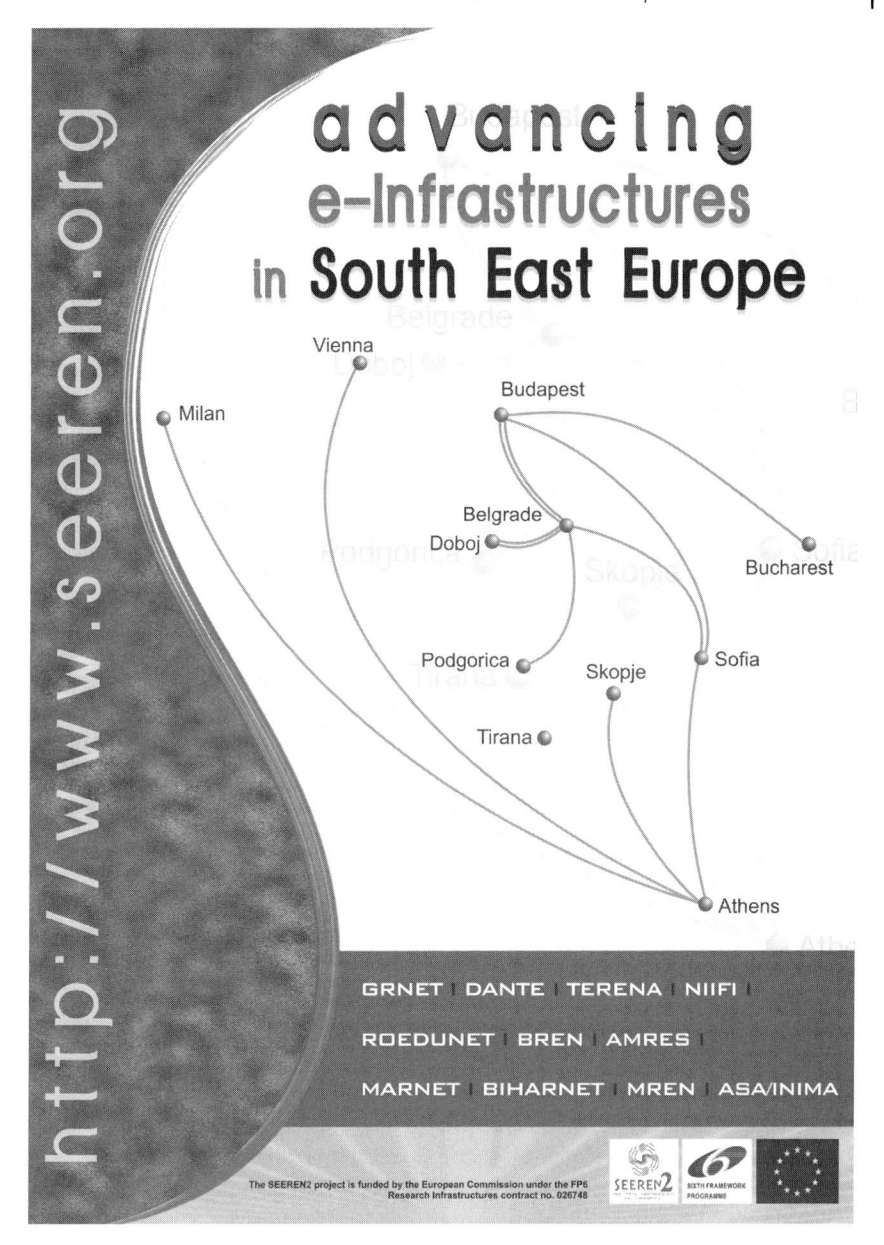

Figure 8.2 SEEREN configuration. There is a color version of this figure in the set at the front of the book.

8.4.2
ILAN/Israel

Israel has been an active participant in European research networking since 1988 when it set up a connection to EARN. When the EARN service closed down, ILAN (the Israeli research network) had to devise its own way of connecting to the emerging Internet and it developed a series of satellite-based links to Internet access points in the United States.

Towards the end of 1997, the Israeli government signed a scientific cooperation agreement with the EU. One of the consequences was that Israeli organizations now qualified to participate in Fourth Framework projects and could receive funding support in the same way as EU organizations.

The terms of the cooperation agreement required the Israeli government to make a financial contribution to the Fourth Framework Programme and Israeli officials started to look for ways of getting a return on the investment. Fourth Framework was well under way by this time and the scope for proposing new projects and finding suitable collaborators was limited. Joining an existing project appeared to offer better returns; TEN-34 and QUANTUM seemed to be ideal candidates. Israeli researchers would get better connectivity to Europe and the EU would pay nearly 50% of the cost.

EC officials welcomed the Israeli initiative and summoned DANTE, as the coordinating partner in QUANTUM, to a meeting with the Israeli Chargé d'Affaires (at the time the most senior representative of Israel in Brussels) to discuss how this might be arranged. The Chargé d'Affaires explained that Israel wished to exercise its right to join the QUANTUM consortium and wanted to know what would be involved in so doing. The DANTE representatives pointed out that neither Israel nor any other non-member had the "right" to join the consortium, that Fourth Framework consortia were made up of groups of organizations which had got together to make research proposals, and that while a request from Israel to join the QUANTUM consortium might well be welcomed, it would be up to the existing consortium members to decide whether or not to accept it. There followed a "dialogue of the deaf" in which each side restated its position over and over again with no movement towards any form of agreement. One EC official left the meeting, dismayed by the impertinence of the DANTE representatives in refusing to accede to the Israeli demands; such an important collaborator should at least be offered special treatment which would make the integration of Israel into the consortium a formality.

With some behind-the-scenes advice at the working level, ILAN submitted a formal request to join the QUANTUM project in February 1998.

The QUANTUM Policy Committee had already made clear that, in principle, it would welcome an interconnection with Israel but some members had reservations about increasing the size of the consortium – other countries were also asking to join – on the grounds of weakened manageability and stability. Earlier discussions on pricing had shown how difficult it was already to devise a charging algorithm which was acceptable to all members of the consortium. Adding further countries from outside the EU, which would inevitably involve expensive new links, would increase these difficulties. Although Israel continued to exert strong pressure via the EC to join the QUANTUM consortium, inconclusive discussions continued for several months.

The solution that was eventually adopted was first suggested by the Chairman of the Policy Committee, Fernando Liello. A proposal for a separate project named Q-MED, complementary to QUANTUM and with the objective of connecting ILAN and CyNet to TEN-34/155, was submitted to and accepted by the EC. GARR and

GRNET were partners providing support and expertise and DANTE was the coordinating partner. The administration of the two projects had to be kept separate; procurement; implementation and eventual operation of the additional links were managed as part of TEN-155.

8.4.3
EUMEDCONNECT

The EU's MEDA (Mediterranean economic development area) program which started in 1996 had the general objective of promoting economic development in those countries which border the Mediterranean but which are not members of the EU. As part of the MEDA program, the EC in 1998 launched the Euro-Mediterranean Initiative for the Information Society (EUMEDIS) to extend the development of the information society in the Mediterranean region by supporting a range of infrastructure, applications and technical support programs.

The principal infrastructure project funded by EUMEDIS was EUMEDCONNECT[1], coordinated by DANTE, which had the ultimate objective of giving researchers in the MEDA countries access to other research networks via GÉANT.

Preparing the ground for EUMEDCONNECT was, however, not straightforward and progress was initially slow; several obstacles had to be overcome and patient discussion and diplomacy was needed to do this. For example, one of the first difficulties was that MEDA governments would not pay for their staff to travel abroad until they were convinced that the journey was certain to bring compensating benefits. More seriously, MEDA sought to promote use of the Internet generally, including its use for commercial purposes, while the research networks and GÉANT were forbidden from carrying traffic between commercial organizations. Diplomatic restrictions on cooperation between certain pairs of countries did not help. These and other issues were resolved by a bootstrapping-style process, that is, taking a small step that was feasible and that would establish the conditions in which the next bigger step became possible. It was only in December 2001 that the EUMEDCONNECT project began, and even then it proceeded in two phases. In the first phase, feasibility and planning studies were conducted. They highlighted the "digital divide" between the Mediterranean region and more advanced regions such as Northern Europe. Before EUMEDCONNECT, there was almost no direct Internet connectivity between Mediterranean countries, and little research and education linkage between the Mediterranean area and Europe. The weakness of the Internet infrastructure discouraged market use of network services and concealed the potential for growth.

---

1) EUMEDCONNECT is the first research and education network for the Mediterranean region. Starting in 2004, 11 project partners are now connected and benefiting from a high capacity network dedicated to users of the research and academic community. This infrastructure is helping to bridge the digital divide between the Mediterranean and European regions, and increase academic collaborations between the regions. It was co-funded by the European Commission's EUMEDIS Program up to 2007; partners are continuing the network while options for a replacement program are being discussed. For more information: www.eumedconnect.net.

This, in turn, hindered the growth and development of research networking. The need for the EUMEDCONNECT network was clear. Phase 1 also established that the EUMEDCONNECT network was technically feasible.

Phase 2 involved the actual development and operation of the EUMEDCONNECT network infrastructure. After completion of a specification and tender process, contracts were awarded and installation work carried out for the first connections which came into service on April 11 2004. 11 of the 12 EUMEDCONNECT Mediterranean partners were now connected to the EUMEDCONNECT network. See Figure 8.3 for the network configuration in May 2005.

The EUMEDCONNECT network was originally contracted to operate until June 2006, but in January 2006 its funding was extended to July 2007. After an interim period when network development and related activities were constrained by the need for them to be fully funded from national sources, a follow-on project, EUMEDCONNECT2, was launched in November 2008. Like its predecessor, EUMEDCONNECT2 benefits from a financial contribution from the EU with further EU support and is committed to improving Internet services for the research and education community in the Mediterranean region.

8.5
Latin America

The deployment of RedCLARA, the Latin American regional research and education network operated by CLARA (Cooperación Latino Americana de Redes Avanzadas), the Latin American research networking association, began in 2004, and by July 2007 had interconnected research networks in 13 of the 18 countries in Latin America (Argentina, Bolivia, Brazil, Chile, Colombia, Costa Rica, Cuba, Ecuador, El Salvador, Guatemala, Honduras, Mexico, Nicaragua, Panama, Paraguay, Peru, Uruguay, and Venezuela), meeting a target originally set by the @LIS (ALliance for the Information Society), one of the EuropeAid programs which implement the EU's external aid policies.

RedCLARA is directly connected to the European GÉANT research GÉANT2 R&E network and interconnects more than 750 universities throughout Latin America with more than 3500 universities across Europe.

RedCLARA is the direct outcome of the ALICE (América Latina Interconectada Con Europa) project (2003–2008). ALICE received generous financial support from the @LIS program of the EU, and was coordinated by DANTE with the participation of research networks from France, Italy, Portugal and Spain, and of national research networking initiatives from the 18 countries listed above. The aim of ALICE was to provide connectivity between GÉANT and these national initiatives in Latin America, in order to enable closer collaboration in research and education between Europe and Latin America.

This is based on the creation of a regional backbone network within Latin America, RedCLARA, to which research networks can connect via a backbone PoP using a relatively short spur link. The aggregated traffic to Europe then uses a single

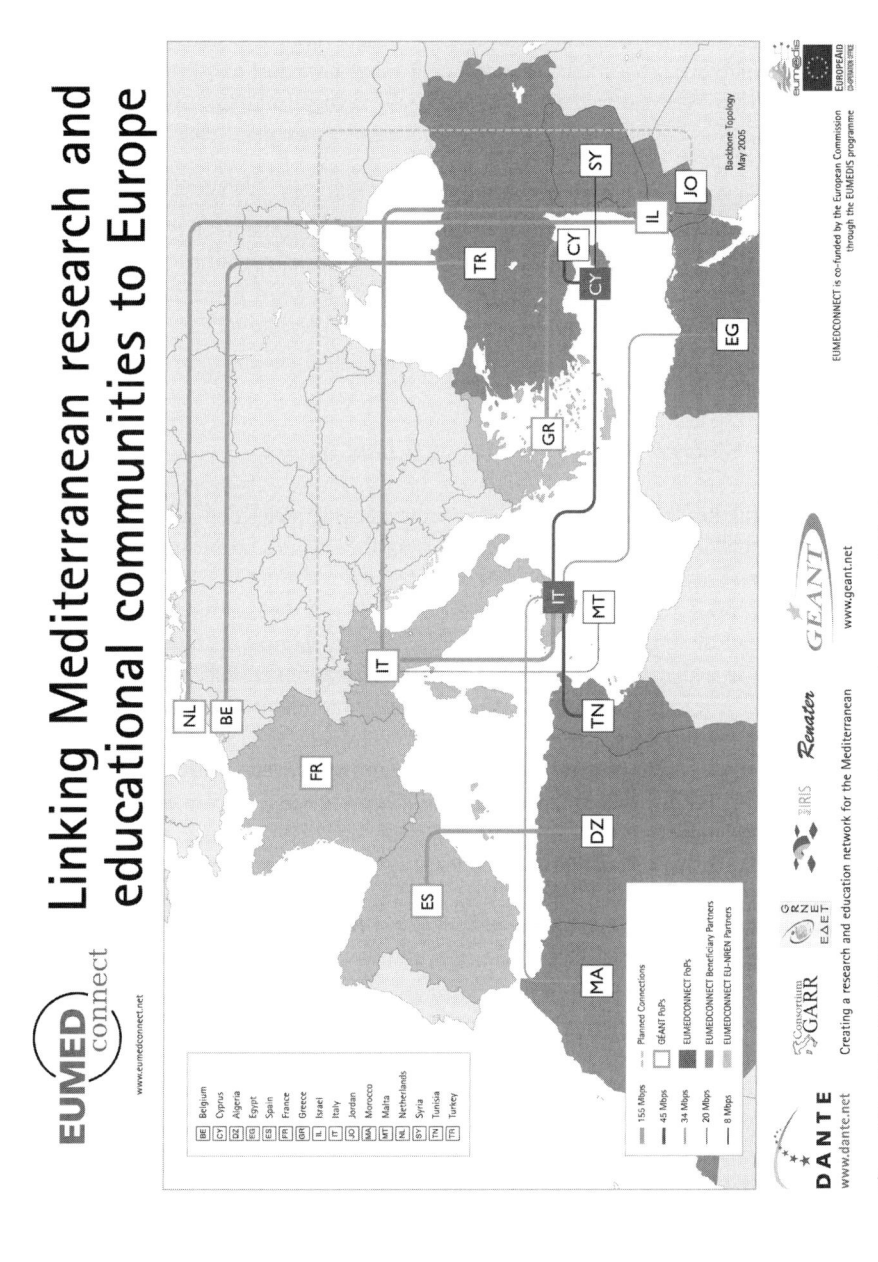

Figure 8.3 EUMEDCONNECT configuration. There is a color version of this figure in the set at the front of the book.

transoceanic link to reach GÉANT. Details of the roll-out of RedCLARA and its external links are described below.

The ALICE project has catalyzed the development of new research networks in Latin America. Before ALICE, only eight of the @LIS target countries (Argentina, Brazil, Chile, Costa Rica, Cuba, Mexico, Uruguay and Venezuela) had functioning research networks – in the other countries Internet connectivity available to research and education institutions was provided by commercial Internet service providers. This situation has altered significantly with the setting up of new research networks connected to RedCLARA in at least a further eight countries (Bolivia, Colombia, Ecuador, Guatemala, Nicaragua, Panama, Peru and Salvador).

Some of the larger research networks, especially in Brazil and Chile, have also been experimenting with, or deploying, new networking technologies, including their own optical networks.

Many benefits of international cooperation in research and education resulted from the setting up of the RedCLARA network and its international connectivity to GÉANT. These can be seen in approved Sixth Framework Programme and Seventh Framework Programme projects involving partners in Latin America which have been made possible by the interconnection of RedCLARA and GÉANT. CLARA has been an active partner in a number of these projects.

8.5.1
A Very Brief History of Academic Networking in Latin America

In Latin America, one can observe the same general pattern of development of academic networking services as in other parts of the world, beginning with e-mail networks, such as BITNET and UUCP, installed between 1986 and 1994, and migrating to an IP network some time afterwards (between 1989 and 1996) as shown in Table 8.1.

The spread of commercial or commodity Internet services in the latter part of the 1990s had a significant impact on the development of the research networks of Latin America, leading to the disappearance of most of them by the end of the 1990s, either because they could no longer compete with the new ISPs, or because the academic networks themselves began offering commodity service. By the year 2000, only eight functioning research networks remained in Latin America, either through the financial support of government (in Brazil, Costa Rica, Cuba, Uruguay and Venezuela) or of private industry (in Mexico), or by having built up a sustainable

Table 8.1 Introduction of international connectivity for e-mail (BITNET/UUCP) and IP networks (various sources).

	MX	CL	BR	NI	UY	PY	VE	AR	CR	CO	EC	PE	BO	CU	PA	GT	SV	HN
e-mail	86	86	88	88	88	89	90	90	90	90	91	91	91	91	92	92	94	94
IP	89		92	91	94	94	95	92	93	93	94		92	94	95	96	94	95	96	95

MX, Mexico; CL, Chile; BR, Brazil; NI, Nicaragua; UY, Uruguay; PY, Paraguay; VE, Venezuela; AR, Argentina; CR, Costa Rica; CO, Colombia; EC, Ecuador; PE, Peru; BO, Bolivia; CU, Cuba; PA, Panama; GT, Guatemala; SV, Salvador; HN, Honduras.

membership organization to maintain the networking infrastructure and its operations (in Argentina and Chile).

Connectivity between research networks in Latin America and the global research networking fabric which developed in the mid-1990s was implemented during the late 1990s. The CUDI (Corporación Universitaria para el Desarrollo de Internet) network in Mexico established several cross-border connections to the neighboring United States. The three advanced research networks of the Southern Cone of South America (RETINA – Red Teleinformática Académica – in Argentina, RNP – Rede National de ensino e Pesquisa – in Brazil, and REUNA – Red Universitaria National – in Chile) could only be connected adequately after the first of the new high-capacity submarine cables had been installed in the region by Global Crossing in 2001. Before this, most research networks in Latin America had maintained international connections by geosynchronous satellite links, usually to the United States. Thus, starting in 2001, the first connections to the new global research infrastructure were made using the Global Crossing cable to Miami, where Florida International University (FIU) was developing the AMPATH (Americas path) project to build an Internet exchange point for Latin American R&E connectivity. By 2003, research networks in Latin America served by the AMPATH project included REUNA (Chile), RNP and ANSP, Academic Network at São Paulo (Brazil), RETINA (Argentina) and REACCIUN, Red Académica de Centros de Investigación y Universidades Nacionales (Venezuela).

In 2002, the EC financed the CAESAR (connecting all European and Southern American researchers) project to carry out a feasibility study to set up direct connectivity between GÉANT and research networks in Latin America. The CAESAR project was coordinated by DANTE and supported by the research networks in Portugal and Spain. CAESAR provided the spark needed to ignite the process of cooperation within the R&E community in Latin America, in order to build a regional network which could be part of the solution built by the ALICE project. As a direct result of the contacts made between the participants from 12 countries in Latin America at a CAESAR workshop held in Toledo in June 2002, the CLARA organization was set up in 2003 to develop interconnections between research networks in Latin America and provide connections to the global research Internet.

Today CLARA has members in 15 of the 18 target countries of @LIS, maintains a registered office in Montevideo, Uruguay, and has a small full-time staff, many of them co-located with member research networks. CLARA also provides the forum for the participation of Latin American research networks in the regional backbone network project, and has contributed substantially to the development of this project by participating in the design of the RedCLARA network architecture, and by taking on technical responsibility for the engineering, operation and future technical development of this network.

8.5.2
The ALICE Project and the RedCLARA Network

The ALICE (América Latina Interconectada Con Europa) project started in June 2003 and was originally planned as a 36-month project to last until the end of May 2006.

However, as a result of better-than-anticipated connectivity prices in Latin America and a delay in the roll-out of the RedCLARA network, the ALICE partners applied for an extension of the project until March 2008, to make use of all available funding from the EC EuropeAid. The extension was granted and this enabled the ALICE partners to work towards the consolidation of the RedCLARA network and its connection with research networks across Latin America.

The main objective of the ALICE project was the creation of a regional research infrastructure to interconnect the research networks in Latin America and to provide a link to the pan-European GÉANT network. It has always been the aim of ALICE to ensure that this regional Latin American network would be operated and managed by the Latin American partners, and that it would provide the basis for an exchange of training and expertise among the Latin American partners and between Latin America and Europe.

So ALICE is more than just an infrastructure project. Training courses and workshops funded by ALICE have been developed for Latin American university networking engineers, to share knowledge and expertise on topics including network deployment, advanced routing technology, network measurement systems, security, IPv6, VoIP and video-conferencing. By means of these training courses and workshops, ALICE has laid the foundation for the creation of a sustainable future for Latin American research networking. There has been a real desire in the Latin American and European research networking communities to educate and share best practices amongst a growing community of networkers.

ALICE has achieved its objectives. Instrumental for this achievement was the setting up in 2003 of CLARA modeled loosely after TERENA. Since its creation, CLARA has taken responsibility within the ALICE project and more specifically for the operation and management of the RedCLARA network through the CLARA Network Engineering Group (NEG), CLARA NOC and CLARA-TEC (CLARA-Technical Forum).

The establishment of the RedCLARA Network is the main achievement of the European ALICE project. Starting on September 1 2004 with an interconnection between the Chilean research network, REUNA and the GÉANT PoP in Madrid, the network evolved during 2004/5 into a complete ring interconnecting five main PoPs in Latin America and offering spur links to nine countries in Southern and Central America as well as a direct link to the GÉANT2 PoP in Madrid.

However, with ALICE funding coming to an end in early 2008, the year 2007 saw major changes in the RedCLARA topology needed to operate within a reduced budget. Various formerly ALICE-funded links were replaced by cheaper connectivity provided to CLARA via FIU. In many cases these new links supported connections to RedCLARA at a new PoP established in Miami. For example, the Central American countries no longer connected to one of the five original RedCLARA PoPs located in Latin America, but to the new PoP in Florida.

The architecture of the RedCLARA network and its changes over time have been designed by CLARA-TEC taking account of what was available in the Latin American telecommunications market in 2003 when the tender for connectivity was first issued and, subsequently, dealing with the budget restrictions in 2007. The configuration of the RedCLARA network in July 2007 is shown in Figure 8.4.

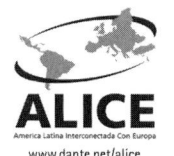

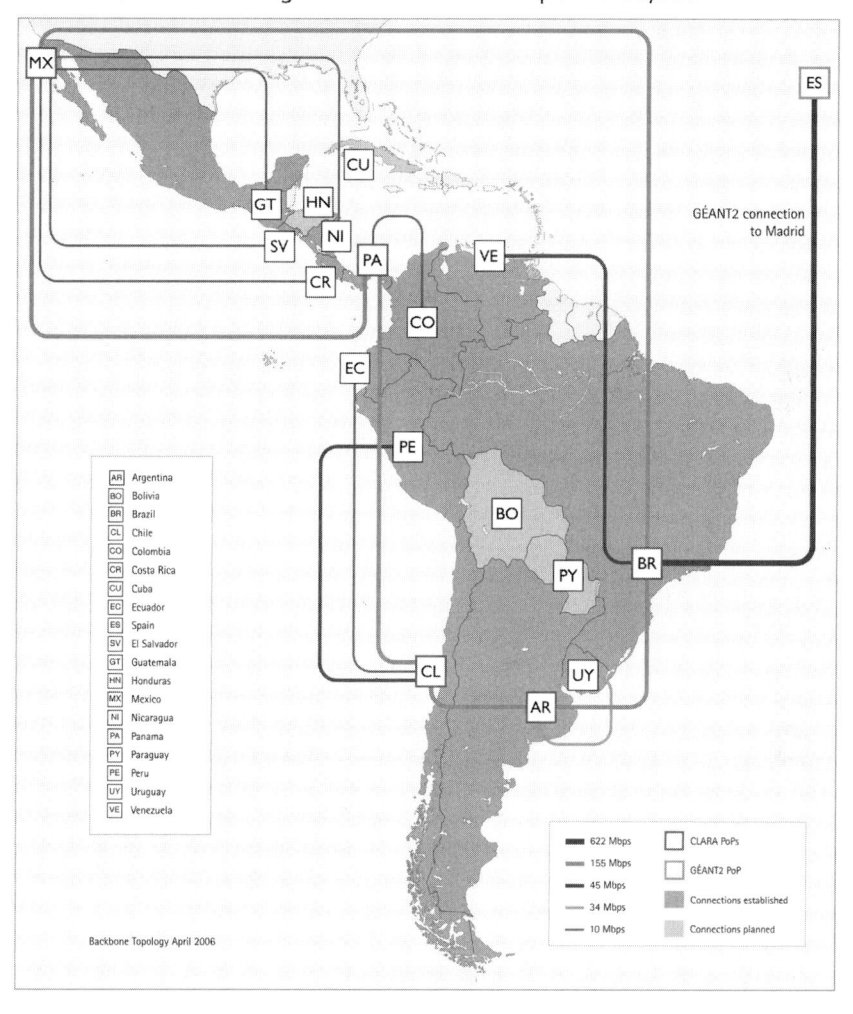

Figure 8.4 RedCLARA topology map, July 2007. There is a color version of this figure in the set at the front of the book.

Since 2005, the RedCLARA network has also been connected to research networks in the United States by means of links provided by the WHREN/LILA (Western hemisphere research and education networks/links interconnecting Latin America) project, jointly financed by NSF and FAPESP (Fundação de Amparo à Pesquisa do Estado de São Paulo), with the participation of FIU (Florida), CENIC, Corporation for Education Network Initiatives in California (California), CLARA, CUDI (Mexico), and RNP and ANSP (Brazil). By 2006, RedCLARA had a dedicated 1 Gbps link from Tijuana (Mexico) to Pacific Wave in Los Angeles, and shared a 2.5 Gbps connection from São Paulo (Brazil) to Atlantic Wave in Miami. The Level 2 infrastructures provided by Pacific Wave and Atlantic Wave allow direct peering by RedCLARA with all other participating networks, including national and regional networks from the United States, Canada, the Pacific Rim and Europe.

The limitations of the Latin American telecommunications market are also the limits of the RedCLARA network. As is obvious, the highest capacity links are the transatlantic link, which is also the part of the network with the lowest price per Mbps per year and the links to the United States. The main RedCLARA PoPs are in locations that have well developed and competitive telecommunications markets, with the possible exception of the PoP in Tijuana which was chosen for its proximity to the United States. Higher capacity links are available to those research networks located in the more developed countries where better telecommunications services are available. Low bandwidth links had to be chosen by the research networks in locations that still suffer from restrictions in their national telecommunication markets which make bandwidth scarce and therefore expensive, or in which prices are kept artificially high by providers and as a result are unaffordable.

It is expected that RedCLARA will be able to follow a growth path similar to that of the European research infrastructure, leading to dramatic increases in capacity between the main RedCLARA PoPs and towards Europe and the United States. However, as telecommunications markets across Southern and Central America vary greatly, it is not certain that all Latin American research networks will be able to benefit from these capacity increases.

Following a tender carried out within the Latin American research network community, the CLARA NEG was contracted by the ALICE project to the Brazilian research network, RNP, and the NOC was contracted to the Mexican research network, CUDI. Both CLARA NEG and the NOC started their operations in June 2004. The preparation for the roll-out of the RedCLARA network began in June 2004 and was coordinated between members of DANTE staff, the CLARA NEG and the CLARA NOC. Technical coordination was achieved then, as it still is today, via bi-weekly video-conferences between all the involved parties.

The task of CLARA NEG, run by RNP is the operation of RedCLARA as a state-of-the-art backbone network, offering services that are typically available to advanced regional networks in other parts of the world. The engineers working for the CLARA NEG exercise overall responsibility for network operations, including oversight of the CLARA NOC. This oversight includes the definition of how several of the CLARA NOC functions are to be carried out, as well as the choice of appropriate software or hardware to be utilized.

CLARA NOC, run until 2008 by CUDI, is responsible for the real-time monitoring of availability and performance and the immediate response to fault notifications, including their follow-up until correction. CLARA NOC also provides a single point of contact with the RedCLARA network, passing on outsider queries to the appropriate person or institution.

ALICE also aimed at the exchange of knowledge and know-how between the European and Latin American project partners. This objective has been addressed by CLARA through the creation of CLARA-TEC and its associated technical working groups, modeled loosely after the TERENA technical task forces. The name CLARA-TEC is given to the group of engineers of those research networks with membership in the CLARA organization. The ALICE project supported a twice-yearly meeting of participants in CLARA-TEC to ensure smooth communications within the technical community of RedCLARA, and such meetings continue to be held after ALICE's termination. During these technical meetings, updates are presented by members of CLARA NEG, CLARA NOC, CLARA itself, and, during ALICE, by the European research networks which were ALICE partners and DANTE. In addition, the Latin American research networks are given the opportunity to present the latest developments in their countries.

With initial support from ALICE, CLARA-TEC also organizes training and capacity-building during these twice-yearly meetings, which have so far included training on network deployment, advanced routing technology, network measurement systems, security, IPv6, VoIP and video-conferencing. Supported by members of the CLARA NEG and NOC, CLARA-TEC has also been able to provide special training for the Bolivian, Venezuelan and Ecuadorian research networks, addressing the special training needs of engineers working in these research networks or their connected universities and institutions.

8.5.3
New and Greatly Improved Research Networks in Latin America

The ALICE project not only created the RedCLARA network, it also gave great impetus to research networking on the national level in Latin America, with immediate benefit to the students and researchers in several countries: thanks to the momentum created by ALICE, CLARA and RedCLARA, new national R&E network initiatives have been created across Latin America, in countries such as Bolivia, Colombia, Ecuador, El Salvador, Guatemala, Nicaragua, Panama and Peru. It is thanks to these newly created research networks that are all connected to RedCLARA. RedCLARA can truly be called a regional Latin American network.

In both Chile and Brazil, considerable experimentation in optical networking has recently been carried out by government-funded test-bed networks supporting R&D in networking technologies and applications. In Chile, the G-REUNA (Gigabit-Red Universitaria National) project established a 250 km darkfiber network connecting Valparaíso to the capital, Santiago, interconnecting 3 universities and REUNA, the Chilean research network. The fiber was lit up using DWDM equipment, and separate lambdas supported Gigabit ethernet communication between the participating institutions. This experiment, begun in 2001, went on for one year.

A technologically similar network was established in Brazil in 2004, and was still in operation in 2009. Known as Project GIGA (gigabits networking research), the research test-bed interconnects more than 20 universities and research institutions in the neighboring states of Rio de Janeiro and São Paulo, and uses more than 750 km of dark fiber provided free of charge by telecom providers. This project is jointly coordinated by RNP and by Fundação CPqD (Centro de Pesquisa e Desenvolvimento em Telecomunicações), a telecommunications R&D center, which formerly belonged to the now extinct state monopoly. Project GIGA has involved research groups from more than 50 universities in 15 of the 26 states in Brazil, and there is great interest in technology transfer to Brazilian companies. In particular, the WDM (wavelength division multiplexing) equipment used in the test-bed is manufactured in Brazil, and has more recently been put to use in commercial networks. The test-bed network has also supported national and international scientific collaborations, such as participation in the demonstrations at the annual supercomputing events by a high-energy physics group from Rio de Janeiro. A successor project is currently being negotiated.

With the experience gained through project GIGA, RNP has engaged in the process of upgrading its production networks throughout Brazil. In November 2005, the core of the national backbone network, which interconnects 10 capital cities, was upgraded to 2.5 and 10 Gbps links, based on unprotected DWDM lambdas. In all, about 12 000 km of lambdas were contracted commercially by RNP in order to provide its IP service at these transmission rates. The current plan for 2007–2010 includes upgrading links to nearly all the other 17 capitals to at least 1 Gbps. At the same time, RNP is carrying out a nationwide program of building metropolitan optical networks in the 27 capital cities, where it provides access to the national backbone network. These networks are based on darkfiber infrastructures, almost always built and owned by RNP, and supporting 1 and 10 Gbps ethernet networks operated by local consortia of universities and research centers. Frequently, the fiber infrastructure is being shared with government departments, at local, state and national levels, who operate their own separate networks. The first of these metropolitan networks was inaugurated in May 2007 in Belém, capital of the state of Pará. This network uses 50 km of fiber-optic cable, and provides connectivity to 32 sites belonging to 12 local institutions. By 2010, it is expected that more than 300 universities and research centers located in capital cities will have at least 1 Gbps connectivity between the national backbone and all of their campuses.

Since early 2007, responsibility for the research network in Argentina, formerly RETINA, has been assumed by the national government, and the network is now known as INNOVA|RED. Besides providing full support for the CLARA/ALICE initiative, the INNOVA|RED is also engaged in extensive improvements in the network, based on a DWDM optical infrastructure shared with a local telecommunications company. These improvements involve the provision of an extensive 10 Gbps national backbone, and the simultaneous provision of a 10 Gbps CLARA link between Argentina and Chile, as well as a link to the Pierre Auger Cosmic Ray Observatory, near to Mendoza, Argentina. This new network will become operational in 2009. This is the first known case in Latin America of such an agreement between a research network and a fiber owner, jointly to invest in and share the resulting optical networking capacity, and is considered a good augury for future research network and CLARA developments.

8.5.4
Collaborative Networked Applications in Latin America

Examples of collaborative projects between Latin America and Europe which have come about thanks to the creation of the RedCLARA network and its interconnection to GÉANT can be found as early as 2004, when RedCLARA was first implemented. For the 2004 edition of Supercomputing, in November 2004, a group of high-energy physicists from the State University of Rio de Janeiro (UERJ, Universidade do Estado do Rio de Janeiro) used the RedCLARA network to transmit up to 500 Mbps to CERN in Europe, and 400 Mbps to Pittsburgh (via the GÉANT links provided to the Abilene network in the United States). A few days later, at the RedCLARA launch event in Rio de Janeiro, Brazil, a demonstration was given of simultaneous transmission and visualization of multiple streams of compressed HD video-on-demand, where the video streams were transmitted across the GÉANT -RedCLARA link from i2CAT (Internet2 Catalunya) in Barcelona, Spain.

The value of this new European-Latin American connectivity is increasingly coming to be recognized by the establishment of formal joint research projects, financed by the EU's IST program, and involving partnerships between research groups in Europe and Latin America. A number of such projects started during 2006, including EELA (E-science grid facility for Europe and Latin America), AugerAccess (cosmic ray physics), RINGrid (remote instrumentation in next-generation grids) and EXPReS (e-VLBI). EELA is a two-year project, involving CLARA, CERN and a further 19 partners from R&E institutes in three European and seven Latin American countries, and is coordinated by CIEMAT (Centro de Investigaciones Energéticas, Medioambientales y Tecnológicas) from Spain. Briefly, EELA seeks to set up a pilot grid network between Europe and Latin America, compatible with the EGEE grid in Europe. In 2008 the successor EELA-2 project was begun to extend the reach of EELA to more countries, and to establish sustainable grid organizations within the region.

In the field of astrophysics research, the Southern Cone countries of Argentina, Brazil and Chile have long housed radio, optical and cosmic ray observatories, many built as a result of European investment. Recently, remote network access has assumed an increasingly important role in their utilization, permitting rapid access to observational results, such as in e-VLBI, or even in permitting remote, real-time instrument control, possibly assisted by human technical staff. The RINGrid project dealt generically with remote network access to large instruments, such as optical telescopes in astrophysics and electron microscopy. CLARA is also a participant in the RINGrid project, coordinated by PSNC (Poznań Supercomputing and Networking Center), Poland, and the optical observatory involved is the Southern Astrophysical Research (SOAR) Telescope, built and operated by a consortium with significant Brazilian participation.

The involvement of CLARA in these European joint research projects, representing the Latin American research networks, has been an excellent means of providing close and continuous communications support to advanced users, as well as harmonious development and improvement of the networking infrastructure, through the introduction of appropriate networking services and management tools.

The creation of RedCLARA and CLARA has been a huge step forward for Latin American R&D in general, and for Latin American research networking in particular. Until ALICE, there was no direct connectivity between the research networks of Latin America, and all traffic had to be exchanged via the United States. Since the creation of RedCLARA and its interconnection to GÉANT, European and Latin American scientists are able to collaborate using an advanced network infrastructure, with a fast and direct link between them.

Collaborative research between Latin America and Europe has already benefited from this, as can be seen in the use of RedCLARA and its interconnection to GÉANT by the EU's IST projects, EELA, EELA-2, RINGrid, AugerAccess and EXPReS (e-VLBI).

8.5.5
The Future of the Latin American Regional Network

An important aspect in the success of the ALICE project has been the amount and percentage of EU funding. The project budget of €12.5 M allowed the creation of a reasonably dimensioned regional Latin American research network and its interconnection to Europe. The 80% funding from Europe and 20% from Latin America has ensured actual implementation of the project, but has also ensured the commitment of the Latin American partners.

EC funding of the Latin American RedCLARA network and its interconnection to GÉANT was available through ALICE until March 31 2008. In late 2008, the ALICE2 project was approved, with a budget of €18 M, of which €12 M will be financed by the EU during a period of four years. ALICE2, coordinated by CLARA will seek to use this time to establish a self-sustaining regional network with a facilities-based infrastructure and lower operating costs than the traditional model, in order to be truly self-sufficient when the project ends.

In order to achieve this aim, CLARA is seeking to reproduce, in as many cases as possible, the development of network infrastructure being pioneered in Argentina, Brazil and Chile, where agreements are being reached with fiber owners for the joint development of DWDM networks. When such schemes involve cross-border fiber, as in the case between Argentina and Chile, then CLARA itself becomes a party to the partnership, and RedCLARA will have access to greatly increased network capacity.

There is currently great optimism in the Latin American region about the perspective of the growth and integration of research networks by developing such partnerships. Similar initiatives are being pursued in all countries within the region.

8.6
Russia

As in many other countries, the history of the Russian Internet began with research and education networking before the establishment of any official research network structure. The first Internet channel from Russia to the global Internet was a dial-up connection from Moscow to Helsinki University. The connection was established in August 1990 by enthusiasts from Demos, the first Russian "capitalist-type" scientific research cooperative which had been organized by the specialists from the Kurchatov Institute, a Russian scientific center. The connection was limited to UUCP access which allowed e-mail and news services, but that was only the beginning. After the official August 28 1990 birth date of the Russian Internet, events moved increasingly rapidly and the .su domain was registered before the end of the year.

To get an understanding of the influence of the social and political environment on the development of the Internet and research networking in Russia, one must recall the main events of the early 1990s in the country. Mikhail Gorbachev had become President of the USSR (Union of Soviet Socialist Republics), censorship was canceled by the State Law (1990), there was an unsuccessful coup in Moscow, the USSR disintegrated (1991), prices were set free and skyrocketed, citizens' bank deposits were wiped out (1992), and there were armed crises between government and parliament (1993). In addition, there was huge state foreign debt, no remaining national gold stock, and the price of oil (the main component of Russian exports) was ten times lower than nowadays.

In spite of all these difficulties, the aspirations and desires of Internet enthusiasts were so huge that several research networks were created in those years. As a result, the main feature of Russian research network history and its current state is the existence of several research networks within one country. The main reason for such a multi-network structure is the existence of several ministries and other funding bodies, each with their own responsibilities, specific areas of interest, and financial constraints. Nevertheless, research network activities and funding were always coordinated by special agreements and state programs such as Universities of Russia (1992–1997), Creation of Research Network of Computer Telecommunications for Science and Higher Education (1995–2000), Development of Unified Educational Environment (2001–2005), Development of Education System (2002–2010), Research and Development of Priority Directions of Science and Technology (2002–2006) and others. Coordination of these programs is provided by a special public council set up in 1996.

8.6.1
The Origins of the Main Russian Research Networks

FREEnet (network for research, education and engineering) was established in 1991 on the initiative of the Institute of Organic Chemistry of the RAS (Russian Academy of Sciences). Initially, an e-mail service making use of a gateway with EARN/BITNET was the only one provided. IP Internet access was established within FREEnet in

1993. In 1995, the ac.ru (academic) domain was organized and supported by the FREEnet NOC. It should also be mentioned that several universities and research institutes began to offer UUCP mail services independently to their employees and students in 1990–1991. Most of them used Relcom (Reliable Communications), a pure research and education network at the time. Relcom Ltd. was established as a network operations organization in 1992.

The RSSI (Russian Space Science Internet) project was established in April 1993 following a joint decision of the Russian co-chairmen of the working group on space research and NASA. In February 1994, the first phase of the project had been completed. A 256 kbps satellite link connected RSSI with NASA's Goddard Space Flight Center in the United States and allowed the first RSSI member organizations to gain access to the Internet. The RSSI NOC was set up at that time. The RSSI operator is the Space Research Institute of the RAS. In mid-1997, RSSI increased its channel capacity to 512 kbps.

RUHEP/Radio-MSU (Russian HEP/Radio-Moscow State University) started up in 1993 and was based on radio-relay lines connecting MSU and several HEP research centers. In the same year, the Moscow-Hamburg satellite channel was established. Since 1999 RUHEP has participated actively in the Virtual Silk Highway project, which provides global Internet connectivity to the Caucasus and Central Asia (Armenia, Azerbaijan, Georgia, Kazakhstan, Kyrgyzstan, Tajikistan, Turkmenistan, and Uzbekistan) through satellite technology.

RUNNet (Russian university network) was established in 1994 on the initiative of the State University of Fine Mechanics and Optics by the State Committee of Higher Education as a very important branch of the Russian Universities program. In the same year, an Agreement on Cooperation between RUNNet and NORDUnet was signed. The network operator VusTelecomCentre (Universities Telecommunication Centre) was created for the purposes of RUNNet development and support. Initially, RUNNet was mainly based on satellite technologies. In 1995, satellite nodes were established in Moscow, Saint Petersburg, Ekaterinburg, Novosibirsk, Saratov, Ulianovsk, Nizhni-Novgorod, Rostov-on-Don, Tambov, Tomsk, Krasnoyarsk and Irkutsk. In 1996 Vladivostok, Izhevsk, Perm, Barnaul and Pereslavl-Zalesski were integrated into the satellite infrastructure. In 1997 Khabarovsk, Nalchik, Mahachkala and Stavropol were added to the picture. Bandwidth was limited to 64–128 kbps due to the limitations of early satellite technologies. Functioning of this satellite infrastructure was supported by RUNNet's own teleport in Saint Petersburg. Several Russian satellites have been used; the typical bandwidth for a single university now is 2 Mbps, but only a few universities still use the satellite service.

Changes are the result of improvements in terrestrial structures (most of these universities use satellite channels in parallel with terrestrial ones). Terrestrial RUNNet infrastructure was actively developed from 1995 onwards. The first international RUNNet link operating at 256 kbps between Saint Petersburg and the Supercomputer Centre in Espoo (Finland) was established with NORDUnet in early 1995. In 1996, it was upgraded to 1 Mbps and in 1997 to 2 Mbps. Also in 1997, a new international 4 Mbps channel was installed between Saint-Petersburg and the New York PoP of Teleglobe. Thus, the aggregate RUNNet international connectivity rose to 6 Mbps. 1998 saw a further step in international connectivity with RUNNet–

NORDUnet capacity increasing to 4 Mbps and RUNNet–Teleglobe to 6 Mbps. In the same year, new satellite nodes were installed in Vladikavkaz, Orenburg and Moscow. In subsequent years there were several upgrades in the capacity of the RUNNet–NORDUnet connection; in 2001 to 34 Mbps, in 2002 to 155 Mbps, in 2003 to 622 Mbps, and in 2004 to 2.5 Gbps.

The RUNNet operator is now the State Institute of Information Technologies and Telecommunications (SIIT&T) "Informika". The RUNNet NOC is supported by SIIT&T "Informika" Saint-Petersburg branch which was set up in 2000. RUNNet has PoPs in Moscow, Saint Petersburg, Samara, Novosibirsk, Khabarovsk, Ekaterinburg, Nizhni-Novgorod, Rostov-on-Don, Vladivostok, Stockholm and Amsterdam. Universities and research institutes in 56 regions of Russia have links to these PoPs.[2] RUNNet now operates international connections Moscow-Saint-Petersburg-Stockholm (STM-16), Stockholm-Amsterdam (STM-4), and Moscow-Helsinki (STM-4). An upgrade of the Moscow-Saint-Petersburg-Stockholm connection to STM-64 is on the way.

The backbone infrastructure of RUNNet has been based on SDH technology since 2005. The RUNNet NOC has provided support of the edu.ru (education) domain since 1998, as well as governmental domains mon.gov.ru (in Russian spelling, the Ministry of Education and Science), ed.gov.ru (education, Federal Agency of Education), and fasi.gov.ru (Federal Agency of Science and Innovations). In 1999, the group of RUNNet organizers was awarded a state prize by the Russian Government.

RBNet (Russian backbone network) has been basically constructed in the framework of the Inter-Agency program Creation of National Computer Network for Science and Higher School (1996–2002). The RBNet operator is the Russian Institute of Public Networks (RIPN). As a result of the program, RBNet PoPs were set up in Moscow, Samara, Novosibirsk Khabarovsk, Ekaterinburg, Nizhni Novgorod, Rostov-on-Don, Kazan, and Dubna. RBNet has PoPs abroad in Amsterdam and Chicago.

At the end of 1998, A 6 Mbps ATM channel to STARTAP (Chicago) was organized, connecting Russian research networks to the new generation networks in North America. This MirNET project was run by a consortium composed of the University of Tennessee, Knoxville (UTK), MSU, RIPN, "Friends and Partners"Foundation[3], the RAS, RUNNet and others. In 2002, in cooperation with Telia, RBNet set up the Moscow-Chicago 155 Mbps channel. In 2007 RBNet obtained international connectivity with STM-64 capacity between Moscow and Amsterdam, making use of NORDUnet DWDM infrastructure between Amsterdam and Stockholm. RBNet and RUNNet participate in GLORIAD, coordinated in Russia by the Kurchatov Institute. The GLORIAD advanced science Internet network was launched in January 2004 by the United States, China and Russia, and, in 2005, it expanded its reach to Korea, Canada and the Netherlands. In 2006 it connected the five Nordic countries. It provides an optical network ring encircling the northern hemisphere with individual network circuits at up to 10 Gbps and promotes new opportunities for cooperation for

---

[2] Satellite RUNNet segment is still operated by VusTelecomCenter.
[3] "Friends and Partners" Foundation promotes contacts between people in the West and in the countries of the Former Soviet Union.

scientists, educators and students. The network topology expanded in 2006 to provide several ring redundancies; it now represents a true ring of rings around the earth, offering richer bandwidth and redundant network paths for improved reliability. The GLORIAD path in Russia passes through Saint Petersburg, Moscow, Samara, Novosibirsk and Khabarovsk and now has 155 Mbps capacity – which is a limitation of course.

RASNet (Russian Academy of Sciences Network). As its title indicates, this network is oriented towards the Russian research institutes of the Academy of Sciences. RASNet activity is provided under the supervision of the Joint Supercomputer Centre of RAS. In 1999, the Russian Academy of Sciences together with MSU, the Joint Institute of Nuclear Research (JINR) and RIPN signed an agreement aimed at establishing connections with TEN-155, and corresponding negotiations with DANTE were held in 2000. As a result of joint efforts supported by DANTE, RASNet established connectivity with GÉANT in 2002 via a STM-1 Moscow-Stockholm channel carried on RBNet's infrastructure. In 2004 DANTE set up a GÉANT PoP in Moscow with connections, each of 2.5 Gbps, to Frankfurt and Copenhagen. The GÉANT PoP in Moscow is now actively used by the Russian research and education community for access to the European research networks.

RELARN-IP (Russian electronic academic and research network-IP) and UMOS (South Moscow backbone network), established in 1994, are examples of regional networks serving mainly the Moscow region. Between 1998 and 2000, networks based on fiber-optic channels were set up in most large Russian cities with more than 1M inhabitants.

MSUNet (Moscow State University Network) was set up in 1994. It participated actively in the RUNNet and RBNet projects and now has a 10 Gbps campus network connecting buildings in different parts of Moscow.

Other large users of telecommunication technologies are the Kurchatov Institute and JINR situated in Dubna. Including the Russian Federation, 18 member states from Eastern Europe and Asia participate in the JINR, which also collaborates extensively with other HEP projects around the world. Like CERN, the JINR has significant demands for international network capacity. It provides its own local service on its site at Dubna but depends on the national research and education networks, specifically RBNet and RUNNet, for its wide area and international connectivity.

Until 1996, almost all traffic between Russian networks (not only research networks) travelled abroad. The need for an Internet exchange point became evident and the first one was set up in Moscow in 1996 on the initiative of the research networks. Now Internet exchanges are also functioning in Saint Petersburg, Samara and Novosibirsk.

The International channel capacities from Russia in 1997 were:

- RUNNet-NORDUnet, 2 Mbps
- Radio-MSU-DESY (DFN),128 kbps
- RSSI-NASA Internet, 256 kbps
- MSUnet-Ebone, 256 kbps
- FREEnet-Deutsche Telekom, 256 kbps.

Two years later (1999) RUNNet and RBNet, together with the JCS Metrocom Company, organized a 34 Mbps Moscow-Saint-Petersburg ATM channel that connected PoPs in these cities – at that time a huge step ahead for Russia. Implementation of new information technologies was proceeding in parallel with the infrastructure development of R&E networks.

Almost all opening ceremonies of new Internet centers in universities from 1996 onwards were accompanied by video conferences. From 2002, Russian research networks were able to use the MBONE (multicast backbone) Exchange at STARTAP/StarLight in Chicago. (An internal multicast Internet exchange, Multicast-IX, had been organized some years earlier). Starting in 2003, multicast educational IP-TV-channel broadcasting systems were developed within the RUNNet infrastructure. In 2004 IP-telephony was established as a service for Russian research networks. In 2000 RUNNet organized a reflector for RTP (real time protocol) video conferencing and in 2006 RBNet opened a VRVS (virtual room videoconferencing system) reflector.

The first experiments with IPv6 in Russia began between RUNNet, RBNet and FREEnet in 2002. The first IPv6 native international connectivity was established between RUNNet and NORDUnet (Stockholm) in 2003 and between FREENet, RBNet and Internet2 (Abilene, Chicago). Now IPv6 is widely used in communication between Russian universities as a second IP stack on the basis of tunneling technology.

Russian research networks provide the communications base for grid projects. Several research institutes and universities such as the Russian Scientific Centre, Kurchatov Institute, JINR, the Institute of Theoretical and Experimental Physics, the Institute of HEP and others have participated actively in European EGEE projects since 2004. In 2005 RDIG (Russian data intensive grid) with its own Russian operation centre (ROC) began functioning. Russian research network infrastructure allows Russian universities and research institutes to participate in a number of international projects in several scientific disciplines.

The Russian research network structure, and RUNNet in particular, is an important source of information resources for secondary schools and universities. In 2002, the special state project for the creation of an Internet portals system with free information educational resources – electronic libraries, lectures, videos, test programs, and so on, was launched and by 2007, 12 Internet portals devoted to different areas of knowledge were in operation.

9
Transatlantic Connections

This chapter looks at what has happened and what is happening today to connect the United States with Europe. It gives examples of some of the projects currently in progress that are developing the network infrastructure and supporting collaboration between research groups which have very demanding requirements for network services. What they intend to achieve and some of the successes so far are highlighted.

9.1
The "Welcome Guest" Period

Network developments in the United States have always been an important element in European research networking. Much of the hardware and software that was necessary to create the Internet was developed in North America and technical progress in the United States has been followed keenly by European engineers. American equipment is widely used to build networks throughout the world. The additional challenges associated with the operation of transatlantic circuits are of great interest to engineers in both continents and, for many European research groups, effective communication with their United States counterparts is important. Geography and, to a lesser extent, competition have influenced costs of communicating with the United States in different European countries. Added to these factors is the question of "who pays?" The involvement of United States funding bodies in transatlantic connectivity, welcome though it was, did bring new administrative difficulties. For example, the procurement procedures (referred to earlier) of the organizations managing the two ends of a circuit, while being entirely consistent in themselves, could include procedures which made them incompatible with each other. Additional effort was then needed to find a compromise acceptable to everyone involved.

Circuits which cross oceans are inherently more expensive than terrestrial circuits. The cables must be sufficiently robust to withstand the rigors of survival on the ocean bed; they are subject to additional stress and to abrasion where they cross the ridges of submerged mountain ranges. Repeaters need electrical power which can only be provided from one or other of the landing sites. Cables must therefore carry power as

A History of International Research Networking. Edited by Howard Davies and Beatrice Bressan
Copyright © 2010 WILEY-VCH Verlag GmbH & Co. KGaA, Weinheim
ISBN: 978-3-527-32710-2

well as the telecommunications circuits, maintenance and repair are much more difficult, and operational planning, including the provision of back-up, must take account of the length of time needed to locate and repair a damaged cable in mid-ocean compared to a fault on a terrestrial cable, especially when repair ships are stuck in harbor because of bad weather.

Before European telecommunications liberalization in 1998, the cost of transatlantic connectivity was significantly lower in countries with an Atlantic or North Sea coast. Just as with international circuits within Europe, transmission capacity was provided in the form of two half-circuits by two telecoms operators, one at each end. Since the European half link had to be provided by the national monopoly telecoms operator, the cost of extending the transatlantic circuit from its eastern landfall to the premises of a customer in the same country was relatively small and could be included in the half link price. In other countries, however, the customer's national operator provided an international circuit to extend the transatlantic segment to the customer and added the (high) cost of this to the transatlantic cost. The cost differential was greatly reduced after liberalization, when companies operating transatlantic cables were able to acquire and re-sell transmission capacity within Europe. At that point, they could offer to terminate transatlantic links at the customer's location using their own European infrastructure. Although the cost differential between countries has not been completely eliminated, charges are now more closely related to the actual costs of provision.

For customers operating at a European level, as is the case with the research networks acting collectively, there has always been an element of competition between the telecom operators which could be exploited. An organization with a network covering several European countries and which has sufficient capacity to support the collection/distribution of traffic to/from the United States could choose in which country to terminate its transatlantic connection. Although the national telecoms operators' charges were universally high, there could still be a significant difference between the cheapest and the most expensive. PTT Telecom, for example, set its prices at a level which made the Netherlands an attractive endpoint for transatlantic circuits.

For many years, the capacity of transatlantic connections was a major bottleneck and caused serious congestion, resulting in poor performance for user applications. It often happened that when a new circuit was brought into service, it would be running with greater than 90% load within a few days or even hours. It was also the case in the early days of the WWW when the United States was a major source of information; general Web traffic formed a high proportion of the total transatlantic load. This was particularly the case for Central European countries where there were few local or national information servers for several years. During the early 1990s there was an imbalance between the traffic loads in two directions across the Atlantic: the average data rate in the West-East direction was generally three or four times that from Europe to the United States. Nowadays the balance is much more even when calculated over a 24-hour period; the traffic patterns do, unsurprisingly, vary during the day, peaking in the east-west direction during European working hours and in the other direction when Americans are at work.

The imbalance of traffic flows in the early days of transatlantic communications tended to reinforce the inherent United States view that the Internet is an American artifact and that people from other continents are welcome to use it as long as they pay the full cost of connecting to it. European efforts to negotiate more equitable cost-sharing arrangements were unsuccessful for many years, and progress was only made after Europe's own telecoms pricing became more rational in the years following liberalization.

The first transatlantic connections, open for general use by European researchers, were those provided by EARN and its links to BITNET in the United States. DARPA supported a link between ARPAnet and Norway and the United Kingdom with an onward connection to INRIA (Institut National de Recherche en Informatique et Automatique) in France, but the use of these links was restricted to people involved in specific research projects. UUCPnet, which was used mainly by the computer science community, had a link from Amsterdam. The first connection between a European research network and the Internet in the United States was made by NORDUnet in November 1988 shortly after its commissioning as a star network configuration centered on Stockholm and in advance of its first connection internationally in Europe to SARA (Stichting Academisch Rekencentrum Amsterdam) in Amsterdam in January 1989.

In the early 1990s, individual research networks made their own arrangements for United States connectivity and adopted different strategies which depended on the amount of money they could make available, the charging regime in their country, and their choice of either a European service provider or a United States partner organization.

When DANTE was set up in July 1993 and took responsibility for EMPB, the network had no connection to the United States. In order to establish its credibility as an organization capable of providing the full range of international services required by its research network customers, including the handling of both research and so-called "commodity" traffic to and from the United States, DANTE needed to make transatlantic capacity available quickly. The United States research networks were forbidden by their funding agencies from handling commodity traffic – but this was well understood by everyone involved – so connection to one of the United States ISPs was essential both for handling traffic to and from commercial organizations in the United States and because of their ability to offer global connectivity, that is, the ability to route any IP packet to the correct destination anywhere in the world. The ISPs were prepared to offer these services, but took the view that their customers should pay the full cost of making a connection to a United States PoP as well as their network access charges. The United States research networks took a more cooperative approach, at least in theory; the CCIRN had adopted a policy of equitable cost-sharing between the organizations responsible for each end of any transatlantic link in 1990. In practice, however, they were not rushing to join forces with DANTE if that involved a financial commitment on their part. In the absence of any willingness on the part of possible United States partners to pay even part of the cost, DANTE felt obliged to pay the full cost of the links itself. This represented a serious drain on the already limited working capital of the company, which in turn limited its freedom to develop new services

Table 9.1 Transatlantic Links (February 1994).

	EU end Location	Responsible	US end Location	Responsible	Speed (kbps)
1	Stockholm	NORDUnet	Washington	NSF	2048
2	London	JNT	Washington	DARPA, NASA, NSF	2048
3	Duesseldorf	DFN	Princeton	ESNET	512
4	Amsterdam	DANTE	Washington	DANTE	2048
5	Paris	RENATER	Washington	NSF	1536
6	Geneva	DANTE	Washington	DANTE	1536
7	Geneva	L3	New York	L3/ESNET	512
8	Bologna	INFN	Chicago	ESNET	512

during the first months and years of its existence. Many people outside the United States were unhappy with this situation and wanted to see a fairer system of dividing the total cost between all the countries that benefited.

In February 1994, the set of transatlantic links used by the research community was as shown in Table 9.1.

The London-Washington link was split by TDM equipment into three channels so that capacity could be guaranteed to each of the three United States agencies involved. The L3 link was available only to participants in the L3 experiment at the LEP collider at CERN. There were also two links connecting NASA and ESA sites but they were not available for general use.

There was a significant development in May 1994, when the United States NSF offered to make a contribution to the costs of new capacity to NORDUnet, France and the United Kingdom. This offer was warmly welcomed by many people who saw the new connections as a means of promoting the use of TCP/IP in Europe. Others were concerned by the way in which NSF had selected its partners without consulting other European organizations. The move was seen by these people as at best unhelpful and at worst United States interference in European affairs, which set back a European campaign for equitable cost-sharing by several years. An NSF claim that it was providing connections to Europe as a whole could hardly be justified by a configuration which offered no connection to Germany, Italy and Spain as well as a number of smaller European countries.

Although the added capacity resulting from the NSF action was significant at the time, it did not come anywhere near to satisfying the inherent demand from European users, and the research networks all made determined efforts to increase the capacity available to them.

DANTE's introduction of its second United States circuit in February 1994 had brought the aggregate capacity of all the circuits between European research networks and organizations in the United States to 10.5 Mbps. During the following five years, the aggregate capacity increased rapidly to 219 Mbps in August 1997 and to just over 1.2 Gbps in March 1999, with a further addition of 332 Mbps planned for installation during the course of that year.

This rapid expansion took place within a set of constraints that applied throughout this period and was characterized by the following:

- Each research network acquired its capacity according to its own priorities and requirements. The capacity might be supplied directly by a telecoms operator, by sharing with a neighboring research network, by using a shared service provided by DANTE or Ebone, or some combination of these.
- The principal criterion in its choice of circuit provider and circuit capacity was cost, with resilience as an important secondary factor.
- Compared to international circuits within Europe, availability of capacity was not a real problem. Transatlantic circuit costs were lower than the cost of international circuits within Europe but were still high. The capacity selected by each research network was more likely to be limited by what it could afford to spend than by capacity availability.
- Everyone understood that prices were being reduced rapidly and that this would continue for as far ahead as anyone could see. Nobody made commitments lasting longer than 12 months, and there were frequent changes of supplier, as each research network selected the best available replacement deal when its current contract expired.
- There was competition between providers of the United States half-links, but it was limited by the organizational structure which had been set up to install and operate transatlantic cables.
- Each group of cables was owned by a separate company. Manufacture and installation of the cable would typically be funded and managed by a company set up for the purpose by a consortium of telecoms operators. These and other telecoms operators would buy 25-year leases on circuit capacity which they would then use to support their services to customers. As in the case of international terrestrial circuits within Europe, customers would normally lease two half-circuits, one from an operator at each end.

"Acceptable use" was an important factor in each research network selection of the best option. Funding bodies on both sides of the Atlantic had policies which allowed them to fund services which supported R&E activities, but forbade the carriage of commercial traffic or any other form of subsidy of commercial activities. This led to the question: what is a commercial activity? Even if you succeed in establishing criteria for labeling a packet stream as commercial or non-commercial, how can you make sure that the commercial traffic does not violate the funding bodies' conditions for supporting the service? (Nowadays it is generally accepted that any traffic which has a research or education institution as its source or destination is considered to be non-commercial).

In order to provide global connectivity to their users (i.e. the possibility of communication with a device anywhere in the world which has a valid IP address), the research networks (and DANTE) were obliged to subscribe to one of the top level services which hold routing tables covering the whole Internet. For a long time, the service providers offered access only in the United States, and commercial traffic had to be carried across the Atlantic on an expensive United States link. In many cases, the United States half-circuit would be provided by one of the companies that was also a top-level ISP, and the cost of network access including global connectivity was covered by a single charge. In this way, the European research networks paid the whole cost of transatlantic connectivity with no contribution from the United States side.

When 34 and 45 Mbps circuits were introduced, some of the smaller research networks which had been using dedicated circuits could not justify the acquisition of a single 34–45 Mbps circuit. The cost in absolute terms was higher, even though the price-per-unit of capacity was much lower and the research network would also be paying for capacity which it did not use. This provided an incentive for the research network to make use of DANTE's shared service.

In order to do this some means of transporting the traffic between the research network and the European end point of one of DANTE's transatlantic circuits was also necessary. Technically, it would have been simple to install a circuit between the research network and a DANTE PoP which also housed the end of a transatlantic link but the circuit would have been an international one and with prices at the pre-liberalization levels the financial advantage of sharing transatlantic capacity would be lost. An alternative was to use the European network for transit to the most convenient location. Those research networks which had their own transatlantic connectivity were, not unreasonably, unwilling to increase the capacity (and cost) of the European network in ways which gave them no benefit. However, they did agree that the European network could be used for transit of United States traffic, as long as there remained sufficient capacity to handle all European traffic with no degradation of performance and all costs associated with the use of the European network for transit were covered by the research networks which used the service.

ATM technology proved to be extremely useful in managing traffic issues. Research and commercial traffic were carried on different virtual circuits and kept separate. Capacity could be made available for research traffic, even in the case of overload of the virtual circuit carrying commercial traffic. Each research network using the service could be guaranteed the capacity it had paid for. There was even a performance gain resulting from the setting up of a single virtual circuit between the research network's access port to the European network and the access port on a DANTE router in the United States which connected the commercial service provider with no IP router being visible in between.

At times, DANTE was able to offer transatlantic capacity to research networks at prices which were lower than they could get from the same suppliers themselves. The cost of the European half-link was the same but DANTE was able to take advantage of significant volume discounts by acquiring multiple half-links on the western side from the same supplier. At one point before the introduction of 34 and 45 Mbps circuits, DANTE was operating seventeen 1.5 Mbps circuits between New York and four different locations in Europe.

During the earlier part of this period, the connection of the transatlantic circuit to one or more of the United States research networks and to an ISP in the United States was handled by the provider of the United States circuit, as part of its overall service. As time went on and the complexity of the arrangements on the United States side increased, it became attractive for DANTE to establish its own PoP in the United

States. This brought the added difficulty – compared with installing a PoP in Europe – of managing the planning, installation, operation and maintenance of equipment located thousands of kilometers away, but eventually the advantages of being able to manage both ends of the set of transatlantic links as a single logical system and the ability to offer housing and support services to research networks which had their own transatlantic circuits outweighed the extra difficulties and the case for the installation of a PoP was made.

In June 1997, there was a move towards United States funding of transatlantic capacity when the NSF issued a "solicitation" (equivalent to an EC Call for Proposals) for the provision of intercontinental links as part of its HPIIS program. From a European perspective, there were potential difficulties with this solicitation: there was a short deadline (August 1997) for the submission of proposals, the funding which was likely to be available for transatlantic capacity was small compared with the expenditure that was already being incurred by the European research networks and, most seriously, it followed United States Government procurement procedures – not unreasonably from a United States point of view but taking no account of the policies and organizational structures established in Europe. A response which directly matched European requirements and expectations risked being rejected because it was not in accordance with the NSF specification. A particular difficulty was that any links established as a result of the solicitation would be connected at their United States end to the vBNS and that vBNS access rules would apply. These rules restricted access to organizations which could demonstrate their involvement in advanced research requiring the support of high capacity network services. vBNS should not be used as a transit network and under no circumstances was it to be used to carry commodity traffic. The European research networks nevertheless agreed that they should submit a coordinated response and mandated DANTE to act on their behalf.

The first hurdle to be overcome was the requirement of NSF that the organization providing the formal response must be based in the United States. The University of Illinois at Chicago (UIC) agreed to play this role in respect of the European submission, subcontracting the bulk of the work to DANTE which took responsibility for coordinating the relevant European activity (including reporting).

Even though the response submitted jointly by DANTE and the UIC recognized the mismatch between the European and United States situations and included proposals on how to deal with them, it was judged by NSF's evaluators to be non-conformant on the grounds that it did not meet the requirement that there should be some selection of the European sites that were permitted to access vBNS. Discussion with NSF officials of alternative ways forward lasted for several months but failed to find a solution which would allow all of the European research networks to make use of the planned transatlantic capacity and the proposal prepared by DANTE made no further progress.

The fundamental mismatch between European and United States procedures was eventually overcome by both sides agreeing to acquire and share equal amounts of transatlantic capacity and each side using its own procurement procedures for the acquisition. It would be several years before this arrangement was put into place;

in the meantime, HPIIS funds were used to support the US-based Euro-Link initiative to improve connectivity between the US and a sub-set of the European research networks.

9.2
The Partnership Period

With several organizations on each side of the Atlantic seeking, in the absence of a common solution, to find their own ways of satisfying their priority requirements it was inevitable that a number of alliances between European and US organizations would be set up. It was equally inevitable that each of these alliances would have its own view of how best to provide the services needed by its members and that this would lead to different technical strategies being adopted. With the passage of time, however, the high degree of commonality of the requirements and the rapidly improving price/performance ratios of data transmission systems meant that more general approaches to the provision of transatlantic connectivity could be adopted.

9.2.1
Euro-Link

In 1999, the NSF HPIIS program funded UIC to facilitate high-performance connections between the United States and Europe. UIC created the Euro-Link consortium with several research networks in Europe and Israel. There were four research networks which were charter members – the Netherlands' SURFnet, the Nordic countries' NORDUnet, France's RENATER and Israel's IUCC – with CERN joining mid-year as the fifth member.

The Euro-Link funding covered a period of five years. Initially, UIC used it to contribute to the expenses incurred by European research networks connecting to the United States. However, by 2001, the cost of transatlantic networking was coming down, the demand for bandwidth was increasing and it was time to look for new ways of matching available capacity with demand.

The dramatic increase in affordable transatlantic bandwidth became evident when the iGrid (international grid) workshop took place in Amsterdam in 2002. Participants supplied an aggregate capacity of 25 Gbps into Amsterdam (compared to the 155 Mbps connection between Amsterdam and Chicago the year before!) This capacity was provided by SURFnet (2.5 Gbps between Amsterdam and Chicago, and 2.5 Gbps between Amsterdam and CERN), IEEAF (Internet Educational Equal Access Foundation, 10 Gbps between Amsterdam and New York), and Level3 (10 Gbps between Amsterdam and Chicago), plus additional bandwidth from EU DataTAG, Research and technological development for a Data TransAtlantic Grid (2.5 Gbps between CERN and Chicago).

In parallel with these increases in available bandwidth, there were major developments in the technology available to exploit them; the first steps could be taken towards the use of optical networking on an intercontinental scale.

9.2.2
GLIF - Global Lambda Integrated Facility

"Lambdas" are considered by many to represent the next major phase in the network evolution. Lambda networking is based on the use of different wavelengths of light, "lambdas", to make separate connections between two end points connected by optical fiber. Since it is possible to transmit several wavelengths on one fiber with no interference between them, each user community can have its own individual network of lambdas and several user networks of different configurations can share an underlying set of fibers.

As in the early days of the Internet, experimental work and the development of new innovations is fostered by research networks. The history of global lambda collaboration began in September 2001, when SURFnet, TERENA, Internet2, CANARIE, US/HPIIS, CERN, NORDUnet and others organized the first LambdaGrid Workshop in Amsterdam. By summer 2002, the first research-only lambda was set up between the Dutch NetherLight and the American StarLight in Chicago.

At the third annual Global LambdaGrid Workshop, which was arranged adjacent to the NORDUnet conference in Reykjavik, Iceland in August 2003, it was agreed to continue the collaboration under the name GLIF (Global lambda integrated facility). GLIF is a worldwide virtual organization that aims to promote the paradigm of lambda networking. The participants in GLIF are national research and education networking organizations, consortia and institutions that, having acquired enough bandwidth for their production traffic, have spare capacity which can be used for scientific application and middleware development purposes. Dark fiber, with its ability to carry many more lambdas than are required for production traffic, usually has the surplus capacity needed for development purposes.

GLIF collaboration seems to grow every year: in 2004 the GLIF meeting in Nottingham, England, organized by JISC (Joint Information Systems Committee) and JANET, was arranged by invitation only to emphasize that it was a "workshop" and not a "conference". Sixty people were invited, including networking managers, engineers, application developers and industry representatives from major institutions all over the world. There was strong interest in future collaboration and GLIF asked TERENA to provide it with secretariat functions on a more permanent basis.

The infrastructure provided by the organizations participating in GLIF consists of a number of GLIF open lightpath exchanges (GOLEs) and lambda connections between them, made available by the GLIF participants. GOLE sites at the end of 2008 included CERN (Geneva), CzechLight (Prague), MoscowLight (Moscow), NetherLight (Amsterdam), NorthernLight (Copenhagen) and UKLight (London) in Europe; AMPATH (Americas path, Miami), MAN LAN (MANhattan LANding, New York), NGIX-East (Next Generation Internet Exchange-East, Washington DC), Pacific Wave (Los Angeles, Seattle and Sunnyvale) and StarLight (Chicago) in the United States; SouthernLight (Sao Paulo) in South America; and, HKOEP (Hong Kong Open Exchange Portal, Hong Kong), KRLight (Daejeon), T-LEX (Tokyo Lambda Exchange, Tokyo) and TaiwanLight (Taipei) in Asia.

9.2.3
TransLight/StarLight

In 2003, to meet the ever-increasing demand for production networking and to increase capacity between the United States and Europe, Euro-Link funds were used to purchase a 10 Gbps transatlantic circuit between Chicago and Amsterdam, in partnership with SURFnet. This circuit provided the United States and European research and education communities with both packet-switched routed paths for many-to-many usage; and circuit-switched lightpaths for high-speed, few-to-few usage. That is, half the capacity was configured as a routed infrastructure for Internet2 and GÉANT interconnection, and half was configured as a switched infrastructure to support LambdaGrid application and middleware experiments between national research networks that had lightpaths connected to StarLight or NetherLight.[1] The Euro-Link organizers considered this an experiment, called "TransLight", consisting of a routed/switched network architecture and a governance model for how the United States and international networking collaborators could work together.

In September 2004, as more countries started sharing bandwidth with one another, TransLight participants dissolved its governance body in favor of having GLIF assume this role.

NSF funding of Euro-Link (including, the TransLight experiment during the final two years of the award) continued through 2005, when NSF replaced HPIIS with its International Research Network Connections (IRNC) program and awarded a new five-year grant for the 2005–2010 period to UIC to establish TransLight/StarLight.

TransLight/StarLight's mission is to best serve established United States and European production science. It does this by supporting scientists, engineers and educators who have persistent large-flow, real-time, or other advanced application requirements. It provides networking and supporting infrastructure to connect research networks in the United States to their counterparts in Europe, as well as supplementing bandwidth provided by other countries.

The transition from Euro-Link to TransLight/StarLight as the NSF HPIIS program was phased out and was replaced by the NSF IRNC program was one of evolution, maintaining the most diverse possible connectivity among international networks, matching capability to each research and education community served. Hybrid network services are necessary if e-science is to advance. TransLight/StarLight uses lambdas to advantage, using packets when expedient, and dedicated circuits when necessary. To show the advantages afforded by network diversity, the iGrid 2005 event, held in September 2005 in San Diego, California, demonstrated the latest advances in scientific collaboration and discovery which had been made possible by GLIF partners and research teams.

Since its inception in 2005, TransLight/StarLight provides two connections between the United States and Europe for production science: a routed connection

---

1) Euro-Link also contributed support for the EU DataTAG link between Chicago and Geneva, managed by CERN.

that connected the United States Internet2 network, the National LambdaRail (NLR) network, and the DoE's ESnet to the pan-European GÉANT2 (between MAN LAN in New York and the GÉANT2 exchange in Amsterdam), and a switched connection (between StarLight in Chicago and NetherLight in Amsterdam) that is part of the LambdaGrid fabric being created by participants of GLIF. These links are paid for by NSF, and procured and operated by UIC and SURFnet, thus complementing the funding by DANTE of the other transatlantic links.

In July 2006, the StarLight facility in Chicago and the PNWGP (Pacific NorthWest Gigabit Point of Presence) in Seattle were directly connected through a 10 Gbps Ethernet lightpath, called TransLight. The connection, donated by Cisco Systems and deployed by NLR, provides more direct connections between Europe, the United States and Asia, as needed. In addition, Internet2, NLR, ESnet and Canada's CANARIE network all connect to the major United States exchanges, notably those in New York (MAN LAN), Chicago (StarLight) and Seattle (PNWGP). These locations support the vast majority of international connections to the United States and form the fabric by which most international networks peer and exchange traffic with North American networks.

TransLight/StarLight's approach is based not just on backbone connectivity, but on end-to-end connectivity and activism in advanced networking and applications. It has a proven track record in attracting new technologies and stimulating collaborations, especially among leading domain scientists at end sites.

Besides TransLight/StarLight, the NSF IRNC program supports four additional international networking initiatives: network links between the United States and Latin/South America (WHREN); between the United States and northern hemisphere countries around the world, notably Canada, China, Korea, the Netherlands, the Nordic Countries, Russia and the United States, called GLORIAD; between the United States and the Asia-Pacific region (TransPac2); and support for a distributed open exchange along the United States west coast, from Seattle to San Diego, to interconnect North American, Asian, Australian and Mexican/South American links (TransLight/Pacific Wave).

9.2.4
GLIF, Grids and the Future

TransLight/StarLight's switched infrastructure is a United States component of GLIF (Global lambda integrated facility). GLIF is a virtual organization of networking infrastructure, network engineering, system integration, middleware, applications, that has been organized to accomplish real science and engineering; the GLIF community shares a common vision of building a new grid-computing paradigm, in which the central architectural element is optical networks, not computers, to support this decade's most demanding e-science applications. Grid applications ride on dynamically configured networks based on optical wavelengths concurrent with normal Internet paths for the remaining traffic mix.

Only through deployment of an integrated research and production infrastructure at network Layers 1 through 3 will the various technical communities be able to address large-scale and complex systems research in peer-to-peer systems, grids, collaboratories, peering, routing, network management, network monitoring, E2E QoS, adaptive and *ad hoc* networks, fault tolerance, high availability, and critical infrastructure to support advanced applications and grids.

September 11th
The terrorist attack on New York City on September 11 2001 had immediate repercussions many thousands of miles away. The people in Europe who were affected suffered only minor inconvenience compared with the loss of life and serious injuries in New York City, but people still felt the impact in a minor way. The effect on the research networks' services provides a small example of the disturbance to their normal activity.

At the time of the attack, DANTE's transatlantic connectivity was provided by T-Systems, a subsidiary of Deutsche Telekom (DT), in the form of a protected SDH circuit between Frankfurt and the DANTE PoP at 25 Broadway, New York. The New York end of the circuit included a "local loop" between the DT primary PoP at 60 Hudson St (which acted as a switching center for many transatlantic circuits) and 25 Broadway, DT's secondary PoP. This local loop was carried on a diversely routed metropolitan ring passing through several buildings which housed interconnections with other telecoms operators and with major customers. The circuit configurations of the research networks which had their own transatlantic connectivity were similar.

In conformance with the SDH specification for protected circuits, the working path was complemented by a second circuit for protection which followed a different geographic path between the two end points. If a problem was detected on the working path, the management system would automatically switch from working to protection path in less than 50 ms. It so happened that the local loop of the working path for DANTE was carried by a cable which passed through the basement of the World Trade Centre North Tower and was destroyed when the building collapsed. The protection path automatically restored connectivity; however, this circuit was routed through the basement of World Trade Centre South Tower and all connectivity was lost when this building was destroyed.

25 Broadway is fairly close to Ground Zero and was inside the exclusion zone set up to control access to the disaster area, and, against expectations, the equipment it houses was undamaged. When the power grid to the area was destroyed, battery systems provided power until the back-up power generator started up. Engineers and operations staff already in the building were able to start work immediately to review the impact to their hosted services, and to work out ways of repairing them as quickly as possible. Unknown to the staff, more problems were to come.

When the area was evacuated, operations staff were faced with a dilemma. They could leave the building and the area along with other evacuees, not knowing when they would be able to return, or they could stay at work to help with the recovery process, support for the emergency services having top priority. Most chose the latter option – and found that they had to live for several days with the building's vending machines as their only source of food and drink.

The stock of diesel oil used to fuel the generator was sufficient for only 70 hours of operation. Telecommunications services were given some priority over other activities because of their importance in managing the rescue and recovery operations that were going on. Exercising this priority, the site management was able to arrange refueling before stocks ran out, giving the site the capacity to continue operations autonomously for a further four days.

Unfortunately, there was a further interruption when the water pumps for the generators at 25 Broadway failed because the air filters had become blocked by the dust and debris which covered the area. It took some time before spare parts could be flown in and specialist engineers could get authorization to enter the site to carry out the cleaning and repairs necessary to restart operation. However, it was not long before a second generator and reserve fuel tanks were installed so that the PoP could again function.

There was hectic activity in Europe as well as in New York to re-establish connections using previously spare capacity and, given the urgency of the situation, to bring into service circuits which were already planned but not yet operational. The telecoms operators chose cooperation over competition and worked closely together, to do the best job they could to restore services to customers and to keep information flowing.

Operations staff found an alternative route between 25 Broadway and 60 Hudson Street which enabled them to restore DANTE's lines. Some of the research networks which had their own transatlantic capacity to alternative locations were still able to use a previously established back-up route. A supplier of transatlantic connectivity to one of the research networks rushed to complete the installation of a new STM-4 circuit and made this new capacity available to other network operators, with the result that other research networks could again communicate with the United States using the European network for transit. As DANTE had lost its connection to the commodity Internet in the United States, another PNO offered to provide global Internet access from London (the offer was not taken up because DANTE's normal connectivity was quickly restored).

The result of this cooperative activity was that all European research networks had stable United States/global connectivity in place within three days of the attack, although the situation in some cases was somewhat precarious. Given the hurried nature of the reconstruction, several component circuits had not undergone the normal pre-operation testing and had no form of back-up if they failed.

Normal documentation procedures were by-passed, so we shall never know how new fiber routes appeared, where critical equipment came from, or who made what changes in configurations. In all, this incident provided an excellent example of how effective and dedicated people can be when times get tough and they are offered a genuine opportunity to help and make a difference.

10
A European Achievement

This chapter is to some extent a summary of what has been covered so far. It concentrates on the successes that have been achieved (between the numerous failures already highlighted) and how the network is continually moving forward to provide the connectivity required by the end users. It looks at some of the services currently being supplied and the specialist equipment used to do this, some of which was specially built. It also looks at how the research establishment, as opposed to commercial operators, was responsible for much of this.

10.1
GÉANT

As was the case with earlier generations of European research networks, planning of its eventual replacement started soon after TEN-155 came into service. Taking into account the conclusions of a requirements action group (RAG), the EC's publication of its Fifth Framework programme for the year 2000 included two topics, "High-Level Requirements for Broadband Interconnection of National Research, Education and Training Networks" (RN1) and Test-beds (RN2) with a March 31 2000 deadline to submit proposals.

The research networks requirements to be covered in the proposal to the EC would include implementation of a 2.5 Gbps "core" as soon as possible, continuity with TEN-155, and using capacities measured in tens of Gbps before the end of the Framework program in 2000. There should be support for "disruptive" testing, that is, experimentation with low-level services which could put an operational service at risk. There should be connections to all the countries covered by the EC's Sixth Framework program and EU funding would now be available to Switzerland and Cyprus.

This GÉANT network would be composed of a set of core nodes linked by Gbps circuits using IP as the transport protocol, probably carried over SDH. ATM interfaces operating at these speeds were not available (and would not become available). Further development work to provide guaranteed quality of end-to-end service would still be needed despite the expected abundance of bandwidth. Intercontinental circuits and some campus facilities were still likely to become bottlenecks. The provision

A History of International Research Networking. Edited by Howard Davies and Beatrice Bressan
Copyright © 2010 WILEY-VCH Verlag GmbH & Co. KGaA, Weinheim
ISBN: 978-3-527-32710-2

of quality of service management across multiple management domains was seen to be particularly important.

The set of core nodes would also support the European distributed access, that is, interconnections with networks in other world regions could be made at the most convenient GÉANT nodes, independently of traffic flows to individual research networks. The choice of transmission technology would depend on suppliers' offers in an open procurement. An issue that was discussed in the early planning stages was whether to use the consortium agreement that had been developed for QUANTUM. This agreement included provisions for its re-use in future projects, with the specific aim of eliminating the need to spend time and effort in creating a new agreement for each new project that the research networks wished to carry out. Adding new members to the consortium and dealing with the consequences of members leaving the consortium were both covered. There was a view, expressed strongly by SURFnet in particular, that the existing consortium agreement required major changes. Making such changes would inevitably take time, and after long discussion a majority of the members of the Policy Committee felt that the best way forward was to make use of the existing consortium agreement and, in parallel with the procurement and implementation of GÉANT, to work on improvements and preparation of a new agreement. When the chairman tested the level of support for this proposal, the result of the show of hands was 17 in favor and 1 against, which gave an ominous warning of difficulties that lay ahead. The following meeting of the Policy Committee put to the vote (using the weighted voting scheme specified in the consortium agreement) a formal resolution to invite the research networks which qualified for participation in any EU-funded project, but which were not yet members of the consortium, to join. The result was 16 research networks (with 211 votes) in favor, 1 research network (12 votes) against and no abstentions. Since the consortium agreement required unanimity for certain actions that included the acceptance of new parties, the resolution failed. This decision had a number of consequences, none of them positive.

Besides the effort required on the part of the research networks in setting up the new consortium agreement, many questions from the EC and other involved bodies as to why one research network was not prepared to go along with the others had to be answered: was there a potentially difficult issue which could lead to failure of the project? Representatives of the research networks which would have been invited to join the consortium felt a sense of rejection; they had also the difficult task of explaining to their colleagues and superiors at home why they were not allowed to join and why they seemed to be treated like second-class citizens. They also had to deal with the unspoken but inevitable question as to why they had failed to get their country into the premier league of EU-funded projects and the implied reflection on their competence.

There were also consequences for technical planning. In the initial stages, plans were made on the assumption that SURFnet would eventually return to the fold. Contingency plans were made in case this did not happen, since the installation of one of the proposed core nodes in any country could not be justified if there was no participation from the country's research network. As time passed with no change in the situation, the planning was switched; a revised configuration design was based on the assumption that SURFnet would not be connected – though with a contingency plan in case it changed its mind at the last-minute. Despite being put under pressure from several directions (presentations showing a map of Europe with the participating countries highlighted on a map of Europe with a small hole in the middle), it was only two months before the start of the service that SURFnet abandoned its lone campaign, continuing to insist that it wanted to join the consortium for this project only, without any commitment to continue as a member if any further project was undertaken.

The general view amongst the other consortium members was that circumstances under which a research network could opt out were being built into the EC contract for GÉANT so there would be no real problem if any research network wished to leave the consortium because it disagreed with what was being done within the project; for example, the first deliverable under the contract was to be a detailed specification of the network to be implemented; a research network unhappy with the proposal would have the option of leaving the consortium and the EC contract at that point.

(It was rumored at the time that the formal project manager, who is responsible amongst other things for all communications between the consortium and the EC, had to spend 20% of his time over a six-month period to deal with different aspects of the affair. These rumors have never been denied).

While all this organizational confusion was being sorted out, the technical and administrative work associated with the procurement and implementation of a new network service proceeded in parallel. By now, the effects of telecommunications liberalization were obvious. It was well known that there were many competing suppliers of transmission capacity between the main centers of European economic activity, namely Amsterdam, Frankfurt, London and Paris. What was less obvious was what the telecoms operators would be prepared to offer in terms of circuit capacity, how many newcomers large and small would take advantage of liberalization of the market, and to what extent competition had reached the more peripheral areas of Europe.

The ideal solution would seem to be one based on dedicated fiber and wavelengths, but the tender had to answer a number of questions: is dedicated fiber available (throughout)? Is equipment to manage wavelengths ready for operational service? Is the equipment affordable? For what length of time would the telecoms operators be prepared to make firm commitments in a rapidly changing market?

A Call for Expressions of Interest was issued in May 2000 and generated 88 responses. An Invitation to Tender covering connectivity (with a target of at least 2.5 Gbps between 8 locations), PoP housing and facilities management was issued on July 7 2000, with a September 29 2000 deadline for responses. The specification of requirements for transmission capacity was left open and, since TEN-155 contracts continued till November 30 2001, the Invitation to Tender indicated a December 1 2001 target start date for the new service.

Forty four tenders were received, of which 29 offered bandwidth, 17 offered network management and 37 offered PoP housing. Of the 29 bandwidth offers, 12 came from pan-European carriers, 6 from regional carriers and one from a systems integrator. Twelve offers of PoP housing came from research networks. It was immediately clear that the initial bandwidth target (2.5 Gbps in 8 countries in 2001) could be met; indeed, it would be possible to set up the initial configuration of 6 nodes linked by 10 Gbps circuits and a further 3 connected at 2.5 Gbps. On the other hand, it was also clear that devising an equitable charging scheme would be even more difficult than for previous networks, since the disparity between the cost of connection in the cheapest countries in Europe and the cost in the more expensive countries had widened even further.

The total number of circuits offered was over a thousand and the evaluation of tenders for connectivity was therefore complex. The potential suppliers were divided into three groups; those that offered pan-European coverage, those that covered several countries in one region of Europe (for example Central Europe), and those that offered a single circuit or just one or two circuits to peripheral countries. The factors taken into account in the connectivity evaluation were: price, reach, upgradability, robustness of infrastructure, physical presence of infrastructure, and financial viability of the supplier.

The first three of these factors are conventional and well understood; ownership of the infrastructure had not previously been an issue but liberalization had introduced new complications. For example, a small and under-capitalized company is free to make offers in competition with established operators, but with fewer resources to support its proposal. For instance, one operator might offer three circuits on separate fibers along the sides of an ABC triangle, while a second operator might also offer three circuits, AB, BC and AC, the last of these being implemented by taking two more AB and BC circuits and connecting them together at the switching center at B. Since the AB and BC circuits share the same fibers with the AC circuit, a line-break will have much more serious consequences. As another example, assuming that telecoms operator A owns ducts and fibers and sells capacity to operator B and that A and B then make competing offers to an end-user, all other things being equal, the end-user does better to contract with operator A, since operator A will have the responsibility of dealing with incidents that effect its fiber system and operator B will be dependent on the ability of A as its supplier to deal with the incident.

The selection of PoP locations was also complicated and had to wait until conclusions of the connectivity evaluation were available, since the choice was based mainly on the total lifetime cost, including space rental (if any), the cost of local loops to extend international circuits to the PoP, and local loops to extend the research network's configuration to the PoP site. These costs at each location were very dependent on the possibilities offered by the chosen connectivity suppliers. Although there was some commonality between sites, each country had to be considered separately.

The end result of the tender evaluation was that COLT Telecommunications was awarded a contract for seven circuits linking six countries, Telia was contracted to connect the Nordic countries and Deutsche Telekom was awarded a contract for circuits linking central European countries

A separate router tender was won by Didata, a sales agent for Juniper. There was some discussion amongst the research networks as to whether the opportunity should be taken to start off with a 10 Gbps core immediately.

The advantages of this option were:

- It would avoid the need for an early upgrade with its associated migration and the upheaval this would cause.
- It should solve the capacity problem for quite a while.
- Although the cost would be higher, it looked affordable and the 10 Gbps offers gave reasonable value for money compared with 2.5 Gbps.
- It would provide a justification for a longer contract period.
- It would put European research networking at the forefront of global developments and provide the research networks with material that they could use to justify their funding.

The disadvantages were:

- Added cost for unnecessary capacity
- Riskier technology (though the risk was not judged to be high)
- Less (connectivity) supplier experience
- More limited choice of router equipment
- Less (router) supplier experience, and, in general, a greater risk of technical problems

In the end, the balance came down on the side of the 10 Gbps option.

It is noteworthy that while the three principal contractors supplied over 99% of the aggregate capacity, the three contracts represented only 70% of the total annual cost.

The charging algorithm for the research networks was eventually based on one with two components, with 60% of the total cost being shared according to access capacity independently of geography, and 40% based on the cost of connection to each country. The 60/40 split was devised empirically in preparing a scheme which was fair to all the participants and which allowed changes to be made – for example to a particular research network's access capacity – with all other research networks charges remaining stable. Implementation of the network was largely straightforward and included the usual number of scares and nail-biting moments when news of some unexpected problem was announced.

The contract with KPN/Qwest for services used in TEN-155 expired on November 30 2001, and KPN warned that the contract with their suppliers would be terminated unless DANTE gave three months notice of its wish to extend the contract period. The decision to stick with the planned start date for GÉANT of December 1 2001 put pressure on both the research networks and the GÉANT suppliers.

The implementation of 19 PoPs, 37 international trunk circuits and 45 access connections to national and other networks during the three month period September-November 2001 proceeded according to plan except for two problems. First, it proved extremely difficult to import routers into both Hungary and Poland; in the latter case, the router was delivered more than four months after the contracted delivery date. Secondly, contingency measures had to be invoked when suppliers failed to deliver SDH connectivity to Greece and Portugal on time.

All of the research networks were nevertheless moved to GÉANT before the November 30 2001 deadline for switching off TEN-155. The aggregate trunk capacity when the service started was more than 130 Gbps and the network was carrying more than 1 Petabyte of data per month by the end of 2002. After some (relatively minor) upgrades, the network configuration in April 2004 was as shown in Figure 10.1.

Much more attention was given to satisfying user requirements than with earlier networks. The development of performance development tools and techniques which could be used to guarantee quality of service end-to-end (i.e. across the local area and research networks that transport traffic to and from the access ports of the international inter-research network) continued. A "Premium IP" service was piloted in collaboration with a number of user groups which required guaranteed service quality in terms of parameters such as delivery delay and jitter. A virtual PERT (performance enhancement and response team) was made available to support the users of GÉANT – from over 3500 R&E institutions in 34 countries – by fine-tuning network performance and troubleshooting performance issues.

The GÉANT infrastructure was used to support other telecommunications projects. The most important of these was 6NET which was set up to investigate the operational issues associated with an IPv6 network.

The version of the IP protocol in common use is IPv4 which suffers from a shortage of address space. Although in theory the IPv4 address length of 32 bits provides roughly 4 billion addresses, address allocation procedures (especially those used in the early days of the Internet) which involve handing a large block of addresses to a single organization are very wasteful. As the Internet has grown, there have been a number of address-related issues such as the size of routing tables when the possibility of further expansion has been threatened.

The long-term solution to these addressing problems has been the specification of a new version of the Internet protocol, IPv6, which provides for an address length of 128 bits (plus a number of other improvements on IPv4 relating to performance and security) but its introduction into service required a major effort. The idea of closing down the global IPv4 Internet one day and starting up a new IPv6 Internet is unthinkable so, in addition to checking that a closed network based on IPv6 will work correctly (including interworking between the implementations of different equipment suppliers), a number of complex issues need to be addressed in order to manage the transition: routers and network interfaces to servers and user computers must be able to handle both IPv4 and IPv6 traffic streams simultaneously, it must be possible to switch a network application from use of IPv4 to IPv6 in an orderly fashion, network applications which support IPv6 must still be accessible to users of Ipv4-based workstations, and so on.

The 6NET project was initiated in 2001 by networking company Cisco Systems, Inc., DANTE and a number of national R&E networks with funding support from the EU. The goal of the project was to operate an international IPv6 network to gain more knowledge and experience of using IPv6 by testing new applications and services and by seeing how IPv6 would work in realistic conditions when used in a large-scale international research network.

The 6NET project started at the beginning of 2002 and continued until July 2005. During these years, the project built an IPv6 network connecting 16 countries, much of it using GÉANT infrastructure. Over 30 partners, both institutions and organizations from the research sector and private companies took part in the project.

GÉANT. The world's most advanced international research network

GÉANT: The Multi-Gigabit pan-European Research Network

Delivered by DANTE for the benefit of European research and education

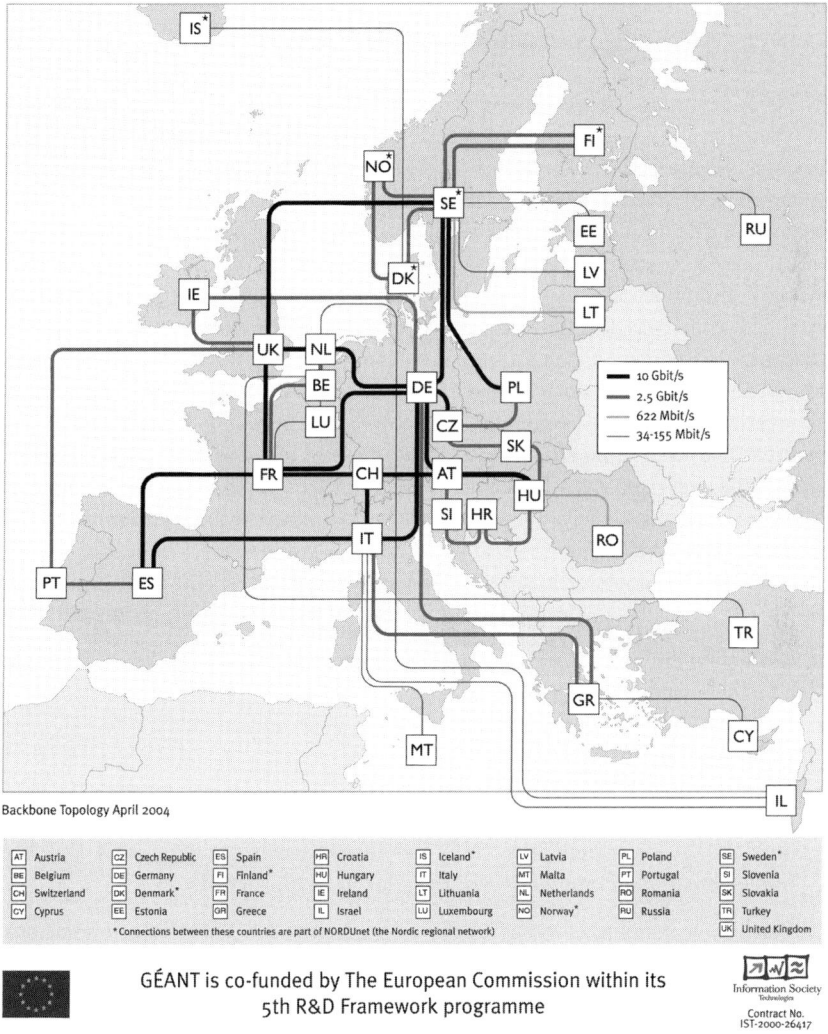

Backbone Topology April 2004

Legend:
- 10 Gbit/s
- 2.5 Gbit/s
- 622 Mbit/s
- 34-155 Mbit/s

AT Austria	CZ Czech Republic	ES Spain	HR Croatia	IS Iceland*	LV Latvia	PL Poland	SE Sweden*
BE Belgium	DE Germany	FI Finland*	HU Hungary	IT Italy	MT Malta	PT Portugal	SI Slovenia
CH Switzerland	DK Denmark*	FR France	IE Ireland	LT Lithuania	NL Netherlands	RO Romania	SK Slovakia
CY Cyprus	EE Estonia	GR Greece	IL Israel	LU Luxembourg	NO Norway*	RU Russia	TR Turkey
							UK United Kingdom

*Connections between these countries are part of NORDUnet (the Nordic regional network)

GÉANT is co-funded by The European Commission within its 5th R&D Framework programme

Information Society Technologies
Contract No. IST-2000-26417

Figure 10.1 GÉANTconfiguration, April 2004. There is a color version of this figure in set at the front of the book.

Because of the large installed base of equipment using IPv4 and the effort required to convert network services to run over IPv6, the coexistence of IPv6 with IPv4 will continue for decades. One of the immediate results of the 6NET investigation, however, was that the experience gained could be applied to GÉANT itself (as well as to many of the research networks) and the GÉANT service was upgraded to a dual-stack (IPv4 and IPv6) service in November 2003.

10.2
GÉANT2, Creation of the First International Hybrid Network

By 2003, a number of trends and requirements had been identified that would determine the future of European research networking for several years to come. One was the emergence of optical networking, which had already been introduced by a number of research networks on a national level. A second was the technical and organizational impact of new and very demanding applications, for example ones which use the combined processing power of two or more specialist high performance computers and which depend on the rapid exchange of large quantities of data. The third was the emerging requirement for end-to-end services, besides ensuring that performance requirements would be met on links which traversed several networks in addition to GÉANT, concerns about the adequacy and consistency of security, privacy and confidentiality features across multiple management domains would have to be addressed. More generally, users were demanding more predictable and guaranteed performance, both for traditional IP and for end-to-end based services. Ways of dealing with these issues provided the background to the planning for GÉANT2.

GÉANT2, the successor to GÉANT, had several objectives:

- First and foremost to provide a multi-Gbps infrastructure with emphasis on developing an "end-to-end" approach to the provision of service across multiple interconnected networks.
- Gaining an improved understanding of user needs and providing direct support to deal with performance issues.
- The traditional network architecture, based purely on IP service, was to evolve to a more flexible structure based on a combination of routing and switching, building on experimentation with the management of light paths and the implementation of emerging standards for network control.

Both the geographic coverage of the network and the global interconnections already in place were to be expanded and enhanced.

10.2.1
The Gestation Period

Planning for GÉANT2 began in the fourth quarter of 2002. A project proposal was submitted to the EU's Sixth Framework Programme in May 2003, even though the EC was not expected to sign a contract until September 2004; expenditure would begin in 2005.

The participating research networks established five working groups to plan particular aspects of the proposal and set up an Editorial Board to ensure consistency and timely delivery of the proposal with DANTE taking responsibility for production of the final text and for project management.

A revised management structure was proposed for GÉANT2. A sub-set of the Policy Committee members, including representatives of DANTE, would form an Executive Committee; a Technical Committee would include leaders of all technical activities.

The GÉANT2 project comprised three main elements:

- The **Service Activities** (SAs) addressed scenarios for the evolution of the network from a service portfolio and an architectural perspective. They focused on procurement, network operations and basic services, end-to-end quality of service and connections to other world regions.
- The **Joint Research Activities** (JRAs) were carried out to provide future network enhancements. Priority areas were performance monitoring, security, bandwidth-on-demand, provision of a test-bed facility, mobility and roaming, and the provision of global connectivity.
- The **Networking Activities** were designed to manage the GÉANT2 project, to coordinate with other projects and disseminate GÉANT2's results. In addition, effort was devoted to improving ways of meeting user demand and supporting research network development.

The GÉANT2 project began in September 2004. The GÉANT and GÉANT2 projects ran in parallel until January 2006, when the building of GÉANT2 Phase One was completed. Thirty-two partners were involved: DANTE, TERENA and 32 research networks (including NORDUnet).

10.2.2
Complex Procurement

The procurement of components of the GÉANT2 network was complex and the tender procedures lasted from December 2003 to July 2005. The intention was to deploy the first international hybrid network which combined routed IP traffic with switched point-to-point circuits. This was quite a challenge as, at the time of planning, 10 Gbps leased capacity was still state-of-the-art. But it was generally recognized that a simple model based on leased connectivity was not one that would fit GÉANT's successor. Therefore a full range of possibilities had to be explored.

A lack of available services had been an issue in the procurement of previous networks but the liberalization of the international telecommunications market in Europe had made it possible for any organization to acquire rights to exploit fiber, bringing significant cost savings. The increasingly widespread availability of different transmission media or methods across Europe (dark fiber, managed fiber, lambdas, SDH, ethernet, etc.) meant that the range of possibilities was very wide.

The procurement of the necessary equipment and services made use of two separate tenders, one dealt with transmission services, the other covered both operational management and the supply of transmission and switching equipment. The DANTE Board of Directors established an Evaluation Committee to assess the proposals, consisting of five experts from the research networks and four experts from within DANTE. The Committee was chaired by Robin Arak (UKERNA).

The first Call for Expressions of Interest with respect to the transmission tender was issued on December 11 2003. Sixty responses were received from major pan-European as well as regional carriers; this was judged to be a good result.

The Tender Invitation was sent out on January 16 2004 and 34 responses were received. There was a limited number of dark fiber offers; they varied considerably in price and quality as well as the ability and experience of suppliers to act as integrator.

Determining the choice of transmission medium and equipment which would be most cost-effective – dark fiber or leased lambda/wavelengths – was complex. Cost models for equipment and a cost sharing algorithm were needed to support an informed recommendation for procurement decisions. The cost model had to project break-even dates (within and beyond the four year project duration) between dark fiber and leased lambda services. Furthermore, the research networks' wish to deploy as much dark fiber as possible, especially in countries hosting the Tier-1 computing centers associated with the LHC being built at CERN had to be taken into consideration.

In February 2005, it was clear which countries would be in the "dark fiber cloud" (i.e. dark fiber would be brought into a PoP serving the research network) and which countries would receive a 10 Gbps service. Contracts for some of the links were ready for approval at the end of March 2005 but as there were more suppliers in GÉANT2 than in GÉANT, more time was needed to complete negotiations with them. In order to manage cost and cash flow issues, it was decided to concentrate first on the acquisition of dark fiber, and then to proceed to deal with the choice of leased capacity; the lead time for acquiring dark fiber was also much longer. A minimum of four suppliers (pan-European and regional) and a maximum of eight were to be contracted as dark fiber providers.

In May 2005, the preferred suppliers for all routes were approved by the GÉANT2 Policy Committee and the first GÉANT2 contracts could be signed in July. GÉANT2 uses a larger set of vendors across its topology than GÉANT which lowers the risk of problems arising from any provider's insolvency.

Assessment of equipment tender offers took place in August 2004 after more information on the fiber offers had been obtained. To assist in the decision process, DANTE organized three architecture workshops on optical transmission and switching technology options in December 2004, March and April 2005. The aim of the first two workshops was to discuss possible GÉANT2 services, architecture and access options for research networks and to make recommendations. The third architecture workshop was held in order to confirm that the (by then) chosen solution would work and meet technical requirements.

The equipment offers were evaluated in relation to their ability to support the two fundamental requirements, to light the dark fiber that was being procured separately, and to provision end-to-end Gbps services. In May 2005, Alcatel was selected to turn GÉANT's transmission infrastructure into a converged optical and IP network running over a single platform. The addition of a new optical network layer would provide direct optical connectivity to the existing IP network and would enhance service performance. The solution presented an optimized combination of DWDM and optical cross-connects with integrated management. In particular the Alcatel 1678 MCC (Metro Core Connect) equipment was amongst the first to market with a solution for transporting Ethernet VLANs (Virtual LANs) over an optical network.

Following a public Call for Expressions of Interest, a tender for the supply of network operations services for GÉANT2 was issued in July 2004. The tender was divided into two lots, one dealing with switching and associated services, the second lot covering transmission and associated services. From a shortlist of three, DANTE's recommendation was to award a three year contract for both parts of the service to the operator of the GÉANT network, Communication et Systèmes.

10.2.3
Roll-Out and Migration

The roll-out of the new network was carried out in five phases after careful calculation of risks and contingency planning to deal with them. The first phase of the deployment was completed in January 2006, with 13 of the network's 44 routes fully installed and operational, and 5 out of 18 dark fiber routes live.

The initial portfolio of services consisted of four types: a standard IP service, supporting all conventional applications that are based on the use of the IP protocol; IP multicast; a limited offering of IP QoS to support applications for which this technology is appropriate; and static VPNs. The complete configuration is shown in Figure 10.2.

10.2.4
Switched Point-to-Point (p2p) Connections

One of the main objectives of GÉANT2 was the establishment of switched point-to-point (p2p) services. The ability to switch data streams between two defined points on the network enables the creation of paths which are dedicated to specific users and which carry only their traffic.

GÉANT2 offers p2p ethernet services using label switched paths (LSP) as specified in MPLS and ethernet private lines (EPL) over next-generation SDH. While LSPs are preferred for transmission rates up to 1 Gbps, EPL services are offered for Gbps circuits. These services are manually configured by the NOC; however, bandwidth-on-demand (BoD) services are being researched in JRA3 (AutoBAHN, automated bandwidth allocation across heterogeneous networks) to automate their provisioning and configuration across multiple domains.

In July 2007, as part of a demonstration of the AutoBAHN architecture, a 1 Gbps ethernet circuit was set up dynamically between two end-user workstations, one in Greece and the other in Ireland. The circuit spanned the infrastructures of

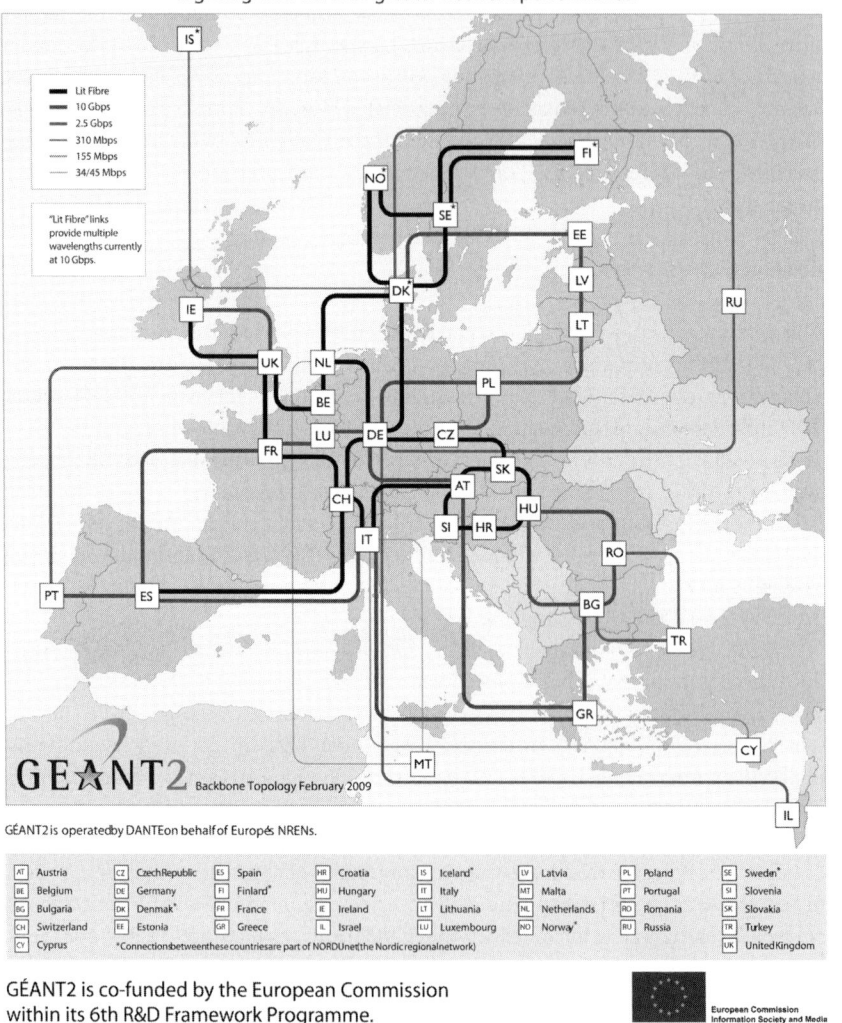

Figure 10.2 GÉANT2 configuration. There is a color version of this figure in the set at the front of the book.

GRNET, GÉANT2 and HEAnet, and, for the first time, a true E2E connection was in place.

The setting up of E2E connections between organizations located in different countries, crossing the networks of several different providers requires complex and intensive collaboration between all the partners involved. To manage this collaboration, DANTE created – with research network support – the GÉANT2 end-to-end coordination unit (E2ECU) in 2007. The functions of the unit include: monitoring of the multi-domain point-to-point links; providing a single point of contact to report faults and to announce scheduled maintenance; and issuing trouble tickets to report on fault resolution to all parties involved in the multi-domain link. The E2ECU function is performed by the GÉANT2 NOC. E2ECU enables staff of the research networks to concentrate their effort on operating their own networks, while working together with GÉANT2 and other research networks to improve the management and monitoring of end-to-end circuits.

10.2.5
Cost Sharing

Because of the network's advanced architecture, the principles on which cost sharing in GÉANT2 is based are more complex than for GÉANT. The basic principles of the GÉANT cost-sharing model were that it should be fair and equitable, it should encourage the use of lambdas, charges should bear a reasonable relation to underlying costs, and the research networks should not pay significantly more than they had been doing previously.

The initial model made a distinction between "on-fiber" and "off-fiber" research networks. The location of a GÉANT2 PoP in a particular research network determined if it was a candidate for the use of the "fiber cloud"; it was then up to the candidates to decide whether or not they wished to be a member of the fiber cloud.

On-fiber research networks all had to subscribe to the GÉANT+ (with access to the IP service at 10 Gbps and access at 10 Gbps to the p2p service). The first lambdas implemented in the network on each dark fiber would provide those two services.

Off-fiber research networks were connected by leased circuits. They would be primarily using the IP service at a chosen bandwidth. The off-fiber networks could utilize a portion of their existing access capacity for dedicated p2p links. These links are extended across the dark fiber cloud at no additional charge. If more p2p capacity is required and technically possible, off-fiber research networks can use a separate leased circuit to access the cloud. In this case, the contribution of off-fiber research networks was the cost of the additional leased circuit to the applicable GÉANT2 PoP on the fiber cloud.

The approach established for the on-fiber networks was for them to share equally a base cost of 40% of the total, while the remaining 60% was allocated in proportion to a weight based on country size, GDP (gross domestic product) and level of network development of each research network. To avoid the problems that can arise if there are large changes in individual subscriptions from one year to another, a 20%

cap was introduced to limit the increase in a research network's annual subscription. The off-fiber networks were to share 40% on the basis of the bandwidth capacity they subscribe to while 60% was based on the actual costs of the links to the research network. For each group the total subscriptions are then the sums of these two elements.

In October 2007 the Policy Committee decided to make a number of changes to the cost-sharing model based on input from the research networks. The most significant elements of the adjusted model were: the removal of separate calculation tables for "on-" and "off-" fiber-connected research networks; the introduction of cost allocation to different service elements (service-based cost allocation); the retention of 10 Gbps IP and 10 Gbps p2p (GÉANT+) access capacity requirements for research networks connected by lit fiber-based infrastructure; the weighting factors to also take account of the research networks ability to use additional lambda service. The changes have the effect of reducing fees reflecting the IP service access level of contribution research networks are likely to require.

The new model reflected the development of the GÉANT2 network service portfolio. Specifically, the costs were now apportioned between the different service elements making it clearer which service is being allocated which cost.

10.2.6
Cross Border Initiatives

As a complement to GÉANT2 connections, direct links between two neighboring research networks can be established using so-called cross border fiber (CBF) which may also be concatenated with the research networks' own CBF links to different neighbors. Through this mechanism, it is possible for research networks to access a wide area optical network infrastructure that is, for the most part, physically separate from the set of fibers used by GÉANT2 and over which E2E links can be provisioned.

In 2005 the Research Network Policy Committee set up a sub-committee to deal with CBF arrangements in the context of GÉANT2. The general idea was to develop a framework – technical, organizational and financial – to facilitate the building of additional pan-European network elements. CBF was seen to contribute to GÉANT2 in several ways: reducing project cost; enlarging the GÉANT2 fiber footprint; refining the wavelength mesh and shortening back-up routes.

There are two categories of CBF-based connectivity services within GÉANT2. Type-A CBF services are between GÉANT2 PoPs. They are integral components of the GÉANT2 backbone network on top of which IP or circuit services are delivered. Type-B CBF services are multi domain end-to-end circuits, which instead of using the GÉANT2 backbone as the pan-European component, make use of border crossings arranged directly between adjacent research networks. Type-B CBF services deliver wavelengths for the benefit of individual end sites in selected projects. While they are typically financed by end-customers, partial funding of (project-related) Type-B CBFs via the cost sharing pool is possible.

10.2.7
Global Connectivity

Additional connectivity projects, not part of GÉANT2 itself, have led to interconnections between Europe and research networks in other world regions. These projects cover the countries bordering the Mediterranean (EUMEDCONNECT), Asia-Pacific (TEIN2 and 3), Latin America (ALICE) and China (CERNET, Chinese education and research network, and CSTNET, China science and technology network). Connectivity has been implemented with ERNET in India and the African UbuntuNet Alliance via European GÉANT2 access points. The work in this area will continue. TEIN3 in Asia-Pacific will extend into Southern Asia; in the future there will be funding available to connect Central Asia and South and Eastern Africa to GÉANT2.

GÉANT2 operates distributed access facilities to encourage connectivity from other world regions, rather than *ad hoc* connections to individual countries within the regions. This has led to a significant expansion of the global research and education coverage as a result of which GÉANT2 has become a global leader for regional interconnections.

Connections to North American research networks and to SINET in Japan are made via the GÉANT2 PoP in New York where 2×10 Gbps capacity is available for general IP traffic and a further 2×10 Gbps for point-to-point circuits with Internet2 and ESnet. GÉANT2 and these two North American networks continue to collaborate following the principle of reciprocity in the implementation of transatlantic point-to-point circuits. In the context of DICE (DANTE-Internet2-CANARIE-ESnet), there is a continuing dialogue that is leading to the creation of a seamless operational multi-domain environment for p2p connections, a challenging task in such heterogeneous conditions.

In 2006 DANTE installed the very first transatlantic p2p connection, thereby supporting the work of physicists at Fermilab in the United States and IN2P3 (Institut National de Physique Nucléaire et de Physique des Particules) in France with two OPNs operating between Paris and Chicago. This connection between the two laboratories was a service trial that enabled DANTE and Internet2 to start tackling the operational questions raised in multi-domain environments.

10.2.8
Conclusion

GÉANT2 is the largest research and education network ever built for the European academic community. It has succeeded in its main objectives: to establish a hybrid network infrastructure offering both packet-switched and circuit-switched connections, and to develop and utilize new optical technologies focused on end-to-end connections. While previous pan-European network projects were characterized by commercial and organizational complexities between the research networks, DANTE, the EC and telecoms suppliers, the GÉANT2 era is dominated by changes in network technology and, in particular, the possibility for the European research community to acquire and operate services on its own fiber.

These technology changes present opportunities (and challenges) to explore new technical and operational approaches. They include a number of components, such as optical transport, end-to-end QoS, and point-to-point connectivity. The implementation of the new technology has also had a profound impact on the relationship between the research networks, their customers and the GÉANT2 core network, and has required closer cooperation between the parties involved, both technically and operationally.

The development of new services has been accompanied by changes in the network's cost-sharing arrangements which distinguish between the costs of operating established services and other non-service-related activities (e.g. test-bed).

Further consolidation of GÉANT2 into a robust and stable operational multi-domain hybrid network is the challenge for the future.

10.3
The Impact of Research Networking

Research networking created the Internet. Rarely in history has the academic community done something which has had such a dramatic and profound impact on the economy, the life of citizens, and society at large.

The setting up of a world-wide information network, based on global standards, is the result of publicly funded research: the Internet is an indirect product of universities and laboratories that not only invented the technology but – a rare outcome – made use of it on a world-wide scale, demonstrating its value and promoting its adoption in other areas of human activity.

10.3.1
The Impact on Individuals

The creation of the Internet, with its combination high-speed data transmission, accessible user interface and powerful applications, has provided a new means of communication. It supplements – and does not completely replace – the traditional services based on voice telephony and the transport of paper documents.

The Internet supports person-to-person communication, most commonly in the form of e-mail which, if carefully used, offers a powerful set of tools which allow the rapid interactions between pairs or groups of individuals whilst avoiding the interruptions which are an inherent feature of telephone calls. Powerful applications software allows users who have little interest in the underlying technology to prepare complex documents and send them quickly to collaborators almost anywhere in the world. This makes group working on a national, international and global scale much more effective than was previously the case.

Voice over IP is an Internet facility that, in principle, could supersede the technology used in traditional voice telephony. Despite the very low marginal cost of making telephone calls in this way, however, the population of VoIP users has not yet grown to the critical mass which would make it the preferred technology to support classical telephone transmissions.

A major feature of the Internet and particularly of the World Wide Web is the provision of access by individuals to huge amounts of information covering all conceivable topics. The ease and speed with which this information can be accessed, especially with the assistance of powerful search engines, give individual users the ability to obtain information in seconds which previously might have been hidden behind barriers requiring days or even weeks to break down.

The World Wide Web also supports interactions between individuals and computer systems, particularly those incorporating large databases and for which most data input is handled by filling in forms. Many such systems support online purchasing which gives consumers a wider range of choice of supplier since distance to the supplier's premises is no longer relevant.

10.3.2
The Impact on Commerce

The effect on commercial organizations of the arrival of Internet facilities complements that on individuals. Commercial organizations have a strong need to provide information to customers and potential customers and the World Wide Web provides an excellent means of satisfying this need. At least in those countries where a large proportion of the population has Internet access, no company these days is without at least a minimal Web site which provides pointers to other sources of information about the company, including ways of making direct contact. At the other extreme, the company's operations may be managed almost entirely by means of an extensive database which is accessed via the World Wide Web and is connected to automated purchasing, stock control, scheduling, payment, accounting and other systems.

In some of the more complex applications, for example airline reservations which were previously operated exclusively by the airline's own staff or by specialist agents, much of the workload of investigating alternatives, deciding between options, and entering the data needed to handle the transaction has been shifted to the customer. The resulting efficiency gains may help the supplier to retain his competitive edge. In some areas, completely new services or restructuring of the ways in which a specialist service is provided have been set up to take advantage of Internet technology; eBay and Amazon are prominent examples.

10.3.3
The Impact on Entertainment

The Internet has opened up a wide range of new forms of entertainment, including computer games (solo player vs. computer and multiple players in real time), as well as improved access to traditional forms. High data rates are essential if a network is to be used for the delivery of videos which have the same (or better) quality as broadcast television, as are short response times for interactive applications. The availability of high speed networking has been used to improve the quality of graphic presentations but it seems likely that even the present levels of performance will be insufficient to deal with user demand as an increasing proportion of the general population exploits the benefits of greater choice, of both material and timing, offered by video-on-demand services. (The research networks still have work to do.)

By making the exchange of data files and data streams so easy for users, the Internet has created difficulties for companies which hold the rights to creative material and which have difficulty in asserting those rights in the face of small-scale piracy by a large number of people who are not fully aware of their obligations to respect copyright or, even worse, of the activities of small number of people who deliberately ignore the law and make significant profits by selling cheap copies of copyrighted material. The entertainment industry has been obliged to consider new ways of protecting its interests (as well as continuing to use the traditional method of taking miscreants to court). It needs to devise methods of tightly controlling access to the material it owns while at the same time exploiting together with its customers the new possibilities offered by Internet technology. The issues raised in maintaining a balance between the entertainment industry and its customers will continue to multiply and be the source of considerable discussion as more and more entertainment alternatives are offered by a combination of high definition video material, massive amounts of local and remote storage and very high-speed network connections.

10.3.4
The Impact on the Telecommunications Industry

It is difficult to disentangle the roles played by the legislation which resulted in liberalization of telecommunications services in Europe and by the introduction of Internet services based on a telecommunications infrastructure which is very different from that of the 1980s. It is certain that the Internet in its current form would not exist if liberalization had not been introduced. A further complication in distinguishing between cause and effect is that some of the casualties of the dot.com boom in the late 1990s were caused by poor (or even fraudulent) financial management of the companies which suffered, examples being WorldCom and KPN/Qwest.

The effect of the telecommunications industry of developments in research networking has nevertheless been considerable. The research networking community has challenged and eventually undermined the succession of technical strategies adopted by the telecoms operators. One by one, the various levels of telecoms hierarchy put in place by the operators have been replaced; data transmission services by leased lines which the customer could use as he wished, connection-oriented data transmission systems based on the X.25 protocol by the connectionless IP service. These changes have been followed by the use of IP directly over SDH, then IP over wavelengths. The final step, the acquisition and use of dark fiber, has reduced the role of the telecoms operators (in relation to the research networks) to that of suppliers of fiber over which the research networks have complete technical control.

The large traditional telecoms operators have reacted to the advent of the Internet by setting themselves up as ISPs. Because of their overall size, their continued control (in some countries) of the "last mile" circuits between exchanges and customer premises, and to some extent inertia on the part of their established telephone customers, they tend to be major players within their home country. There is, nevertheless, a competitive market with many new companies offering alternative services. Price competition between the ISPs is very keen and, for customers who choose their ISP carefully, quality of service is an important parameter.

A more significant impact on the telecommunications industry as a whole has been the creation of a new branch of manufacturing industry, namely the production of specialist equipment such as routers, and the formation of a completely new industry which provides information management services across a wide range of activities, from the specialist setting up a Web site for a small company to the provision of search facilities which are used by almost every Internet user.

Traditional manufacturers of telecoms equipment were generally slow to change from their often privileged position as suppliers to the monopoly telecoms operators. For a long time, their development activities continued to be geared to the perceived requirements of the telecoms operators as their customers, and they missed the opportunity of participating in the new Internet-related developments.

The result is that most equipment needed to support the operation of the global Internet is provided by companies which did not exist 30 years ago and for which the Internet is almost the sole raison d'être. The position is similar in the case of the information management companies which have been created purely to exploit the Internet's capabilities. The scale of their activities is now considerable. Many hundreds, if not thousands, of companies are active in these fields. The largest of them – Cisco, founded in 1984 as a router supplier, and Google, set up even more recently in 1998 – have market capitalizations counted in hundreds of billions of US dollars.

10.3.5
The Impact on Education and Research

In the more advanced economies where the Internet is already firmly established, a large majority of children is now exposed to Internet services both at home and at school. The long-term impact of a generation of children for whom use of the Internet has always been part of their way of life remains to be seen but it is bound to lead to social change of some kind. Already there are ways in which Internet services are being exploited. Access to a wide range of information is an obvious improvement on the facilities previously available to students. Sharing of teaching materials improves the quality of teaching; the best teachers can apply their skills to a larger student population through the use of videoconferencing. Specialist teaching can be extended; an example is improvement in the training of doctors by making it possible for trainees to observe surgical procedures as they are carried out and even to interact with the surgeon as his work proceeds.

In the case of research, the research network community has already demonstrated the effectiveness of the Internet in enabling information sharing and collaboration between widely dispersed researchers (individuals or groups). Workers in other academic disciplines have copied the procedures and techniques and have already benefited substantially from their availability.

10.3.6
The Impact on the Environment

The effects of introducing Internet services have not been wholly beneficial and the environment is one area that has suffered. The amount of equipment now in use for activities solely related to the Internet is already considerable and will increase. Although the power required to support a typical domestic installation of two or three computers, a router and a printer is quite small, a very large number of such domestic installations collectively consumes a significant amount of power that requires a sizeable power generation capacity. All this energy is eventually dissipated in the form of heat and is lost to the atmosphere. The effect is exacerbated by two factors. First, this equipment does not replace older, obsolete devices and the power it consumes represents an additional load on power generation facilities. Secondly, much of the equipment is often left switched on permanently which increases the energy demand even more.

For telecoms operators, power consumption and heat dissipation are significant factors that have to be taken into account in the design and construction of points of presence (as they are for operators of other kinds of computer center). Equipment suppliers are being pressed to include reduction in power consumption as an important target in the design of new devices. More generally, governments may take steps to require suppliers of many types of domestic equipment to include the facility of switching automatically to a standby mode if it is not used for a certain length of time. Even the switching off of pilot lights would give a small but not insignificant benefit to the environment.

10.3.7
The Political Impact

The political impact of research networking is difficult to measure. It varies between countries and in some of them it is certainly significant. In the countries of Western Europe, the research networks stand roughly in the middle of the hierarchy of governmental responsibilities. The people driving the development of research networking full-time are equivalent in rank to the heads (or senior research staff) of university departments, the leaders of research groups in commercial organizations, and middle-range civil servants who interact directly with Ministers only occasionally. They obtain funds in competition with other research groups, often discipline-oriented, and judgment of the quality and effectiveness of their output is made by their peers. They have wide discretion concerning the use of the funds under their control and they are free to take new initiatives and to embark on new projects as long as overall budget limits and organizational ground rules are not breached.

In such an environment, the main impact of research networks' activity is felt by their partner organizations in the research and education communities and by the funding bodies that support them. Occasionally, there will be some recognition at a higher level of government of a research network's activity, most commonly when there is something to celebrate and a politician is willing to associate himself with a success story. It is certain, however, that issues involving research networks do not appear regularly on the daily briefing notes sent to heads of government and senior Ministers.

There has been one important exception to this general picture. Before they were joined by the research networks from the CEEC in the early 1990s, the services of Western European research networks were aimed primarily at researchers; support of educational activities was incidental – academic staff in universities which had network connections to support their research were able to use them for teaching purposes as well. The CEE networks, in contrast, had from their beginning the support of teaching at all levels from primary schools to higher education as an objective and national policies were in place to provide the necessary resources.

10.3.8
The Impact on Standard Development Method

The Internet protocols adopted by the European academic networks in the early 1980s have two important properties: they are open, that is, they do not belong to any particular manufacturer and can thus be implemented on any type of computer; they are public, that is, everyone has access to their specifications. In this respect there is no difference from the OSI protocols. The fundamental difference lies elsewhere.

The Internet protocols are delivered via an (initially light) structure, open to all: the IETF. The Internet designers set up this structure so as to benefit from contributions from all over the world, from universities, researchers and engineers in the public or private sector. There is no need to belong to a standards organization in order to propose an idea, an improvement or a new norm: any individual or group of individuals, at whatever rank or qualification, from a mere student to a group of experts, can propose an idea: it will be analyzed by volunteers from the IETF and will be retained if it is considered pertinent. This work method, focused on the individual and, by extension, based upon a certain notion of individualism – the author's name remains attached to his/her contribution – is fundamentally different from the hierarchical procedures in force in official standards organizations such as ISO or ITU which, historically, promulgate the rules for telephony, television and radio communication. Contributions by individuals were not only hampered by the

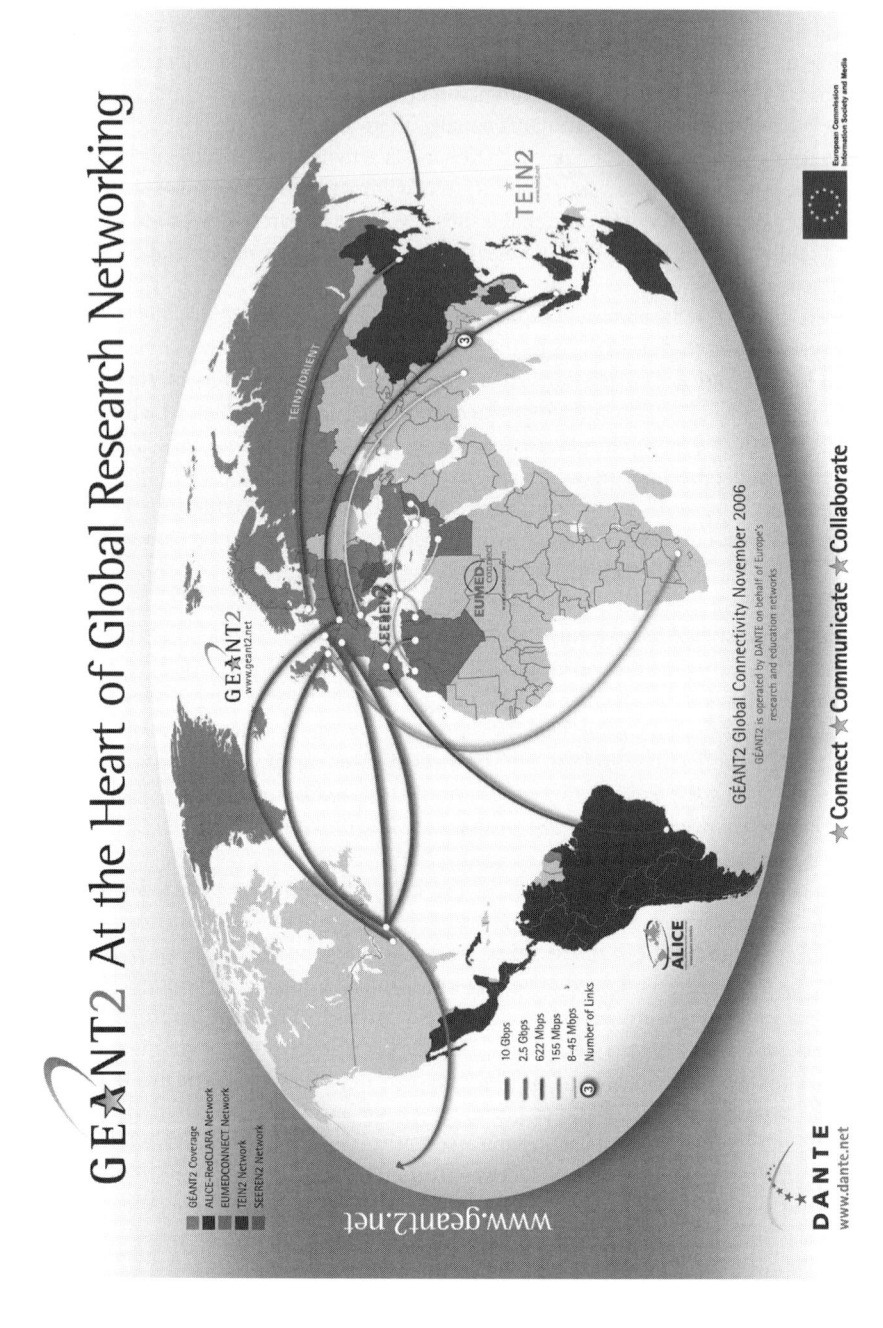

Figure 10.3 Global connectivity. There is a color version of this figure in the set at the front of the book.

obligation to channel inputs via national structures but also by the fact that, in the case of the ITU, the standards themselves were not publicly available free-of-charge. "No-one is deemed to ignore the law" but knowing what the "law" said was significantly expensive for ordinary citizens.

The IETF work method demonstrated that standards can be developed quickly (the traditional pace of ITU standards pre-dating the Internet revolution was based on 4-year ratification cycles). It also showed that by publicizing standards free-of-charge, allowing bottom-up initiatives and, when appropriate, giving personal recognition to individuals rather than to their country or company, the development of standards can mobilize a considerable work force from both academic and industrial spheres.

Standards will no longer be developed exactly as they were before!

10.3.9
Conclusion

The successful deployment by the research academic community of its global networking infrastructure, with European organizations playing a leading role, is an unprecedented event in the history of science, because it has had unprecedented impacts: on the economy, on politics, on everyday life.

Most importantly, for the academic and research community, it is now viewed as being capable of developing and delivering professionally operated systems which can revolutionize the economy in a few years and permeate all levels of society.

Given the differences in language and culture, in historical background and in economic development between the countries of Europe, the full involvement of more than 30 national organizations in setting up a network infrastructure which serves them all as well as forming an integral part of the global research network represents a major achievement of which everyone who has made a contribution can be proud.

There have been difficulties and disagreements on the road to this success; there will continue to be difficulties and disagreements in future as the research networks continue to lead the way in developing, testing, implementing and operating new technologies

The first generation of network engineers and managers is reaching an age at which retirement beckons. It is to be hoped that the next generation will not only continue the successful advance of European research networking over the last 30 years but will also avoid the inevitable pitfalls by learning from the experience of their predecessors (Figure 10.3).

Vision and Pragmatism
In the history of research networking in European user communities, government and industry all played an important role. Yet the interests of the many stakeholders were not always aligned and they had many different views and

approaches. In particular, the incumbent telecom operators, mostly state-owned monopolies operating in protected national markets in the 1980s and most of the 1990s had great difficulty understanding and accepting the paradigm shift in networking introduced by data communications, and later by the Internet. At the same time, governments in Europe had difficulty deciding where their loyalty should be: with "their" national operators and equipment suppliers, or with the users in research and higher education. A number of user communities believed that they had special needs, and, therefore, needed special networks that had to be superior in performance and would enable international data traffic. The use of the term "protocol wars" illustrates the fact that it was no simple matter to align the different views. The emerging research networks could only survive in this environment with a flexible combination of vision and pragmatism. Vision was needed to create a basis for long-term funding and a stable organizational set-up, pragmatism was necessary to cope with rapidly evolving technologies and user needs, but also with the ever-changing political views on how national telecommunication markets would evolve. The challenges that had to be overcome included financial, technical and organizational issues. As a result, many important changes did not derive from extensive studies and reports, but from pragmatic, mostly bottom-up or even "sneaky" introduction of new technologies, services and organizational structures; and often only as "interim" facilities until the "officially" targeted and politically correct final solutions would be ready. The vision-pragmatism combination holds for many aspects, but is best seen in the way the international fragmentation was overcome and in the struggles to provide pan-European international research network services. We now all take for granted global connectivity at speeds that can hardly be supported by today's computers. Society as a whole can no longer function without what we now call "the Internet". The R&E community played and continues to play an essential role in shaping the network future. These results did not come free of charge. In a fruitful combination of vision and pragmatism, the coordinated efforts of many parties were needed to shape the networking landscape we all enjoy today.

Further Reading

Aiken R., Boroumand J., and Wolff S., Back to the Future, *Communications of the ACM, CACM*, Volume **46**, No. 1, January 2004.

Carpenter B.E., (1986) Computer Communications at CERN, *Proceedings of the Conference on Computing in High Energy Physics*, Amsterdam, June 1985, ed. L.O. Hertzberger and W. Hoogland, North-Holland, 1986.

Carpenter, B.E., (1989) Is OSI Too Late? RARE Networkshop 1989, *Computer Networks and ISDN Systems*, **17**, 284–286.

DeFanti T.A., de Laat C., Mambretti J., Neggers K., and St. Arnaud B., (2003) TransLight: A global-scale lambdagrid for e-science, *Communications of the ACM, CACM*, **46** (11), 34–41.

DeFanti T.A., Brown M.D., Mambretti J., Silvester J., Johnson R., (2005) TransLight, a major US component of the GLIF, *Cyberinfrastructure Technology Watch (CTWatch) Quarterly*, **1** (2) Number 2, May 2005.

DeFanti T.A., Brown M.D., and de Laat C., eds, (2003) iGrid 2002: the international virtual laboratory, *Journal of Future Generation Computer Systems (FGCS)*, **19** (6), 803–804.

Fluckiger, F., (2000) Le réseau des chercheurs Européens, *La Recherche*, **328**.

Glenn K., (1993) Profile: EUnet InterOp ConneXions, *The Interoperability Companion*, **7** (11).

IEEE Standard Computer Dictionary, A Compilation of IEEE Standard Computer Glossaries, (1990) IEEE, New York.

Jennings D., (1987) Computing the best for Europe, *Nature*, **329**, 775–778.

Lehtisalo, K. (2005) *The History of NORDUnet*, NORDUnet A/S publisher, Vammala, Finland, ISBN 87-990712-0-7.

Leiner, B.M., Cerf, V.G., Clark, D.D., Kahn, R.E., Kleinrock, L., Lynch, D.C., Postel, J., Roberts L.G., Wolff S., *A Brief History of the Internet*, http://www.isoc.org/internet/history/brief.shtml, Internet Society. Last revised 10 December 2003.

Malamud, C., (1992) *Exploring The Internet - A Technical Travelogue*, PTR Prentice Hall, Englewood Cliffs, ISBN 0-13-296898-3.

McKie J., *Where is Europe. USENIX Conference*, Toronto, Summer 1983.

Newman N. and Tindemans P., The place of OSI in communications between researchers, *The EUREKA COSINE Project*, Proceedings of the 5th International Conference for Open Systems Interconnection, Tokyo, Japan, 1989.

Postel J., *Internet Protocol*, RFC 791, September 1981.

Postel J., *Internet Control Message Protocol*, RFC 792. September 1981.

Postel J., *Transmission Control Protocol*. J. Postel, RFC 793, September 1981.

Scarabucci R.R., Stanton M.A., et al., Project GIGA – High-speed Experimental Network. *First International Conference on Testbeds and Research Infrastructures for the Development of Networks and Communities (TRIDENTCOM'05)*, Trento, Italy, February 2005.

Smarr L., DeFanti T.A., Brown M.D. and de Laat C., eds, (2006) Special section: iGrid 2005: The global lambda integrated facility, *Future Generation Computer Systems*, **22** (8), 849–851.

Stanton M.A., Ribeiro Filho J.L., Simões da Silva N., Building optical networks for the higher education and research community in Brazil, *2nd IEEE/Create-Net International Workshop on Deployment Models and First/Last Mile Networking Technologies for Broadband Community Networks (COMNETS 2005)*, Volume 2, Boston, MA, United States, October 2005.

Stöver C., Stanton M.A., Integrating Latin American and European research and education networks through the ALICE project, *Third Latin American Network Operations and Management Symposium (LANOMS)*, Foz do Iguaçu, Brazil, September 2003.

Tindemans P., (1991) The Status of Support for Research in Europe: Various authors from Europe and the United States, outline of research networking developments in North America, Zoetermeer, January 1991.

Tindemans P., RARE and COSINE: a Pan-European approach to open systems networking for collaborative R&D. *Proceedings of the Nachrichtentechnisches Kolloquium, Institut für Mathematik Universität Bern, Switzerland,* 1988.

Verhoog J., (2008) *SURFnet 1988–2008, Twenty Years of Networking*, SURFnet publication, Spider Media, Voorhout, Utrecht, the Netherlands.

Zimmermann H., (1980) OSI reference model – The ISO model of architecture for open systems, *IEEE Transactions on Communication*, **Com-28**, (4), 425–432.

Appendix A: The People who Made it Happen

The people in the list below have made significant contributions to one or more chapters of this book. Their efforts are gratefully acknowledged by the editors. The Contributors are listed, together with their CVs, in alphabetic order of surname.

Claudio Allocchio is a Senior Manager at GARR, the Italian R&E network, where he is the Policy and Security Advisor responsible for advanced application services. He started in 1981 as a computer graphics and image processing researcher in astrophysics at the Trieste Astronomical Observatory, then moved to CERN, where he started his networking activities in a team which built some of the first network international links, and as developer of the first multiprotocol mail gateway. He moved back to Trieste in 1988 as Network Manager at Elettra synchrotron laboratory, and joined GARR in its early start activities. Since 1991, he has been taking part in the IETF, with various roles: editing many standard RFCs, chairing working groups, and, currently, as Application Area Directorate member. In the early 1990s, he ran the COSINE S2.2 sub-project providing full mail connectivity to the worldwide research community, and joined RARE (now TERENA), where he played various roles: messaging WG member and chairman, TERENA Technical Committee member, from 2001 to 2007 TERENA Vice-President for the Technical Programme and TERENA Executive Committee member. From 1993, he was involved in the creation of the ".it" country code top-level domain (ccTLD) registry. He served as President of the Italian Naming Authority from 1995 to 2005, and as advisor to the Ministry of Communication domain names committee; he is now a member of the ccTLD Registry Advisory Board.

Lajos Bálint is currently the Treasurer of TERENA. He is Vice-President of HUNGARNET, the Hungarian Academic and Research Networking Association, and Director of International Relations at NIIFI (Nemzeti Informacios Infrastruktura Fejlesztesi Iroda), the National Information Infrastructure Development Institute in Hungary. He represents HUNGARNET at TERENA. His key interests are in research networks, information technology, research infrastructures, telecommunications, man-machine systems, and human-computer interaction. He has been a part-time teacher since 1970, and an Honorary Professor at the Faculty of Electronic Engineering of the Technical University of Budapest since 1991. He has presented more than 160 publications (papers, conference contributions, reports, books) between 1969 and 2008.

A History of International Research Networking. Edited by Howard Davies and Beatrice Bressan
Copyright © 2010 WILEY-VCH Verlag GmbH & Co. KGaA, Weinheim
ISBN: 978-3-527-32710-2

Vincent Berkhout is currently a Client Engagement Director at COLT Telecom, working in the financial sector. After completing his degree at the Hogeschool Utrecht, he completed a post-grad at the University of Twente as Technology Designer of distributed information systems. He started at DANTE in 1994 as an application engineer to run the PARADISE (Piloting a Researcher's Directory Service in Europe) project, renamed NameFLOW, directory service, and later coordinated the other application services. He took the role as operations manager in 1996, managing the TEN-34 network. He then became the program leader for the implementation of TEN-155 and GÉANT. He completed a full-time MBA at Cranfield University in 2003, specializing in change and project management. He started at COLT Telecom as a Business Development Manager working on European network propositions for multinational businesses. As a Client Engagement Director, he works as a strategic consultant for a number of banks, designing high-resilient, fully-integrated network solutions.

Josephine Bersee worked as a Publicity Officer for RARE (TERENA's predecessor) from 1990 to 1993. In 1993, she joined DANTE in Cambridge as External Relations Manager until 1998. She moved to Asia in early 2001 and has been involved in freelance activities for DANTE from time to time. She has a Master's degree from the University of Amsterdam.

Beatrice Bressan, after having been the Head of Communications at the Swiss Institute of Bioinformatics (SIB) and at the Physics Department in Geneva University, is now Director of Communications of MAAT-G Geneva (Cloud Computing Company) and responsible for the outreach of the CERN TOTEM (total cross-section, elastic scattering and diffraction dissociation measurement at the LHC) experiment. As a science writer, she has over ten years' experience in the field of scientific and technological communication, with extensive experience in journalism, media publishing and public relations. She is also a Member of the European Union of Science Journalists' Associations (EUSJA). After her university studies in mathematical physics and science communication, she completed her Ph.D. research and carried out a postdoctoral fellowship on knowledge management and knowledge transfer inside the CERN laboratory for the Department of Physical Sciences at Helsinki University. She worked several years in the production of promotional material in the Technology Transfer group of CERN. Through her work as a physicist and science writer, she aims to give a better understanding of complex scientific and technological topics for politicians, industrialists and the general public.

Maxine Brown is an Associate Director of the EVL (Electronic Visualization Laboratory) at the UIC. She currently serves as co-principal investigator of the United States NSF's International Research Network Connections Program's TransLight/StarLight award, and was previously co-principal investigator of the NSF-funded Euro-Link and STARTAP/StarLight initiatives. She is the project manager of the NSF-funded OptIPuter (optical networking, Internet protocol, computer) project. She was one of several American technical advisors to the G7 GIBN (global interoperability for broadband networks) activity in 1995, is a member of the Pacific Rim Applications and Grid Middleware Assembly (PRAGMA), is a founding member of GLIF, and is co-chair of the GLIF Research & Applications working group. She served as an officer of the ACM SIGGRAPH (Association for Computing Machinery's Special Interest Group on Graphics and Interactive Techniques) organization and has been very active in ACM SIGGRAPH and ACM/IEEE (Association for Computing Machinery/Institute of Electrical and Electronics Engineers) supercomputing conferences. She also co-created and co-chaired the international grid workshops. In recognition of her services to UIC and the community at large, she is a recipient of the 1990 UIC Chancellor's Academic Professional Excellence (CAPE) award; the 2001 UIC Merit Award; and the 1998 ACM SIGGRAPH Outstanding Service Award.

Brian E. Carpenter joined the University of Auckland as a Senior Researcher in Computer Science in 2007, and was appointed Professor in January 2009. Before that, he spent ten years with IBM at various locations, working on Internet standards and technology. From 1997, he was at IBM's Hursley Laboratory in England. He then moved to iCAIR, the international centre for advanced Internet research, sponsored by IBM at Northwestern University in Evanston, Illinois. He was most recently based in Switzerland as a Distinguished Engineer and a member of the IBM Academy of Technology. Before joining IBM, he led the networking group at CERN from 1985 to 1996. This followed ten years' experience in software for process control systems at CERN, which was interrupted by three years teaching computer science at Massey University in New Zealand. He holds a degree in Physics and a Ph.D. in Computer Science, and is a Chartered Engineer (United Kingdom). He has been an active participant in the Global Grid Forum, and in the IETF, where he has worked on IPv6 and on Differentiated Services. He has also worked with the CERN Openlab for DataGrid Applications. He served from 1994 to 2002 on the Internet Architecture Board, which he chaired for five years. He also served as a Trustee of the Internet Society, and was Chairman of its Board of Trustees for two years until 2002. He was Chair of the IETF (2005–2007).

Tryfon Chiotis has been the Chief Technical Officer of GRNET, the Greek research and technology network since 1999. Today, he directs a very active research team of more than 15 engineers, while a lot of work is outsourced to a research and academic community of over 150 engineers/developers. He obtained his Diploma in Electrical Engineering from the Electrical & Computer Engineering Department of the National Technical University of Athens (NTUA) in 1992, and a Ph.D. at the Computer Science Division of the Electrical & Computer Engineering Department of NTUA in 1998. He is currently working for GRNET, a company owned by the Greek Ministry of Development, which provides advanced Internet services to Greek universities and research institutes. He is a member of the NREN Policy Committee of the pan-European GÉANT2 project. He is a member of the Scientific Committee of the Greek National Broadband Task Force, and a delegate of the Greek government to the European Space Agency.

Dai Davies is one of the General Managers of DANTE in Cambridge. He studied engineering in Cambridge, and then became a development engineer at British

Telecommunications. He received a post-graduate degree in computer science. After his computer studies, he moved from telephony to data-communications. Starting as a development engineer in packet switching in the United Kingdom, he developed an interest in data-communication protocols working on some of the early protocol designs. He spent two years working for Deutsche Telecom on Germany ISDN development, and then returned to the United Kingdom to work on LAN development. In 1984, he moved into a commercial role, eventually running business development marketing in the international division of BT's marketing group. In 1991, he went to Amsterdam as Director of the COSINE Project Management Unit, working on what was originally the IXI network and subsequently EuropaNET. During the COSINE project, he helped develop the blue-print needed for the establishment of an operational activity to continue the development of networking services that led to the creation of DANTE in 1993.

Howard Davies has a First Class Honours degree in Engineering Science and a D.Phil. from the University of Oxford. From 1964 to 1977, he worked in the Data Handling Division of CERN in Geneva, initially as a Scientific Programmer, later as a Group Leader and Project Manager for CERNET. Between 1977 and 1993, he was Director of the Computer Unit at the University of Exeter, responsible not only for the provision of computing services to all academic departments within the university, but also for the development of network-based services based on the use of JANET and its successors. During this period, he spent a six-month sabbatical leave in 1986 as a Visiting Computer Specialist at the Stanford Linear Accelerator Center (SLAC), Stanford, California; he acted as (part-time) Director of the Interim COSINE Project Management Unit from 1989 to 1991, and from 1992 to 1994 was Vice-President of RARE. He was appointed Joint General Manager of DANTE in 1993. He retired at the end of 2001.

Thomas A. DeFanti, Ph.D., at the University of California, San Diego (UCSD), is a research scientist in electronic visualization at the Calit2, the California Institute of Telecommunications and Information Technology. At the UIC, he is co-director of the EVL (with Jason Leigh), is a distinguished Professor Emeritus in the department of computer science, and the co-director (with Jason Leigh) of the Software Technologies Research Center. He is principal investigator of the NSF International Research Network Connections Program TransLight/StarLight award to UIC, that provides a persistent 10 Gbps networking infrastructure between the United States and Europe, and he is co-principal investigator of the NSF OptIPuter cooperative agreement. He was recipient of the 1988 ACM Outstanding Contribution Award, was appointed an ACM Fellow in 1994, and was one of several United States technical advisors to the G7 GIBN activity in 1995. He shares recognition along with EVL director Daniel J. Sandin for conceiving the CAVE (Cave automatic virtual environment) virtual reality theatre in 1991. He has collaborated with Maxine Brown to lead state, national and international teams to build the most advanced production-quality networks available to scientists, with major NSF funding. He is a founding member of GLIF. In the United States, he established the 10 Gb Ethernet CAVEwave research network between EVL/StarLight, Seattle/PNWGP, UCSD/Calit2, and McLean (Virginia) for OptIPuter and other national/international research uses, as a model for future high-end science and engineering collaboration infrastructure.

François Fluckiger, Director of the CERN Schools of Computing, is the Technology Transfer Officer for Information Technologies at CERN and Manager of the CERN openlab. Before joining CERN in 1978, he was employed for five years by SESA in Paris. At CERN, he has been in charge of external networking for more than 12 years and held positions in infrastructure and application networking, including the management of CERN's World Wide Web team after the departure of the Web inventor Tim Berners-Lee. He is an adviser to the European Commission, a member of the Internet Society Advisory Council and the author of the reference textbook "Understanding Networked Multimedia" as well as more than 80 articles. He is also a computer sciences lecturer at the University of Geneva. He has 35 years of experience in networking and information technologies. He holds an MSc in Physics from the Paris IV University. He graduated from the Ecole Supérieure d'Electricité in 1973 and was awarded an MBA by the Enterprise Administration Institute in Paris in 1977.

David Foster is the Deputy Leader of the IT Department at CERN. He completed a bachelors and doctorate degree in physics at the University of Durham, as well as an MBA at Durham Business School. He is a chartered physicist and fellow of the Institute of Physics, as well as a member of the Chartered Management Institute and Association of MBA's. Joining CERN in 1981 as a fellow, he worked on compiler systems for embedded computers. In 1987 he joined the CERN IBM systems group taking over responsibility for IBM communications including RSCS, SNA, DECnet and TCP/IP. After taking leave of absence to work in California, he became responsible for desktop computing and PCs during the 1990s. He has recently worked on SMS delivery systems for mobile data content providers and on the software architectures for grid computing. After being responsible for all electronic communications systems for several years, he now has responsibilities for international networking and grid computing activities.

Fabrizio Gagliardi is Europe, Middle East, Africa and Latin America director for scientific and technical computing in External Research, at Microsoft Research Corporation. He joined Microsoft in November 2005 after a long career at CERN. There he held several technical and managerial positions starting in 1975: Director of the EU EGEE Grid project (2004–2005); Director of the EU Data-Grid project (2001–2004); Head of mass storage services (1997–2000); Leader of the EU GPMIMD2 (General Purpose Multiple Instruction Multiple Data Machines 2) project (1993–1996). He is co-founder and member of the International Advisory Committee of the Open Grid Forum. He has a doctorate in computer science, granted by the University of Pisa in 1974. He has been an IEEE member since 1985.

Jan Gruntorád is Director of CESNET, the Czech educational and scientific network, in Prague and a member of DANTE's Board of Directors. He holds a diploma in Engineering and a Ph.D. degree from the Faculty of Electrical Engineering of the Czech Technical University in Prague. In 1992 he was awarded a grant by the Ministry of Education for the establishment of an Internet-type network in the Czech Republic: the result was CESNET, an association of all Czech Universities and the Czech Academy of Sciences, founded as a legal body and the formal NREN in March 1996. Since its creation, he has been a member of its Board of Directors and Chief Executive Officer responsible for research and operational tasks within CESNET. From 1998 to 2003, he was Chairman of CEENET. Over the same period, he served on the Board of Directors of Ebone. In 2003, he became a member of the Board of Directors of DANTE. He also represents the Czech Republic in TERENA. Since 1999 he has been a consultant for NATO in the field of computer networks for the R&E community in the Caucasus.

David Hartley went up to Cambridge University in 1956 where he studied mathematics. After his Ph.D., he was involved in developing programming languages and operating systems, after which he was appointed Director of the University Computing Service in 1970, a position he held for over 23 years. One of his most notable achievements was to wire up all the University and College sites, which in effect meant most of the City of Cambridge. This established an underground fiber network stretching from the City's limits north and south, with about 80 separate sites in between. In 1994, the United Kingdom Government transformed the JNT, which ran the United Kingdom research network called JANET, into a separate company, UKERNA. David was appointed its first Chief Executive. In this role, he was instrumental in forming the TEN-34 Consortium and chaired the TEN-34 Management Committee. He retired from UKERNA in 1997 and was appointed Executive Director of the Cambridge Crystallographic Data Centre, a spin-off company from the Cambridge chemistry department. After this, he became Steward of Clare College, Cambridge. He has held a number of other professional and advisory positions, including being an adviser to the United Kingdom Prime Minister in the 1980s, and President of the British Computer Society in 1999–2000. Now more or less retired, he develops IT systems for various organizations in and around Cambridge, and remains a Fellow of Clare College.

James Hutton did his first degree in physics at Cambridge and doctorate in particle physics at the RAL near Oxford. He then joined the Data Handling Group at RAL, working on many aspects of computing in support of the United Kingdom particle physics programme. In 1978 he became head of the Data Handling Group and was active in supporting the use of computer networking. In 1984 he took over as chair of ECFA Sub-group 5 on networking and promoted the first European Networkshop in Luxembourg. In 1987 he became the first secretary-general of RARE, now TERENA. He established the RARE Secretariat in Amsterdam, led the work on the COSINE Project Specification Phase, and then took a leading role in establishing IXI, the first pan-European network interconnecting the national research networks. In 1990, he returned to the United Kingdom and joined the JNT, which later became UKERNA and now JANET. He retired from UKERNA in 2003 as Business Director.

Yuri Izhvanov is a first deputy director of SIIT&T "Informika", responsible for the Russian University Network (RUNNet) functioning. He is also a part-time professor of the Moscow State Institute of Electronics and Mathematics (Technical University) where he studied from 1966 to 1971, and got his Ph.D. degree in computer science (1997). He is a member of the International Association of C/C++ Users (ACCU) and a member of the International Network on Engineering Education and Research (iNEER) steering committee. Recent activities include R&E networking, implementation of new information technologies in education. He is a general manager of several state projects in this field.

Klaus-Peter Kossakowski has been managing director of the DFN-CERT since September 2003. He has worked in the IT security field for more than 18 years. He became visiting scientist of the Software Engineering Institute at the Carnegie Mellon University, Pittsburgh, Pennsylvania, in 1998. He has served on the executive board of the DFN-Verein since 2002. He was previously President of the global forum of security teams and CERTs – FIRST – from 2003 to 2005, and on its board from 1997 to 2005. He obtained his doctorate at the University of Hamburg. He also holds a first-class degree in Information Science from the University of Hamburg. Recent activities include research projects related to early warning and situational awareness carried out in a collaborative effort between heterogeneous organizations and entities.

Glenn Kowack is an entrepreneur and executive in the internetworking and software industries. He was EUnet's (European UNIX network) founding European-level Chief Executive Officer from 1990 to 1995, participated in the founding of the Ebone, and was a member of the Ebone management committee. He was a member of the TERENA General Assembly; a Vice President and board member of the Commercial Internet eXchange (the Internet's first exchange point); a member of the Policy Oversight Committee, whose work led to the founding of ICANN (Internet Corporation for Assigned Names and Numbers); and Vice President for strategy and planning at the Internet Society. He was European managing director for Ipass Incorporated, and founded both NextHop Technologies Incorporated, a leading routing software developer, and Netnostics Incorporated, which did research on new network architectures. During the 1980s he directed UNIX research at Gould Computer Systems and was a founding staff member of UNIX International. He has provided strategic advising to the University of Michigan's Merit Network, Harris Semiconductor, Exodus Communications, and is a presently a member of ICANN's Registry Services Technical Evaluation Panel. He is also an occasional angel investor and author, and a frequent speaker. He wrote one of the early papers on the Internet's impact on the emergence of global civil society. His most recent writing is about influences on Internet evolution. He has degrees in mathematics and computer science, and psychology, from the University of Illinois at Urbana-Champaign.

Peter Linington is Professor of Computer Communication at the University of Kent in the United Kingdom. He studied in Cambridge, taking Natural Sciences and then a Ph.D. in the Metal Physics Group in the Cavendish laboratory. In 1971 he joined the University of Cambridge Computing Service as a Computer Officer, and became involved in protocol design when the University participated in the United

Kingdom Post Office's EPSS pilot. In 1978, he was seconded to the Department of Industry's Data Communication Protocols Unit, promoting the new OSI standards. He left Cambridge in 1983 to become Coordinator of the UNIVERSE project, a large industry and academic collaboration investigating the engineering of interconnected local area and satellite networks. The following year, he became Head of the JNT and Network Executive, responsible for the development and operation of the United Kingdom's newly unified JANET network. During this period, he became the first President of RARE. He moved to the University of Kent in 1987, where he remained until his retirement in early 2008.

Vassilis Maglaris is Professor of Electrical & Computer Engineering at NTUA, teaching and performing research on computer networks. He completed his studies in Athens and New York, and held industrial and academic positions in the United States for ten years before joining NTUA in 1989. In 1994, he was responsible for establishing GRNET, serving as its Chairman from its inception (1995) to 2004. Since October 2004, he has been serving as the Chairman of the NREN Policy Committee. The NREN Policy Committee harmonizes policies amongst 34 NRENs in the extended European Research Area; it is also responsible for governance of their Pan-European interconnect GÉANT/GÉANT2.

Boudewijn Nederkoorn was the Managing Director of SURFnet, the national research and education network in the Netherlands, in Utrecht, for more than 20 years. Immediately after his studies in Mathematics, he worked at Shell Oil. Subsequently, he worked for the University of Nijmegen at the academic hospital, setting up the hospital management information system. In the mid-1980s, he became the Managing Director of the University Computing Centre in Nijmegen, the Netherlands. The University Computer Centre in Nijmegen was one of the computer centers that took the initiative of working on a common national research network in the Netherlands, together with a number of other universities and people interested in the area. Starting in January 1988, he built the entire structure of SURF – the SURF Foundation and SURFnet as a working company of SURF – and managed the implementation of successive generations of SURFnet.

Kees Neggers is one of the founders of SURFnet, the national research and education network in the Netherlands and has been one of its Managing Directors since 1988. He received an Electrical Engineering degree from the Eindhoven University of Technology in 1972. He started his career as a staff member of an advisory committee on computing infrastructure to the Dutch Minister of Science and Education. He worked at the Computing Centre of the University of Groningen between 1975 and 1984. In 1984, he became one of the managing directors of the University Computing Centre in Nijmegen, where his networking career started. Nijmegen became the Dutch national node in EARN and was one of the drivers towards a national research network in the Netherlands. From there on, he became heavily involved in international research networking. He was among the founders of RARE, ISOC (Internet Society) and the RIPE NCC, and served for many years on the Boards of these organizations. During these terms he was involved in many initiatives, notably

COSINE, CCIRN, Ebone, DANTE, Amsterdam Internet Exchange, the merger of RARE and EARN into TERENA and more recently GLIF.

Michael Nowlan is a member of the Board of HEAnet, the Higher Education Authority network. He has a Masters degree in computer applications from the University of Dublin and has worked most of his life in Trinity College Dublin, where he has been the Director of Information Systems Services since 1995. He was a participant in the foundation of the Irish HEAnet NREN from its inception in 1983, and became a member of the Board of HEAnet. As well as being involved in academic networking, participating in several COSINE groups, he was involved in bringing the commercial Internet to Ireland through EUnet, and was a founding member and chairman of the board of the pan-European EUnet network in its early years.

Dorte Olesen has been the President of TERENA from 2003. She received her MSc in mathematics and physics from the University of Copenhagen in 1973. She also holds a Ph.D. in mathematics from 1975, and became an Associate Professor at the University of Copenhagen in 1980. After spending a year at the Mathematical Sciences Research Center in Berkeley, California, she became Dean of the Faculty of Natural Sciences in Copenhagen 1986–88, after which she was appointed full Professor at the University of Roskilde, and in 1989 Director General of the Danish IT-Centre for Research and Education, UNI•C. She has been the President of the Danish Association of the Advancement of Science from 1988. In 1992, she became a member of the High Performance Computing and Networking Advisory Committee of the European Commission, and chaired its Networking Sub-group (the LINKS group). In 1987–93, she was a Member and eventually Co-chair of the Danish Council for Research Policy, an advisory council to the Danish Government and Parliament. In 1991–93 she chaired a Committee on technology-supported learning formed by the Danish Minister of Education and she was a member of the Steering Committee for the Norwegian Scientific Computing Initiative, NOTUR, from 2000–2004. In 2000–2003 she was a member of the Danish Complaints Board for Domain Names. She has been Chair of the board of Roskilde University from 2004–2008, and Member of the Danish Defence Research Council from 1998.

Roberto Sabatino manages the R&D aspects of the GÉANT2 project in DANTE, with emphasis on the ultimate goal of developing usable services. After his degree in computer science from the University of Turin in 1990, he started to work long before he completed his studies, as a software development engineer for telecommunications protocols. In 1995 he moved to Cambridge to take up a Research Associate position in the Cambridge University Computer Laboratory on the performance of high speed networks. At the time, this was 155 Mbps ATM, FDDI (fiber distributed data interface), 100 Mbps Ethernet. In 1997 he joined DANTE as network engineer. In these years has played a key role in the design and development of the TEN-155, GÉANT and GÉANT2 networks. He was appointed Head of Network Planning in 1998 and Chief Technology Officer of DANTE in 2002 in the context of the GÉANT2 project.

Michael Stanton is Director of Innovation at RNP, the Brazilian NREN, and also Technical Coordinator of CLARA, the Latin American regional network association.

After completing his Ph.D. in mathematics at Cambridge University, he started his higher education career in Brazil in 1971, and since 1994 has been Professor of Computer Networking at the Universidade Federal Fluminense (UFF) in Niterói, Rio de Janeiro state. Beginning in 1986, he participated in kick-starting R&E networking in Brazil, which included linking a nascent national network, first to BITNET in 1988, and then to the Internet in 1992. During that period, he helped set up and run both the regional network in Rio de Janeiro state (Rede-Rio) and RNP. After an 8-year absence, he returned to RNP, with responsibility for oversight of R&D and RNP involvement in new networking and e-science projects.

Cathrin Stöver is International Relations Manager in DANTE. She studied European Business Studies in Germany, France and the United Kingdom, and spent some time working for Derby City Council before joining DANTE in 1997. For the last five years, she has focused on the project management of the Latin American ALICE project, which led to the creation of the regional RedCLARA network and also of CLARA, DANTE's counterpart in Latin America.

Peter Tindemans chairs the European Spallation Neutron Source efforts and a European Alliance for Permanent Access to establish a European Digital Information Infrastructure. He is working with the World Bank, UNESCO (United Nations Educational, Scientific and Cultural Organization) and governments on STI (science, technology and innovation) in the Middle East and Africa. He was Chairman of the CPG from early 1987 to April 1991. Until 1999, he directed research and science policy in the Netherlands, chaired the OECD (Organization for Economic Cooperation and Development) Megascience Forum, was a member of the EUREKA High Level Group and involved in the preparation of successive EU Framework Programs. He has a Ph.D. in Theoretical Physics from Leiden University. He now works at Global Knowledge Strategies and Partnerships, in the area of science, technology and society. Recent activities included being Rapporteur-General of the NIH (National Institutes of Health), ESF and EU conference on Research Integrity and the Portuguese EU Presidency conference on the Future of Science in Europe. He is a member of the Governing Board of Euroscience.

Stefano Trumpy is a Research Manager at the Institute of Informatics and Telematics of the Italian National Research Council. In recent years, he has been involved in international aspects of Internet governance. He is the Italian representative in the Governmental Advisory Committee of ICANN; he is a member of the Italian governmental delegation in the Internet Governance Forum and promoter of the dynamic coalition "Internet bill of rights". He was the guest editor of the September 2004 Special Issue of IEEE Proceedings on "Evolution of Internet Technologies". He was also the TERENA President for two mandates, from 1995 through 1999. Manager of the ccTLD ".it" from its creation in 1987 through 1999; at present he is in charge of the international relations of the registry. He was the Director of CNUCE (Centro Nazionale Universitario di Calcolo Elettronico) Institute of CNR (Consiglio Nazionale delle Ricerche), involved in computing and networking, from 1983 to 1996.

Klaus Ullmann has been Managing Director of DFN in Berlin since 1984 and is Chairman of the DANTE Board. He has a diploma in theoretical physics. He began his career in network development at the Hahn-Meitner Institute in Berlin, working with the networking group of the IT department on local and regional networking. Since that time, he has contributed extensively to the development of research networking in Germany and at a European level. He was the project leader of a regional network for the Berlin universities and research establishments, and then head of the Planning Team for DFN. In addition, he was a member of the Executive Committee of the European umbrella organization of national R&E networks, RARE, and later President of RARE from 1986 to 1990, the period when its activities were dominated by the COSINE project. In 2005, he was also elected Chairman of the GÉANT2 Executive Committee.

Jean-Marc Uzé is Technical Director, Product & Technology at Juniper Networks for the European, Middle East and African regions. He has a Master of Science in Network Engineering, and started his career as head of the Data-processing centre of INRA (Institut National de la Recherche Agronomique). Jean-Marc spent 4 years at GIP (Groupement d'Intérêt Public) RENATER. As Project Director, he led the RENATER 2 project, the new generation National Research Network of France. As International Project Manager, he was involved in several projects such as TEN-34, TEN-155 and the United States connectivity. In addition, he led and coordinated the MPLS activities of the European technical TF-TEN (task force on trans-European networking) and TF-TANT (task force testing of advanced networking technologies). He joined Air France Airline Company in 2000 as Network Project Manager in the Department of Strategy for Data-processing and Telecommunications. He finally joined Juniper Networks in 2001, initially as a consultant focusing on Research, Education and Government Networks and Institutions. He has also been a member of the Scientific Committee of the MPLS World Congress since its beginning in 1999.

Karel Vietsch is the Secretary General of TERENA. He studied mathematics and economics at Leiden University, and subsequently worked as a teaching and research assistant at the same university. He obtained his Ph.D. in 1979. After military service as a systems and data analyst, Karel became Manager of the Department of Mathematics and Computer Science at Delft University of Technology. In 1984, he joined the Science Policy Department of the Netherlands Ministry of Education, Culture and Science, where he was involved, among many other things, in the creation of SURFnet and in the COSINE project. He left the Ministry and joined TERENA in 1996. His current duties include being a member of the Executive Committee of the GÉANT2 project and representing TERENA in a number of bodies, including the CCIRN and the ENPG.

David West joined DANTE in 2001 as a Project Manager after spending 15 years at British Telecommunications where he was a senior manager responsible for international product and business development programs. At DANTE, he has led the EUMEDCONNECT project from its inception. Since 2004 this has provided the first Mediterranean regional research and education network connecting North Africa and the Middle Eastern countries. It spawned equivalent programs for other world regions and he has led and managed the Asian TEIN2 program which connects the Asia-Pacific and South Asian regions and a new program for Central Asia (CAREN, Central Asian Research and Education Network). He has extensive experience in the telecommunications field of managing and supporting new projects, and in establishing supplier and partner relationships. He is educated to postgraduate degree level and spent the earlier part of his career in the UK urban development industry.

Appendix B: List of NREN Managers

Austria
Manfred Paul, Chairman of the ACOnet association 1986–1992
Peter Rastl, ACOnet Manager 1992–present

Belgium
Pierre Bruyère, BELNET Director 1993–present

Bulgaria
Kiril Boyanov, UNICOM-B Chairman 1991–1999
Orlin Kouzov, Executive Director of the NREN 1999–2006
Plamen Vatchkov, BREN Chairman 2006–present

Croatia
Predrag Vidas, CARNet Chief Executive Officer 1995–1998
Jasenka Gojšić, CARNet Chief Executive Officer 1998–2004
Zvonimir Stanić, CARNet Chief Executive Officer 2004–present

Cyprus
Agathoclis Stylianou, CyNet General Manager 2001–present

Czech Republic
Jan Gruntorád, CESNET General Manager 1996–present

Denmark
Hans Jørgen Helms, NEUCC Director 1965–1974
Peter Villemoes, NEUCC Director 1974–1983
Hans Ole Aagaard, NEUCC Director 1983–1985
Erik Kofod, UNI•C Managing Director 1985–1989
Dorte Olesen, UNI•C Managing Director 1989–present

Estonia
Enok Sein, EENet Director 1993–1997
Mihkel Kraav, EENet Director 1997–present

A History of International Research Networking. Edited by Howard Davies and Beatrice Bressan
Copyright © 2010 WILEY-VCH Verlag GmbH & Co. KGaA, Weinheim
ISBN: 978-3-527-32710-2

Finland
Matti Ihamuotila, CSC General Manager 1983–2004 and Chairman of the FUNET Steering Group 1983–1989
Ari Rikkilä, FUNET Project Secretary 1983–1985
Panu Pietikäinen, FUNET Project Manager 1985–1986
Markus Sadeniemi, FUNET Director 1986–2004
Lars Backström, Chairman of the FUNET Steering Group 1990–1995
Kimmo Koski, CSC General Manager 2004–present
Janne Kanner, FUNET Director 2004–present

France
Michel Lartail, RENATER General Manager 1993–1998
Laurent de Mercey, RENATER Interim Director 1998
Dany Vandromme, RENATER General Manager 1998–present

Germany
Klaus-Eckart Maass, DFN Managing Director 1984–2006
Klaus Ullmann, DFN Managing Director 1984–present
Jochem Pattloch, DFN Managing Director 2006–present

Greece
Vasilis Maglaris, Chairman of the GRNET Board 1998–2004
Panayiotis Tsanakas, Chairman of the GRNET Board 2004–present
Theodoros Karounos, GRNET Managing Director 2001–2002
Tryfon Chiotis, GRNET Technical Director 2001–2002 and GRNET Chief Technical Officer 2002–present
Zak Koune, GRNET Program Director 2002–2006
Antonis Tzortzakakis, GRNET Program Director 2006–2007

Hungary
Miklós Nagy, NIIFI General Manager 1986–present

Iceland
Jóhann Gunnarsson, SURIS General Manager 1987–1990
Páll Jensson, SURIS General Manager 1990–1991
Þorsteinn I. Sigfússon, SURIS General Manager 1991–1993
Helgi Þórsson, SURIS General Manager 1993–1994
Páll Jensson, SURIS General Manager 1994–1995
Helgi Jónsson, INTIS General Manager 1995–2000
Jón Ingi Einarsson, RHnet General Manager 2001–present

Ireland
John Hayden, HEAnet Network Management Committee Chairman 1983–1992
Dennis Jennings, Michael Nowlan, Gordon Young HEAnet NMC Directorate 1996–1997
Mike Norris, HEAnet Network Coordinator 1992–1997
John Boland, HEAnet Ltd. Chief Executive 1997–present

Israel
Avi Cohen, IUCC General Manager 1985–2008
Moshe Gottlieb, IUCC Director General 2008–present

Italy
Orio Carlini, chairman of GARR Technical-Scientific Committee 1987–present
Antonio Cantore, Director of GARR Network 1990–1994
Enzo Valente, Director of GARR Network 1995–2002 and GARR Chief Executive Officer 2003–present
Claudia Battista, Director of GARR Network 2003-

Latvia
Jānis Ķikuts, LATNET Manager 1992–2007
Baiba Kaškina, SigmaNet Manager 2007–present

Lithuania
Laimutis Telksnys, LITNET General Manager 1991–present

Luxembourg
Antoine Barthel, RESTENA General Manager 1989–present
Theo Duhautpas, RESTENA General Manager 1989–present

Former Yugoslav Republic of Macedonia
Oliver Popov, MARNet General Manager and President of the Executive Board 1995–2002
Boroslav Popovski, MARNet General Manager and President of the Executive Board 2002–2008
Margita Kon-Popovska, MARNet General Manager and President of the Executive Board 2008–present

Malta
Robert Sultana, University of Malta Director of IT Services 1996–present

Montenegro
Božo Krstajić, MREN General Manager 2006–present

Netherlands
Boudewijn Nederkoorn, SURFnet Managing Director 1988–2007
Kees Neggers, SURFnet Managing Director 1988–present
Erwin Bleumink, SURFnet Managing Director 2006–present
Erik-Jan Bos, SURFnet Managing Director 2007–present

Nordic countries
Peter Villemoes, NORDUnet General Manager 1980–2005
René Buch, NORDUnet Chief Executive Officer 2005–present

Norway
Petter Kongshaug, UNINETT Director 1987–present

Portugal
Heitor Pina, FCCN General Manager 1991–1996
Pedro Veiga, FCCN General Manager 1997–present

Romania
Nicolae Gabriel Popovici, RoEduNet General Manager 1998–1999
Radu Valer Gramatovici, RoEduNet General Manager 1999–2000
Eduard Andrei, RoEduNet General Manager 2000–2006
Octavian Rusu, RoEduNet General Manager 2006–present

Serbia
Zoran Jovanović, AMRES General Manager 2001–present

Slovakia
Pavol Horváth, President of the SANET Network Association 1991–present

Slovenia
Marko Bonač, ARNES General Manager 1992–present

Spain
José Barberá, RedIRIS Director 1988–1993
Víctor Castelo, RedIRIS Director 1994–2003
Alberto Pérez, RedIRIS Acting Director 2004–2005 and Deputy Director 2004–present
Tomás de Miguel, RedIRIS Director 2005–present

Sweden
Hans Wallberg, SUNET General Manager 1985–present

Switzerland
Bernhard Plattner, SWITCH Managing Director 1987–1988
Peter Gilli, SWITCH Managing Director 1988–1994
Thomas Brunner, SWITCH Managing Director 1994–present
Karl-Heinz Krebser, SWITCH Managing Director 1995–2000

Turkey
Yasar Tonta, ULAKBİM Executive Manager 1996–1998
Erkan Tekman, ULAKBİM Executive Manager 1998–1999
Tugrul Yilmaz, ULAKBİM Executive Manager 2000–2005
Cem Saraç, ULAKBİM Executive Manager 2005–present

United Kingdom
Roland Rosner, Head of Network Unit 1976–1979 and Head of the JNT 1979–1983
Mike Wells, JANET Director of Networking 1983–1988
Peter Linington, Head of the JNT and Network Executive 1983–1986
Bob Cooper, Head of the JNT 1987–1991 and JANET Director of Networking 1988–1994
Willie Black, Head of the JNT 1991–1994
Geoff Manning, UKERNA Chairman and Acting Chief Executive Officer 1992–1993

David Hartley, UKERNA Chief Executive Officer 1994–1997
Geoff McMullen, UKERNA Chief Executive Officer 1997–2001
Robin Arak, UKERNA Chief Executive Officer 2001–2004
Bob Day, UKERNA Acting Chief Executive Officer 2004–2005
Tim Marshall, UKERNA Chief Executive Officer 2005–2007 and JANET Chief Executive Officer 2007–present

Appendix C: List of Network Names

ACOnet	Akademisches computer netz
ACSNET	Academic computing services network
AMRES	The national research and education network of Serbia
ANSP	Academic network at São Paulo
APAN	Asia-Pacific advanced network
ARIADnet	or ARIADNE network was the main national academic and research computer network of Greece before a reorganization which led to the creation of GRNET
ARNES	Academic research network of Slovenia
ARPAnet	Advanced research projects agency network
BELNET	Belgian research network
BITNET	Because it's there network and later because it's time network
BMEnet	Budapesti Mszaki és gazdaságtudományi Egyetem network
BREN	Bulgarian research and education network
CANARIE	Canadian network for the advancement of research, industry and education
CA*net	The research network in Canada
CAREN	Central Asian research and education network
CARNet	Croatian academic and research network
CEENet	Central and Eastern European network
CERNET	A site-wide network developed at CERN (1976–1988) and also the Chinese education and research network since 1995
CESNET	Czech educational and scientific network
CSNET	Computer science network
CSTNET	China science and technology network
CUDI	Corporación Universitaria para el Desarrollo de Internet
CyNet	Cyprus national research and education network
DATAnet 1	The public switched data network operated by the Dutch PTT Telecom (now known as KPN, Koninklijke PTT Nederland)
DATAPAK	The public packet switched network in the Nordic countries
DATEX-P	Data exchange – packetized
DCS	The public X.25 network in Belgium in the early 1990s
DN1	The Dutch public data network

A History of International Research Networking. Edited by Howard Davies and Beatrice Bressan
Copyright © 2010 WILEY-VCH Verlag GmbH & Co. KGaA, Weinheim
ISBN: 978-3-527-32710-2

EAN	Electronic access network
EARN	European academic and research network
EASInet	European academic supercomputing initiative network
Ebone	European backbone
EENet	Estonian educational and research network
EMPB	European multi-protocol backbone
EMPP	European 2 Mbps multi-protocol pilot
EPSS	Experimental packet switching system
ERNET	Education and research network in India
ESAPAC	European space agency X.25 network
ESnet	Energy sciences network
EUMEDCONNECT	IP research network linking Mediterranean and North African countries
EUnet	European UNIX network
EUROnet	European network
EuropaNET	European multi-protocol backbone network
FORTH	A R&D network in Greece operated by the Foundation for Research & Technology – Hellas
FREEnet	Network for research, education and engineering
FUNET	Finnish University network
GARR	Gruppo Armonizzazione reti della ricerca
GÉANT	Gigabit European academic network technology
GLIF	Global lambda integrated facility
GLORIAD	Global ring network for advanced applications development
G-REUNA	Gigabit-Red Universitaria National
GRNET	Greek research and technology network
HEAnet	Higher Education Authority network
HELLASPAC	Hellenic packet switch service
HEPnet	High energy physics network
HUNGARNET	Hungarian academic and research networking association
i2CAT	Internet2 Catalunya
IBDNS	International backbone data network service
IBERPAC	Servicio Iberico de conmutacion por packets
INFNet	Istituto Nazionale di Fisica Nucleare network
INNOVA/RED	The research network in Argentina
ILAN	The Israeli Research Network, owned and operated by Machba, an association owned by the eight principal universities in Israel
ITN	International transit network
IXI	International X.25 infrastructure
JANET	Joint academic network
JUNET	Japan UNIX network
KOREN	Korea advanced research network
LATNET	Latvian academic and research network
LITNET	Lithuanian academic and research network

LUXPAC	Packet-switched networks offered in Luxembourg
MARNet	Macedonian academic and research network
MDNS	Managed data network service
MPBS	Multi-protocol backbone service
MREN	Montenegrin research and education network
MSUNet	The Moscow State University Network
NLnet	The national branch of EUnet in the Netherlands
NLR	National lambdarail
NORDUnet	Nordic University network
NSFnet	National Science Foundation network
OSIRIDE	The Italian Research Council's heterogeneous OSI compatible network
PSNC	Poznań Supercomputing and Networking Center
PLEASE	The public X.25 network in Hungary in the early 1990s
POL-34	The research network in Poland
PSS	Packet switch stream
RASNet	Russian Academy of Science network
RBNet	Russian backbone network
RCCN	Rede da Comunidade Científica Nacional
REACCIUN	Red Académica de Centros de Investigación y Universidades Nacionales
RedCLARA	The Latin American regional research and education network operated by CLARA
RedIRIS	Red de Interconexión de Recursos Informáticos
RELARN	Russian electronic academic and research network
Relcom	Reliable communications
RENATER	Réseau national de télécommunications pour la technologie, l'enseignement et la recherche
RESTENA	Réseau téléinformatique de l'éducation nationale et de la recherche
RESULB	Réseau informatique de l'Université Libre de Bruxelles
RETINA	Red teleinformática académica
REUNA	Red Universitaria National
RHnet	The national research and education network in Iceland
RNP	Rede national de ensino e Pesquisa
RoEDuNet	The national research and education network in Romania
RUNNet	Russian university network
SANET	Slovak academic network association
SEEREN	South-East European research and education networking
SigmaNet	The national research and education network in Latvia
SINET	Science information network
SingAREN	Singapore advanced research and education network
SIPAX.25	Slovenian national X.25 network
SUNET	Swedish university network

SURFnet	The national research and education network in the Netherlands
SURIS	The national research and education network in Iceland
SwipNet	A commercial IP service operated by Tele2, a Swedish PNO
SWITCH	The national research and education network in Switzerland
TEIN	Trans-Eurasia information network
TEN-155	Trans-European network at 155 Mbps
TEN-34	Trans-European network at 34 Mbps
TIPnet	A commercial IP service operated by Telia, a swedish PNO
UKnet	UK network
ULAKBĪM	The national research and education network in Turkey
UMOS	South Moscow backbone network
UNICOM-B	Universal integrated communication-Bulgaria
USENET	A contraction of user network
UUCPnet	UNIX to UNIX copy protocol network
vBNS	Very high speed backbone network service
WHREN	Western Hemisphere research and education networks
WIN	WissenchaftsNetz
YUNAC	The Yugoslav academic and research network

Appendix D: List of Acronyms

ACCU	Association of C/C++ users
ACM	Association for Computing Machinery
ACM SIGGRAPH	Association for Computing Machinery's special interest group on graphics and interactive techniques
ACTS	Advanced communications technologies and services
ADMD	Administrative management domain
AI	Artificial intelligence
ALICE	América Latina Interconectada Con Europa
@LIS	Alliance for the Information Society
AMPATH	Americas path
AMS-IX	Amsterdam Internet Exchange
ARPA	Advanced Research Projects Agency
ASEM	Asia-Europe meeting
ASN.1	Abstract syntax notation one
AT&T	American Telephone & Telegraph Company
ATM	Asynchronous transfer mode
AUCS	AT&T unisource carrier services
AUP	Acceptable use policy
AutoBAHN	Automated bandwidth allocation across heterogeneous networks
BGP-4	Border gateway protocol version 4
BMBF	Bundesministerium für Bildung und Forschung
BMFT	Bundesministerium für Forschung und Technologie
BoD	Bandwidth-on-demand
BSD	Berkeley software distribution
BSI	Bundesamt für Sicherheit in der Informationstechnik
BSMTP	Batched simple mail transfer protocol
BT	British Telecommunications
B.V.	Besloten vennootschap
CAD	Computer-aided design
CAESAR	Connecting all European and Southern American researchers
Calit2	California Institute of Telecommunications and Information Technology

A History of International Research Networking. Edited by Howard Davies and Beatrice Bressan
Copyright © 2010 WILEY-VCH Verlag GmbH & Co. KGaA, Weinheim
ISBN: 978-3-527-32710-2

CAN	Campus area network
CAPE	Chancellor's Academic Professional Excellence
CAVE	Cave automatic virtual environment
CBF	Cross border fiber
CBR	Constant bit rate
CCIRN	Co-ordinating Committee for Intercontinental Research Networking
CCITT	Comité Consultatif International Téléphonique et Télégraphique
CCTA	Central Computer and Telecommunications Agency
ccTLD	Country code top-level domain
CEE	Central and Eastern Europe
CEEC	Central and Eastern European countries
CEENet	Central and Eastern European Network Association
CENIC	Corporation for Education Network Initiatives in California
CENTR	Council of European National Top Level Domains Registries
CEPIS	Council of European Professional Informatics Societies
CEPT	Conference of European Postal and Telecommunication Administration
CERN	Conseil Européen pour la Recherche Nucléaire
CERT	Computer emergency response team
CERT/CC	CERT coordination center
CIDR	Classless inter-domain routing
CIEMAT	Centro de Investigaciones Energéticas, Medioambientales y Tecnológicas
CIP	COSINE implementation phase
CIPEC	COSINE implementation phase execution contract
CLARA	Cooperación Latino Americana de Redes Avanzadas
CLARA-TEC	CLARA-technical forum
CLNS	Connectionless network services
CNAM	Conservatoire National des Arts et Métiers
CNR	Consiglio Nazionale delle Ricerche
CNRS	Centre National de la Recherche Scientifique
CNUCE	Centro Nazionale Universitario di Calcolo Elettronico
CoA	Council of administration
COCOM	Coordinating committee for multilateral export controls
COM	Component object model
COMECON	Council for mutual economic assistance
COMICS	Computer-based message interconnection systems
CORDIS	Community Research and Development Information Service
COSINE	Cooperation for open systems interconnection networking in Europe
COST	European cooperation in the field of scientific and technical research
CPB	COSINE Policy Bureau

CPG	COSINE Policy Group
CPMU	COSINE Project Management Unit
CPqD	Centro de Pesquisa e Desenvolvimento em Telecomunicações
CSIC	Consejo Superior de Investigaciones Científicas
CSIRT	Computer security incident response team
CWDM	Coarse wavelength division multiplexing
CWI	Centrum voor Wiskunde en Informatica
DANTE	Delivery of Advanced Network Technology to Europe
DARPA	Defense Advanced Research Projects Agency
DataTAG	Research and technological development for a data transatlantic grid
DC	District of Columbia
DEC	Digital Equipment Corporation
DECnet	Network protocol design by DEC
DESY	Deutsches Elektronen Synchrotron
DFN	Deutsches Forschungsnetz
DG	Directorate General
D-GIX	Distributed GIX
DICE	DANTE-Internet2-CANARIE-ESnet
DiffServ	Differentiated services
DIKU	Datalogisk Institut Københavns Universitet
DNS	Domain name system
DoD	Department of Defense
DoE	Department of Energy
DS0	Digital signal 0
DT	Deutsche Telekom
DTE	Data terminal equipment
DWDM	Dense wavelength division multiplexing
DYNACORE	Dynamically configurable remote experiment monitoring & control
E2E	End-to-end
E2ECU	E2E coordination unit
EAT	Ebone action team
EBS	Ebone boundary systems
EC	European Commission
ECCO	Ebone Consortium of Contributing Organizations
ECFA	European Committee for Future Accelerators
ECFRN	European Consultative Forum on Research Networking
ECRC	European Computer-Industry Research Centre
ECU	European currency unit
EdCAAD	Edinburgh computer-aided architectural design
EDFA	Erbium-doped fiber amplifier
EDISON	European distributed and interactive simulation over network
EEC	European Economic Community
EELA	E-science grid facility for Europe and Latin America

EEPG	European Engineering and Planning Group
EFTA	European Free Trade Association
EGEE	Enabling grids for e-science
EMEA	Europe, Middle East and Africa
ENA	Ecole Nationale d'Administraton
ENCART	European Network for CyberART
ENPG	European Networking Policy Group
EOT	Ebone operations team
EPL	Ethernet private lines
ESA	European Space Agency
ESF	European Science Foundation
ESMTP	Extended simple mail transfer protocol
ESPRIT	European Strategic Programme for Research in Information Technology
ETH	Eidgenössische Technische Hochschule
EU	European Union
EUMEDIS	Euro-Mediterranean initiative for the Information Society
EUREKA	European Research Coordination Agency
EuroCAIRN	European cooperation for academic and industrial research networking
EUSJA	European Union of Science Journalists' Associations
EUUG	European UNIX Users Group
EVL	Electronic visualization laboratory
e-VLBI	Electronic transfer very-long-baseline interferometry
EXPReS	Express production real-time e-VLBI service
FAPESP	Fundação de Amparo à Pesquisa do Estado de São Paulo
FCCN	Fundação para a Computação Científica Nacional
FDDI	Fiber distributed data interface
FIPS	Federal Information Processing Standard
FIRST	Forum of incident response and security teams
FIU	Florida International University
FTAM	File transfer and access management
FTP	File transfer protocol
FUDI	FR (France) UK (United Kingdom) DE (Germany) IT (Italy)
G7	Group of Seven
GDP	Gross domestic product
GIBN	Global interoperability for broadband networks
GIFT	General internetwork file transfer
GIGA	Gigabits networking research
GILT	Get interconnection between local text system
GIP	Groupement d'Intérêt Public
GIX	Global Internet exchange
GKS	Graphics kernel system
GMD	Gesellschaft für Mathematik und Datenverarbeitung
GMT	Greenwich mean time

GNP	Gross national product
GOLE	GLIF open lightpath exchange
GOSIP	Government OSI profile
GPMIMD2	General purpose multiple instruction multiple data machines 2
GRIP	Guidelines and recommendations for incident processing
GTS	Global telesystems
HAN	Home area network
HD	High definition
HEP	High energy physics
HKOEP	Hong Kong open exchange portal
HPIIS	High performance international Internet services
HTML	Hypertext markup language
HTTP	Hypertext transfer protocol
IAB	Internet Architecture Board
IANW	International Academic NetWorkshop
iCAIR	International Centre for Advanced Internet Research
ICANN	Internet Corporation for Assigned Names and Numbers
ICEAGE	International collaboration to extend and advance grid education
ICI	Institutul National de Cercetare-Dezvoltare în Informatică
ICM	International connections management
iCPMU	interim COSINE Project Management Unit
ICRF	Imperial cancer research fund
ICT	Information and communication technology
id	Identifier
IDC	International Data Corporation
IDWG	Intrusion Detection Working Group
IEEAF	Internet Educational Equal Access Foundation
IEEE	Institute of Electrical and Electronics Engineers
IEPG	Intercontinental Engineering and Planning Group
IES	Information exchange system
IESG	Internet Engineering Steering Group
IETF	Internet Engineering Task Force
iGrid	International grid
IN2P3	Institut National de Physique Nucléaire et de Physique des Particules
INCH	Incident handling
INCS	Integrated network connection service
iNEER	International Network on Engineering Education and Research
INET	Internet Society's Annual Conference
INFN	Istituto Nazionale di Fisica Nucleare
INRA	Institut National de la Recherche Agronomique
INRIA	Institut National de Recherche en Informatique et Automatique
IP	Internet protocol

IPSF	IPsphere forum
IPv4	Internet protocol version 4
IPv6	Internet protocol version 6
IPX	Internetwork packet exchange
IRIS	Interconexión de los recursos informáticos
IRNC	International research network connections
IRT	Incident response team
ISDN	Integrated services digital network
ISO	International Standards Organisation
ISOC	Internet Society
ISP	Internet service provider
IST	Information Society Technologies
IT	Information technology
ITU	International Telecommunication Union
ITU-T	ITU telecommunication standardization sector
IUCC	Inter-University Computation Centre
JAMES	Joint ATM experiment on European services
JENC	Joint European Networking Conference
JINR	Joint Institute of Nuclear Research
JISC	Joint Information Systems Committee
JIVE	Joint Institute for Very-long-baseline Interferometry in Europe
JMA	James Martin Associates
JNT	Joint network team
JRA	Joint research activities
JRC	Joint Research Centre
KISDI	Korea Information Society Development Institute
KPN	Koninklijke PTT Nederland
KTH	Kungliga Tekniska Högskolan
LAN	Local area network
LDAP	Lightweight directory access protocol
LEP	Large electron positron collider
LHC	Large Hadron Collider
LILA	Links interconnecting Latin America
LISTSERV	Mailing list server
LSP	Label switched paths
MAC	Media access control
MAN	Metropolitan area network
MAN LAN	Manhattan landing
MBA	Master of Business and Administration
MBGP	Multicast border gateway protocol
MBONE	Multicast backbone
MBS	Managed bandwidth service
MCC	Metro core connect
MECCANO	Multimedia education and conferencing collaboration over ATM network and others

MECU	Millions of ECU – European Currency Unit
MEDA	Mediterranean economic development area
MHS	Message handling service
MIC	Ministry of Information and Communication
MIME	Multipurpose Internet mail extensions
MIT	Massachusetts Institute of Technology
MoU	Memorandum of understanding
MPLS	Multi-protocol label switching
MSc	Master of Science
MSDP	Multicast source discovery protocol
MSU	Moscow State University
MTA	Message transfer agent
6NET	Large-scale international IPv6 pilot network
NACSIS	National Centre for Science Information Systems
NASA	National Aeronautics and Space Administration
NATO	North Atlantic Treaty Organization
NCP	Network control program
NCSA	National Centre for Supercomputing Applications
NEG	Network Engineering Group
NEUCC	Northern Europe University Computing Centre
NFS	Network file system
NGI	Next generation Internet
NGIX	Next generation Internet exchange
NICE	National host interconnection experiments
NIH	National Institutes of Health
NIIFI	Nemzeti Informacios Infrastruktura Fejlesztesi Iroda
NIKHEF	Nationaal Instituut voor Kernfysica en Hoge Energie Fysica
NIST	National Institute of Science and Technology
NJE	Network job entry
NLUUG	NL UNIX Users Group
NMC	Network Management Committee
NOC	Network operation center
NREN	National research and education network
NSF	National Science Foundation
NTT	Nippon Telegraph and Telephone
NTUA	National Technical University of Athens
OC-3, 12	Optical carrier level 3, 12
OECD	Organization for Economic Cooperation and Development
OMII	Open Middleware Infrastructure Institute
ONP	Open network provision
OPN	Optical private network
OptIPuter	Optical networking, Internet protocol, computer
OSI	Open systems interconnection
OU	Operational unit
OUSC	Operational Unit Steering Committee

p2p	Point-to-point
PAD	Packet assembler–disassembler
PARADISE	Piloting a researcher's directory service in Europe
PC	Personal Computer
PCR	Peak cell rate
PDH	Plesiochronous digital hierarchy
PEM	Privacy enhanced mail
PERT	Performance enhancement and response team
PGP	Pretty good privacy
PHARE	Poland and Hungary: Assistance for restructuring their economies
PIM-SM	Protocol-independent multicast sparse-mode
PKI	Public key infrastructure
PMDF	PASCAL-based memo distribution facility
PMI	Privilege management infrastructure
PNO	Public network operator
PNWGP	Pacific NorthWest giga point of presence
PoP	Point of presence
POS	Packet over SONET
PRAGMA	Pacific Rim applications and grid middleware assembly
PSPDN	Packet-switched public data network
PTO	Public telecoms operator
PTT	Post, telephone, and telegraph operating entity
PUB	Polytechnic University of Bucharest
PVC	Permanent virtual circuit
Q-MED	QUANTUM in the Eastern Mediterranean region
QoS	Quality of service
QTP	QUANTUM test program
QUANTUM	Quality network technology for user-oriented multi-media
RACE	Research for advanced communications in Europe
RAG	Requirements action group
RAL	Rutherford Appleton Laboratory
RARE	Réseaux Associés pour la Recherche Européenne
RAS	Russian Academy of Sciences
RBS	Regional boundary systems
RDIG	Russian data intensive grid
RECAU	Det Regionale Edb-center ved Århus Universitet
RECKU	Det Regionale Edb-center ved Københavns Universitet
R&D	Research and development
R&E	Research and education
RFC	Request for comment
RINGrid	Remote instrumentation in next-generation grids
RIPE	Réseaux IP Européens
RIPE NCC	RIPE Network Coordination Centre
RIPN	Russian Institute of Public Networks

RIR	Regional Internet Registry
RISC	Reduced instruction set computer
ROC	Russian Operation Centre
RSCS	Remote spooling communications subsystem
RSSI	Russian space science Internet
RTP	Real time protocol
RUHEP	Russian HEP
SARA	Stichting Academisch Rekencentrum Amsterdam
SCR	Sustained cell rate
SDH	Synchronous digital hierarchy
SDN	System development network
SERC	Science and Engineering Research Council
SERENATE	Study into European Research and Education Networking As Targeted by Europe
SGML	Standardized generic markup language
SIB	Swiss Institute of Bioinformatics
SIIT&T	State Institute of Information Technologies and Telecommunications
SINTEF	Selskapet for Industriell og Teknisk Forskning ved Norges Tekniske Hoegskole
SLAG	Stanford Linear Accelerator Center
SME	Small or medium-sized enterprise
SMS	Short message service
SMTP	Simple mail transfer protocol
SNA	Systems network architecture
SNMP	Simple network management protocol
SOA	Service oriented architecture
SOAR	Southern astrophysical research
SoftEng	Software engineering
SONET	Synchronous optical network
SPAN	Space physics analysis network
SSO	Single sign-on
STARTAP	Science, technology, and research transit access point
STI	Science, technology and innovation
STM-1, 4, 16, 64	Synchronous transport module level-1, 4, 16, 64
SVC	Switched virtual connection
TCP/IP	Transmission control protocol/Internet protocol
TDM	Time-division multiplexing
TERENA	Trans-European Research and Education Networking Association
TF-OU	Task force operational unit
TF-TANT	Task force testing of advanced networking technologies
TF-TEN	Task force on trans-European networking
TIFR	Tata Institute of Fundamental Research
T-LEX	Tokyo Lambda Exchange

TMF	Telemanagement forum
TOTEM	Total cross-section, elastic scattering and diffraction dissociation measurement at the LHC
UBN	Unisource business networks
UCD	University College Dublin
UCSD	University of California, San Diego
UDP	User datagram protocol
UERJ	Universidade do Estado do Rio de Janeiro
UFF	Universidade Federal Fluminense
UIC	University of Illinois at Chicago
UKERNA	United Kingdom Education and Research Networking Association
UKUUG	UK UNIX Users Group
ULB	Université Libre de Bruxelles
UNESCO	United Nations Educational, Scientific and Cultural Organization
UNIX	Originally UNICS, uniplexed information and computing system
UREC	Unité Reseaux du CNRS
USENIX	A conflation of USEr and uNIX
USSR	Union of Soviet Socialist Republic
UTK	University of Tennessee, Knoxville
UUCP	UNIX to UNIX copy protocol
UUG	UNIX users group
VAT	Value added tax
VAX	Virtual address extension
VAXPSI	VAX packetnet system interface
VBR	Variable bit rate
VLAN	Virtual LAN
VM	Virtual machine
VMS	Virtual memory system
VNET	Virtual networking
VoIP	Voice over Internet Protocol
VP	Virtual path
VPN	Virtual private network
VRVS	Virtual room videoconferencing system
WAIS	Wide area information server
WAN	Wide area network
WCW	Wetenschappelijk Centrum Watergraafsmeer
WDM	Wavelength division multiplexing
WG	Working group
WIDE	Widely integrated distributed environment
WWW	World Wide Web
XML	Extensible markup language

Appendix E: List of Terms

AMS-GWY is a label for the access port (gateway) in Amsterdam through which traffic to and from the commercial Internet passed.

Backbone is a central conduit designed to transfer network traffic at high speeds. Network backbones are designed to maximize the reliability and performance of large-scale, long-distance data communications. The best known network backbones have been those used on the Internet. Backbones typically consist of network routers and switches connected by fiber optic or Ethernet cables.

Bandwidth, digital bandwidth, or network bandwidth, is a measure of available or consumed data communication resources expressed in bps or multiples of it (kbps, Mbps, etc.).

Browser is a software application which enables a user to display and interact with text, images, videos, music, games and other information typically located on a Web page at a Web site on the World Wide Web (WWW) or a local area network (LAN). Text and images on a Web page can contain hyperlinks to other Web pages at the same or a different Web site. Web browsers allow users to access information provided on many Web pages at many Web sites by traversing these links. Web browsers process HTML (hypertext markup language) information to generate a display, so the appearance of a Web page may differ between browsers.

Cloud computing enables the delivery of personal and business services from a set of remote servers (the "cloud") accessed via a high capacity network. Responsibility for managing the computing resources needed to support the services is shifted from the user organization to the operator of the cloud; users of the service are unaware of the location of the systems that store and process their data.

CSC (IT Center for Science) is a non-profit company, administered by the Ministry of Education, providing IT support and resources for academia, research institutes and companies: modeling, computing and information services. CSC provides Finland's widest selection of scientific software and databases and Finland's most powerful supercomputing environment that researchers can use via the FUNET, the finnish university network.

A History of International Research Networking. Edited by Howard Davies and Beatrice Bressan
Copyright © 2010 WILEY-VCH Verlag GmbH & Co. KGaA, Weinheim
ISBN: 978-3-527-32710-2

Dark fiber or unlit fiber in fiber-optic communications (a method of transmitting information from one place to another by sending light through an optical fiber) is the name given to individual fibers that have yet to be used within cables that have been already laid. They are hence not yet connected to any device, and are only there for future usage. The term was originally used when talking about the potential network capacity of telecommunication infrastructure, but now also refers to the increasingly common practice of leasing fiber optic cables from a network service provider.

Dual-stack refers to a network implementation in which operations at a higher layer of the open systems interconnection model (OSI model) are supported by two discrete services at a lower layer. For example, dual-stack Internet protocol hosts run both the IPv4 and the IPv6 versions of IP and can intercommunicate with computers which use either one of these protocols. If both protocols are available, IPv6 is preferred.

E-carrier, where 'E' stands for European, is a carrier system in digital telecommunications, originally standardized by the Conference of European Postal and Telecommunication Administration (CEPT), which revised and improved the earlier American T-carrier technology. Now it has been adopted by the International Telecommunication Union Telecommunication Standardization Sector (ITU-T). The E-carrier standards form part of the plesiochronous digital hierarchy (PDH) where groups of circuits of E1 (the equivalent of the American T-carrier system format) may be bundled onto higher capacity (multiples of the E1 format) links between telephone exchanges or countries. E2 through E5 are carriers in increasing multiples of the E1 format. The E1 signal format carries data at a rate of 2.048 million bits per second. In practice, only E1 (30 circuit) and E3 (480 circuit) versions are used. Physically E1 is transmitted as 32 timeslots and E3 512 timeslots, but one is used for framing and typically one allocated for signaling call set-up and tear down. Unlike Internet data services, E-carrier systems permanently allocate capacity for a voice call for its entire duration. This ensures high call quality because the transmission arrives with the same short delay (latency) and capacity at all times.

Ethernet is a family of frame-based computer networking technologies for local area networks (LANs). It defines a number of wiring and signaling standards for the physical layer of the OSI (open systems interconnection) networking model, through means of network access at the media access control (MAC) and the data link layer (i.e. the protocol layer which transfers data between adjacent network nodes in a wide area network or between nodes on the same local area network segment), and a common addressing format. Ethernet is standardized as IEEE 802.3, which is a collection of IEEE (Institute of Electrical and Electronics Engineers) standards defining the physical layer, and the MAC sub-layer of the data link layer, of wired ethernet. Physical connections are made between nodes and/or infrastructure devices (hubs, switches, routers) by various types of copper or fiber cable. The combination of the twisted pair versions of ethernet for connecting end systems to the network, along with the fiber optic versions for site backbones, is the most widespread wired LAN technology.

Euroscience is a pan-European association, founded in 1997 by members of Europe's research community, to provide an open forum for debate on science and technology and research policies in Europe, to strengthen the links between science and society, to contribute to the creation of an integrated space for science and technology in Europe, linking research organizations and policies at national and European Union (EU) levels, strive for a greater role of the EU in research, and influence science and technology policies. It represents European scientists of all disciplines (natural sciences, mathematics, medical sciences, engineering, social sciences, humanities and the arts), institutions of the public sector, universities, research institutes as well as the business and industry sector.

Gateway is an internetworking system capable of joining together two networks that use different base protocols. It is a node on a network that serves as an entrance to another network. In enterprises, the gateway is the computer that routes the traffic from a workstation to the outside network that is serving the Web pages. In homes, the gateway is the equipment supplied by the Internet service provider (ISP) that connects the user to the Internet.

GOPHER is an Internet application protocol in which hierarchically-organized file structures are maintained on servers that are part of an overall information structure. GOPHER provides a way to bring text files from all over the world to a viewer on your computer. Popular for several years, especially in universities, GOPHER was a step toward the World Wide Web's (www) hypertext transfer protocol (HTTP). With hypertext links, the hypertext markup language (HTML), and the arrival of a graphical browser, Mosaic, the Web quickly transcended GOPHER. Many of the original file structures, especially those in universities, still exist and can be accessed through most Web browsers (because they also support the GOPHER protocol). GOPHER was developed at the University of Minnesota, whose sports teams are called "the Golden Gophers."

Grid is a conceptually simple idea and yet complex to implement. The aim is to be able to utilize computing resources wherever they are and in whatever form. The simplest view can be depicted in the visionary phrase 'boundaryless computing'. Grid computing is the application of several computers to a single problem at the same time – usually to a scientific or technical problem that requires a great number of computer processing cycles or access to large amounts of data. It is a form of distributed computing whereby a 'super and virtual computer' is composed of a cluster of networked, loosely coupled computers, acting in concert to perform very large tasks. This technology has been applied to computationally intensive scientific, mathematical, and academic problems through volunteer computing, and it is used in commercial enterprises for such diverse applications as drug discovery, economic forecasting, seismic analysis, and back-office data processing in support of e-commerce and Web services.

Host is a computer system that is accessed by a user working at a remote location. Typically, the term is used when there are two computer systems connected by modems and telephone lines. The system that contains the data is called the host, while the computer at which the user sits is called the remote terminal.

Hub is a device for connecting multiple twisted pair or fiber optic ethernet devices together and thus making them act as a single network segment. Hubs work at the physical layer (Layer 1) of the OSI (open systems interconnection) model. The device is thus a form of multiport repeater.

Hypertext is text, displayed on a computer, with references (hyperlinks) to other text that the reader can immediately follow, usually by a mouse click or key press sequence. Apart from running text, hypertext may contain tables, images and other presentational devices. Any of these can be hyperlinks; other means of interaction may also be present, for example, a bubble with text may appear when the mouse hovers somewhere, a video clip may be started and stopped, or a form may be filled out and submitted.

The most extensive example of hypertext today is the World Wide Web (www).

Internet is a global network of interconnected computers enabling users to share information along multiple channels. A majority of widely accessible information on the Internet consists of inter-linked hypertext documents and other resources of the World Wide Web (www). The movement of information in the Internet is achieved via a system of interconnected computer networks that share data by packet switching using the standardized Internet protocol suite (commonly known as transmission control protocol/Internet protocol, TCP/IP). It is a network that consists of millions of private and public, academic, business, and government networks of local to global scope that are linked by copper wires, fiber-optic cables, wireless connections, and other technologies.

Internet2 is a not-for-profit consortium in the United States which pioneers and promotes the use of advanced network applications and technologies. The consortium is made up of over 200 US universities, in cooperation with US government agencies, international partners and commercial organisations. The internet2 network configuration includes a high capacity IPv4, IPv6 and multicast service, a virtual circuit service that provides on-demand, dedicated optical paths between end points, and static point-to-point (p2p) circuits supported by an optical infrastructure.

INTIS is an Internet service provider in Iceland, mainly owned by educational institutions and the Icelandic state.

Lambda is a particular frequency of light, and the term is widely used in optical networking. Lambda-based networking is ultimately about using different "colors" or wavelengths of (laser) light in fibers for separate connections. Lambda networking is the technology and set of services directly surrounding the use of multiple optical wavelengths to provide independent communications channels along a strand of fiber-optic cable. Fiber-optic communications changed fundamentally in the early 1990s as the result of two technology breakthroughs: erbium-doped fiber amplifiers (EDFAs), which have the ability to amplify the communications being carried on a fiber-optic cable independently of the speed or method of signaling; and wavelength division multiplexing (WDM), which allows multiple communications channels over a single fiber by using different frequencies for each channel. Current coding schemes allow for typically 10 Gbps to be encoded by a laser on a high-speed network interface.

Lightpath is any dedicated unidirectional point to point connection in an optical network that provides guaranteed service levels to demanding e-Science applications that cannot tolerate the variations in performance of traditional shared Internet protocol (IP) services. Educational and research networks are now offering dedicated network connections to end users. Such connections are allocated dedicated wavelengths (or lambdas) in the underlying optical networks. Networks architectures that support both lightpaths and routed IP paths are called hybrid networks.

Mail-11 was the native email protocol used by the Digital Equipment Corporation's (DEC) Virtual Memory System (VMS), and supported by several other DEC operating systems. Similar to the internet's Simple Mail Transfer Protocol (SMTP) based mail, Mail-11 mail had To:, Cc: and Subject: headers and date-stamped each message. It was one of the most widely used email systems of the 1980s and was still in fairly wide use until as late as the mid-1990's. Messages from Mail-11 systems were frequently passed via gateways to SMTP, USENET, and BITNET systems, and thus are sometimes encountered when browsing archives of those systems. Mail-11 used two colons (::) rather than an "@" to separate user and hostname, and the hostname came first.

Mailer is a computer that receives and sends mail and also the software that receives and sends mail on a computer.

Mosaic is an application that simplifies accessing documents on the World Wide Web (www). Originally produced by the National Centre for Supercomputing Applications (NCSA), Mosaic has always been distributed as freeware. In 1994, however, the NCSA turned over commercial development of the programme to a company called Spyglass. There are now several varieties of Mosaic, some free and some for sale.

Multicast is a form of communication which involves a single sender and multiple receivers on a network. Typical uses include the transmission of conference presentations to interested people who for some reason cannot attend the conference, updating personnel who work from a home office and, the periodic issuance of online newsletters. Multicast is also used to support the MBONE (Multicast backbone), a system which, if sufficient network bandwidth is available, allows users to receive live video and audio streams.

National hosts were set up by the European Commission (EC) to provide coordinated access to advanced telecoms networks for the ACTS (advanced communications technologies and services) projects.

Network is a group of two or more computer systems linked together. There are many types of computer networks, including: local area networks (LANs), the computers are geographically close together (i.e. in the same building); wide area networks (WANs), the computers are farther apart and are connected by telephone lines or radio waves; campus area networks (CANs), the computers are within a limited geographic area (i.e. a campus or military base); and metropolitan area networks, MANs), a data network designed for a town or city, and home area networks (HANs), a network contained within a user's home that connects a person's digital devices.

OSI model (open systems interconnection model or OSI reference model) is an abstract description of a layered communications and computer network protocol design. It was developed as part of the OSI initiative, an effort to standardize computer networking systems that was started in 1977. In its most basic form, it divides network architecture into seven layers. An important principle is that implementations of functions at any given layer intercommunicate only with entities at the next higher and next lower layers, from top to bottom, the layers are application, presentation, session, transport, network, data-link, and physical. The model is often referred to as the OSI seven layer model.

OTE is the Hellenic Telecommunications Organization.

Packet is one unit of binary data capable of being routed through a computer network. To improve communication performance and reliability, each message sent between two network devices is often subdivided into packets by the underlying hardware and software.

PASCAL is a programming language that was created by Niklaus Wirth in 1970. It was named after Blaise Pascal, a famous French Mathematician. It was made as a language to teach programming and to be reliable and efficient.

QZ (Stockholms Datamaskincentral) is the Stockholm Computing Centre at the University of Stockholm.

Router is a device that connects two networks – frequently over large distances. It understands one or more network protocols, such as Internet protocol (IP) or internetwork packet exchange (IPX). A router accepts packets on at least two network interfaces, and forwards packets from one interface to another.

Server is a computer designed to process requests and deliver data to other computers over a local network or the Internet.

Switch is a computer networking device that connects network segments. The term commonly refers to a network bridge that processes and routes data at the data link layer (Layer 2) of the OSI (open systems interconnection) model. Switches that additionally process data at the network layer (Layer 3 and above) are often referred to as Layer 3 switches or multilayer switches.

T-carrier in telecommunications is the generic designator for any of several digitally multiplexed telecommunications carrier systems. This system, introduced by the Bell System in the US in the 1960s, was the first successful system that supported digitized voice transmission. The basic unit of the T-carrier system is the digital signal 0 (DS0), which has a transmission rate of 64 kbps, and is commonly used for one voice circuit. The original transmission rate (1.544 Mbps) in the T1 line is in common use today in Internet service provider (ISP) connections to the Internet.

Telematics refers to the integrated use of telecommunications and informatics, also known as ICT (information and communications technology).

Tier-1 refers to a network that can reach every other network on the Internet without purchasing IP (Internet protocol) transit service or paying settlement charges. By this definition, a Tier-1 network is a transit-free network. But not all transit-free networks are Tier-1 networks. It is possible to become transit free by paying for peering or agreeing to settlements. Moreover, the term Tier-1 network is used in the industry to mean a network with no overt settlements. An overt settlement would be a monetary charge for the amount, direction, or type of traffic sent between networks. A Tier-2 network is operated by an Internet service provider who engages in the practice of peering with other networks, but who still purchases IP transit service to reach some portion of the Internet. Tier-2 providers are the most common providers on the Internet as it is much easier for a network operator to purchase transit services from a Tier-1 network than it is to peer with it and then to try and justify the Tier-1 status that is implied by the peering. The term Tier-3 is sometimes also used to describe networks that purchase IP transit service from other networks (typically Tier-2 networks) in order to reach the Internet. Most Tier-3 networks are singly- rather than multi-homed and, as a consequence, are vulnerable to peering disputes.

Telecommunication is the assisted transmission of signals over a distance for the purpose of communication. In earlier times, this may have involved the use of smoke signals, drums, semaphore, flags or heliograph. In modern times, telecommunication typically involves the use of electronic devices such as the telephone, television, radio or computer. Early inventors in the field of telecommunication include Alexander Graham Bell, Guglielmo Marconi and John Logie Baird. Telecommunication is an important part of the world economy and the telecommunication industry's revenue was estimated to be $1.2 trillion in 2006.

UbuntuNet Alliance for research and education networking is a non-profit association of African National Research and Education Networks (NRENs). It was founded in the latter half of 2005 by established and emerging NRENs in Kenya, Malawi, Rwanda, Mozambique and South Africa with the goal of securing high bandwidth connections, mainly fiber-based, in gigabits per second instead of the current kilobits per second – at affordable prices, that connect African NRENs to each other, to other NRENs worldwide and to the Internet generally. It was incorporated in 2006 in Amsterdam, the Netherlands, in the Trade Registrar of the Chambers of Commerce and Industry. The Alliance has a close relationship with the Association of African Universities, which appoints the Chairperson. The Chairperson since February 2007 is Zimani Kadzamira.

UNI•C is the Danish IT-Centre for Education and Research.

UNINETT is a Norwegian government-owned company responsible for deploying and maintaining a national research based computer network.

Web (or World Wide Web-WWW) is a set of linked sources of information. The information may be contained in static documents or may be provided by means of applications which deliver material in response to user input requests. Information is normally presented on a client computer by a *Web browser* which is an application able to display information of different forms, for example fixed or animated graphics, text etc. Data are sent across the Internet and this is called *Web traffic*. A *Web site* manages a set of information content structured as *Web pages* which contain formatted text, images, videos or other digital assets. The Web pages on a particular web site are typically inter-related; they are hosted on a *Web server*, a computer that is connected to the Internet. Web servers can run *Web applications* that process stored data provide dynamic information content in response to requests from the client, often made in the form of a selection from a list of options. A search service is one type of Web application. Web browsers, search services and other client applications can request information from Web servers to perform other types of information processing, for example extracting database information used for inventory management. These applications request information through *Web services* which handle requests using standard *Web protocols*. *Web 2.0* is an imprecise term but it has been used to describe a later generation of web applications that have emerged to promote social networking and interaction. Facebook, Blog, Twitter, Flickr and others are examples of Web 2.0.

WHOIS is a term referring to a domain name search or look-up feature, used for querying an official database in order to determine the owner of a domain name.

X.25 is an ITU-T (International Telecommunication Union Telecommunication Standardization Sector) network layer protocol for packet switched wide area network (WAN) communication. It forms part of the suite of open systems interconnection (OSI) protocols and works at the physical (Layer 1), data link (Layer 2), and network layers (Layer 3) of the OSI model. Each X.25 packet contains up to 128 bytes of data. The X.25 network handles packet assembly at the source device, delivery, and then disassembly at the destination. X.25 packet delivery technology includes not only switching and network-layer routing, but also error checking and re-transmission logic to handle any delivery failures that might occur. X.25 supports multiple simultaneous conversations by multiplexing packets and using virtual communication channels.

X.29 is the ITU-T (International Telecommunication Union Telecommunication Standardization Sector) standard specifying procedures for the exchange of control information and user data between a packet assembler–disassembler (PAD), and a remote packet-mode data terminal equipment (DTE) or another PAD. It defines the Level 4 (or session layer in the OSI model) for X.25 communications.

X.400 is a suite of ITU-T (International Telecommunication Union Telecommunication Standardization Sector) recommendations that define standards for data communication networks for message handling systems (MHS) – more commonly known as "e-mail". While X.400 never achieved the universal presence of Internet e-mail, it has seen use within organizations, and as part of proprietary e-mail products such as Microsoft Exchange.

X.500 is a series of computer networking standards for electronic directory services which were developed by ITU-T (International Telecommunication Union Telecommunication Standardization Sector) to support the requirements of X.400 electronic mail exchange and name look-up. The X500 series forms part of the open systems interconnection (OSI) suite of protocols.

X.509 is an ITU-T (International Telecommunication Union Telecommunication Standardization Sector) standard for a public key infrastructure (PKI) for single sign-on (SSO) and privilege management infrastructure (PMI). X.509 specifies, amongst other things, standard formats for public key certificates, certificate revocation lists, attribute certificates, and a certification path validation algorithm.

Appendix F: List of Units

The **Czech crown** or **koruna** is the official currency of the Czech Republic (currency sign: Kč, currency code: CZK). 1 crown consists of 100 hellers (haléř), abbreviated as hal. Heller coins have not been in use as of September 1 2008, but hellers are still incorporated into merchandise prices. The final price is always rounded off to the nearest crown value.

The US **dollar** (currency sign: $; currency code: USD) is the unit of currency of the US and is defined by the Coinage Act of 1792 to be between 371 and 416 grains (27.0 g) of silver (depending on purity). It is divided into 100 cents (200 half-cents prior to 1857).

The **pound** or **pound sterling** (currency sign: £; currency code: GBP) is the currency of the United Kingdom, its Crown dependencies (the Isle of Man and the Channel Islands) and the British Overseas Territories of South Georgia and the South Sandwich Islands and British Antarctic Territory. It is subdivided into 100 pence (singular: penny).

The **euro** (currency sign: €; currency code: EUR) is the official currency of 16 out of 27 member states of the European Union (Austria, Belgium, Cyprus, Finland, France, Germany, Greece, Ireland, Italy, Luxembourg, Malta, the Netherlands, Portugal, Slovakia, Slovenia, and Spain). The name euro was officially adopted on 16 December 1995. The euro was introduced to world financial markets as an accounting currency on 1 January 1999, replacing the former European Currency Unit (ECU) at a ratio of 1: 1. Physical coins and banknotes entered circulation on 1 January 2002.

The term **pico** (symbol p) is a prefix denoting a factor of 10^{-12} in the international system of units (SI). Derived from the Italian *piccolo*, meaning small, this was one of the original 12 prefixes defined in 1960 when the SI was established.

The term **nano** is a prefix (symbol n) in the SI system of units denoting a factor of 10^{-9}. It is frequently encountered in science and electronics for prefixing units of time and length, like 30 nanoseconds (symbol ns), or 100 nanometers (nm). The prefix is derived from the Greek *nanos*, meaning dwarf, and was officially confirmed as standard in 1960.

The term **micro** (symbol μ) is a prefix in the SI and other systems of units denoting a factor of 10^{-6} (one millionth). Confirmed in 1960, the prefix comes from the Greek *mikrós*, meaning small.

The term **milli** (symbol m) is a prefix in the SI and other systems of units denoting a factor of 10^{-3}, or 1/1,000 (one thousandth). Adopted in 1795, the prefix comes from the Latin *mille*, meaning one thousand (the plural is *milia*).

A **bit** is a binary digit (symbol bit or b), taking a value of either 0 or 1. Binary digits are a basic unit of information storage and communication in digital computing and digital information theory. The bit is also a unit of measurement, the information capacity of one binary digit. 8 bits equals one byte.

A **kilobit** is an expression of grouped bits meaning 1000 (10^3) bits. The term kilobit is most commonly used in the expression of data rates (digital communication speeds) in the abbreviated form kbps, meaning kilobits per second.

A **Megabit** is an SI-multiple of the unit of bit for digital information storage or transmission, abbreviated Mbit (or Mb). 1 Megabit $= 10^6$ bits $= 1\,000\,000$ bits. The megabit is most commonly used when referring to data transfer rates of networks or telecommunications systems, for example, a 100 Mbps (megabit per second).

A **Gigabit** is an SI-multiple of the unit of bit for digital information storage, with the symbol Gbit (or Gb). 1 gigabit $= 10^9 = 1\,000\,000\,000$ bits, which are equal to 125 decimal megabytes or 122 binary mebibytes, as 8 bits equal one byte.

A **Terabit** is an SI-multiple of the unit of bit for digital information storage, abbreviated Tbit (or Tb). 1 terabit $= 10^{12}$ bits $= 1\,000\,000\,000\,000$ bits (one trillion, or, using the long scale, one billion). 1 terabit is equal to 125 (decimal) gigabytes or 122 (binary) gibibytes.

A **Petabit** is an SI-multiple of the unit of bit for digital information storage, abbreviated Pbit (or Pb). 1 petabit $= 10^{15}$ bits $= 1\,000\,000\,000\,000\,000$ bits (one quadrillion).

Index of Names

a
Adams, Rick   81
Allocchio, Claudio   43, 261
Alvestrand, Harald   94
Arak, Robin   244
Arvilias, Alexis   50

b
Bakonyi, Peter   54
Bálint, Lajos   261
Barberá, José   50
Bartlett, Keith   27
Beale, John   27
Beertema, Piet   81ff.
Bellovin, Steve   80
Berkhout, Vincent   262
Berners-Lee, Tim   73, 109
Bersee, Josephine   262
Blokzijl, Rob   68, 77
Bos, Erik-Jan   125
Bovenga, Piet   13
Boyles, Heather   186
Bressan, Beatrice   262
Brinkhuijsen, Rob   11, 40
Brown, Maxine   262
Brunell, Mats   13
Bryant, Paul   6, 20
Bulmahn, Edelgard   146

c
Cadiou   32
Carlson, Britta   14, 27, 40
Carpenter, Brian E.   94, 263
Carpentier, Michel   12, 32
Cerf, Vint   107
Chernenko, Konstantin   83
Chiotis, Tryfon   263

Cohen, Avi   20
Collinson, Peter   81
Crowcroft, Jon   94
Csaba, László   20

d
Davies, Dai   43ff., 61, 111, 263
– interview   111ff.
Davies, Howard   50, 61, 143, 264
Deckers, Hans   20
DeFanti, Thomas A.   264
Delcourt, Bernard   43, 57
Delhaye, Jean-Loïc   20
Döbbeling, Hans   61
Dondoux, Jacques   136
Druck, Steve   54

e
Ellis, Jim   80
Eppenberger, Urs   43
Eriksen, Björn   81

f
Fältström, Patrik   94
Fluckiger, François   13, 77, 265
Foster, David   265
Foster, Ian   59, 175
Foster, Jill   43
Fuchs, Ira   15

g
Gagliardi, Fabrizio   265
Gilmore, Brian   13, 54
Goldstein, Steven   183f.
Gorbachev, Mikhail   215
Greisen, Frode   17ff., 42f., 54, 86
Gruntorád, Jan   265

A History of International Research Networking. Edited by Howard Davies and Beatrice Bressan
Copyright © 2010 WILEY-VCH Verlag GmbH & Co. KGaA, Weinheim
ISBN: 978-3-527-32710-2

h

Hagen, Teus 81
Hansen, Alf 13
Harms, Jürgen 40ff.
Hartley, David 135ff., 159, 266
Harvey, Christopher C. 163
Hebgen, M. 18
Hoffmann, Geert 48
Huitema, Christian 94
Huizer, Erik 94, 125
Hünke, Horst 28ff., 68
Hutton, James 6, 40, 57, 266

i

Ippolito, Jean Claude 18
Izhvanov, Yuri 266

j

Jennings, Dennis 17f.

k

Kahn, Bob 107
Kalin, Tomaz 56ff.
Karrenberg, Daniel 68
Kesselman, Carl 59, 175
Kirstein, Peter 107
Kossakowski, Klaus-Peter 267
Kowack, Glenn 84, 267
Kündig, Albert 12f.

l

Le Guigner, Jean-Paul 43
Liello, Fernando 48ff., 141, 202
Linington, Peter 6ff., 40ff., 119, 267
Lord, David 17f.

m

Maass, Klaus-Eckart 43
Maglaris, Vasilis 141, 268
Mahon, Barry 6ff.
Malamud, Carl 88
Martin-Löf, Johan 27
Metakides, Georges 175
Michau, Christian 43, 86
Moi, Arne 27

n

Nederkoorn, Boudewijn 43ff., 118, 268
– interview 118ff.
Neggers, Kees 13, 40ff., 54, 86, 118, 128, 182, 268
– interview 118ff.
Newman, Nicholas 6, 27, 32, 123
Nowlan, Michael 269

o

Oakley, Brian 136
Olesen, Dorte 42, 269

p

Palme, Jacob 7
Parajón-Collada 32
Plattner, Bernhard 54
Pouzin, Louis 107
Prévost, Jacques 13

r

Rastl, Peter 54
Ros, Francisco 14
Rose, Marshall 108
Rosenberg, Hans 11ff., 27

s

Sabatino, Roberto 269
Sanderson 32
Simonsen, Keld Jörn 81
Sommani, Marco 20, 54
Stanton, Michael 269
Stöver, Cathrin 270

t

Tafvelin, Sven 54
Tindemans, Peter 27f., 68, 130, 270
Trumpy, Stefano 18, 42, 270
Truscott, Tom 80

u

Ullmann, Klaus 13, 40ff., 61, 119, 126, 141, 271
– interview 126ff.
Uzé, Jean-Marc 271

v

Valente, Enzo 77
Van Binst, Paul 54
Van Houwelling, Douglas 186
van Iersel, Frank 11, 27
Vandromme, Dany 61
Verrue, Robert 146
Vietsch, Karel 27, 56f., 271
Villemoes, Peter 48, 77, 182ff.

w

West, David 271
Williams, David 42, 59, 127

z

Zimmermann, Hubert 107

Subject Index

a

Abilene   150, 186ff.
ACOnet   93, 189
ACSNET (academic computing services network)   195
ACTS (advanced communications technologies and services) project   137, 297
ADMD (administrative management domain)   173
AI (artificial intelligence)   8
Alliance for the Information Society (@LIS)   204ff.
Alcatel 1678 MCC equipment   245
ALICE (América Latina Interconectada Con Europa) project   204ff., 249
ALICE2   214
AltaVista   121
American StarLight   187
AMPATH (Americas path) project   207, 229
AMS-IX (Amsterdam Internet exchange)   125
APAN (Asia-Pacific advanced network)   150
ARPA (Advanced Research Projects Agency)   4, 183
ARPAnet (Advanced Research Projects Agency network)   2, 15, 107f., 183
AsiaNet   195
ASN.1 (abstract syntax notation one) notation   110
AT&T (American Telephone & Telegraph Company)   79
ATM   127, 136ff.
– STM-1 (synchronous transport module level-1)   149
– VP (virtual path)   140
AUCS (AT&T unisource carrier services)   147
AUP (acceptable use policy)   90
AutoBAHN (automated bandwidth allocation across heterogeneous networks)   245

b

backbone   293
bandwidth   135ff., 293
bandwidth-on-demand (BoD) service   245
basic incident coordination   167
Berkeley UNIX version BSD (Berkeley Software Distribution) 4.2   107
BGP-4 (border gateway protocol, version 4)   92
BITNET   15, 223
– network   180
BITNET/UUCP   206
BMBF (Bundesministerium für Bildung und Forschung)   131
BMFT (Bundesministerium für Forschung und Technologie)   12
browser   293
BSI (Bundesamt für Sicherheit in der Informationstechnik)   166
BT (British Telecommunications)   103ff.

c

CAD (computer-aided design)   8
CAESAR (connecting all European and Southern American researchers) project   207
campus area network (CAN)   298
Canadian research network CA*net   150
CANARIE (Canadian Network for the Advancement of Research, Industry and Education)   58
– network   231
CARNet   147
CBF (cross border fiber)   248
– Type-A service   248
– Type-B service   248
CBR (constant bit rate) services   136

Subject Index

CCIRN (Coordinating Committee for Intercontinental Research Networking) 40
CCITT 171f.
CCTA (Central Computer and Telecommunications Agency) 164
CEE (Central and Eastern Europe)
– network 255
– research network 193
CEEC (Central and Eastern European countries) 96ff., 189ff., 255
CEENet (Central and Eastern European Network Association) 190
CENIC (Corporation for Education Network Initiatives in California) 210
Centernet 6
CENTR (Council of European National Top Level Domains Registries) 125
CEPIS (Council of European Professional Informatics Societies) 160
CEPT (Conference of European Postal and Telecommunication Administration) 10ff.
CERN (Conseil Européen pour la Recherche Nucléaire) 9, 73f., 84ff., 108, 120ff., 140, 175, 188, 229
CERNET (Chinese education and research network) 74, 249
CERT (computer emergency response team) 59, 163
– coordination center (CERT/CC) 164
CERT-IT 166
CESNET (Czech educational and scientific network) 188ff.
CIEMAT (Centro de Investigaciones Energéticas, Medioambientales y Tecnológicas) 213
Cisco Systems 231, 240
CLARA (Cooperación Latino Americana de Redes Avanzadas) 204ff.
– Network Engineering Group (NEG) 208ff.
– NOC 208ff.
CLARA/ALICE 212
CLARA-TEC (CLARA-technical forum) 208ff.
CLNS (connectionless network services) 87
cloud computing 293
CNAM (Conservatoire National des Arts et Métiers) 81ff.
CoA (council of administration) 42
COCOM (coordinating committee for multilateral export controls) 19, 189
colored Book 3
COLT Telecommunications 238
COM (component object model) 7

COMECON (council for mutual economic assistance) 189
COMICS (computer-based message interconnection systems) 75
connection oriented network 108
CORDIS (Community Research and Development Information Service) 147
COSINE (cooperation for open systems interconnection networking in Europe) 12ff., 27ff., 64ff., 112ff., 127ff., 181ff.
– implementation phase (CIP) 21
– implementation phase execution contract (CIPEC) 22
– IXI service 87
– MHS 173
– Policy Bureau (CPB) 27
– project management unit (CPMU) 28ff.
– sub-project 170ff.
COSINE/OU 89
cost sharing 247f.
COST-11 6
CPG 130, 182
CPMU 28ff., 90
cross border initiative 248
CSIC (Consejo Superior de Investigaciones Científicas) 143
CSIRT (computer security incident response team) 59, 168
CSNET (Computer Science NETwork) 4ff., 19, 183
CSTNET (China science and technology network) 249
CUDI (Corporación Universitaria para el Desarrollo de Internet) network 207ff.
CWDM (coarse wavelength division multiplexing) link 200
CWI (Centrum voor Wiskunde en Informatica) 81
CyNet 202
CzechLight 188, 229

d

D-GIX (distributed GIX) 92
DANTE (Delivery of Advanced Network Technology to Europe) 24, 30, 39, 51ff., 91ff., 104, 111ff., 126ff., 136ff., 180ff., 207, 223ff.
– gestation 41ff.
– Shareholders Agreement 44
DANTE/TERENA task force 151
dark fiber 294
dark fiber cloud 244
DARPA (Defence Advanced Research Projects Agency) 163, 183, 223

Data TransAtlantic Grid   228
DataTAGlink   230
DEC (Digital Equipment Corporation)   8, 77
DEC VAX™ machine   74
DECnet   19, 74ff., 107, 128, 172
DESY (Deutsches Elektronen Synchrotron)   73f.
DFN (Deutsches Forschungsnetz)   1, 46, 126ff., 143
DFN-CERT   164
DG I   190
DG III (ESPRIT/Information Technologies)   137
DG XIII   190
DG XIIIB (ACTS - Advanced Communications Technologies and Services/ Communications Technologies)   137
DG XIIIC (Telematics)   137
DICE (DANTE-Internet2-CANARIE-ESnet)   249
DIKU (Datalogisk Institut Københavns Universitet)   81
DNS (domain name system)   20
DoE (Department of Energy)   40
DT (Deutsche Telekom)   232, 238
dual-stack   294
Dutch NetherLight   187
DWDM (dense wavelength division multiplexing)   112
– lambdas   212
DYNACORE (dynamically configurable remote experiment monitoring & control)   149

e

E-carrier   294
e-VLBI (electronic transfer very-long-baseline interferometry service)   122
E2E paradigm   157
E2E QoS   232
E2E (end-to-end) transit   95
E2ECU (end-to-end coordination unit)   247
EARN (European academic and research network)   8ff., 17ff., 39, 52ff., 84, 119ff., 128, 180ff., 223
– constitution   17
EARN/BITNET   171, 189
– mail   174
EASInet (European academic supercomputing initiative network)   84
Ebone (European backbone)   60, 86, 100, 126ff., 179ff.
– action team (EAT)   87
– boundary systems (EBS)   87
– Consortium of Contributing Organizations (ECCO)   87
– operations team (EOT)   87
Ebone92   88ff.
– initial configuration   89
– kernel   87
Ebone93   91
– configuration   91
EC (European Commission)   31
ECFA (European Committee for Future Accelerators)   6, 73
– sub-group 5   73ff.
ECFRN (European Consultative Forum on Research Networking)   29f.
– SteeringGroup   36
ECRC (European Computer-Industry Research Centre)   93
EdCAAD (Edinburgh computer-aided architectural design)   83
EDFA (erbium-doped fiber amplifier)   296
EDISON (European distributed and interactive simulation over network)   149
EELA (E-science grid facility for Europe and Latin America)   213
EELA-2   214
EEPG (European Engineering and Planning Group)   41, 86
EGEE (enabling grids for e-science)   59
EMPB (European multi-protocol backbone)   60, 91ff., 128, 223
– network   22
– network topology   98
– topology   97
EMPP (European 2 Mbps multi-protocol pilot)   90
ENA (meaning Ecole Nationale d'Administration)   11
ENCART (European Network for Cyberart)   149
ENPG (European Networking Policy Group)   36
equipment supplier
– relation   152
ERNET   196
ESA (European Space Agency)   29ff.
– Space Physics Analysis Network (SPAN)   163
ESF (European Science Foundation)   6
ESMTP (extended simple mail transfer protocol)   174
ESnet (Energy Sciences network)   40, 131, 231
– transit   150
ESPRIT (European Strategic Programme for Research in Information Technology)   5, 31, 175

Subject Index

ETH (Eidgenössische Technische Hochschule) 12
Ethernet 109, 294
– private lines (EPL) 245
– service 245
– VLANs 245
EU-DataGrid 175
EUChinaGrid 176
EUIndiaGrid 176
EUMEDCONNECT 203, 249
– configuration 205
– network 204
EUMEDCONNECT2 204
EUMedGrid 176
EUMEDIS (Euro-Mediterranean initiative for the Information Society) 203
EUnet (European UNIX network) 29, 78ff.
EUREKA (European Research Coordination Agency) 12, 27ff., 127
– project 123
Euro-Link 228
EuroCAIRN (European cooperation for academic and industrial research networking) 36, 101, 135
EuroCERT 168
EUROnet (European network) 7
EuropaNET (European multi-protocol backbone network) 21, 101f., 112ff., 128, 185
– configuration 105
– IP service 106
European achievement 235ff.
EurOpen 85
Euroscience 295
EUUG (European UNIX Users Group) 80ff.
EXPReS (express production real-time e-VLBI) project 122, 213
external connectivity 150
external support 189

f

FAPESP (Fundação de Amparo à Pesquisa do Estado de São Paulo) 210
FIRST (forum of incident response and security teams) 163ff.
FIU (Florida International University) 207ff.
forwarding and transport layer 156
FREEnet (network for research, education and engineering) 215ff.
FTAM (file transfer and access management) 28
FUDI (France – FR, United Kingdom – UK, Germany – DE, and Italy – IT) countries 139
FUDI PNO 140
FUDI/Unisource (core) configuration 140
full incident coordination 167
Fundação CPqD (Centro de Pesquisa e Desenvolvimento em Telecomunicações) 212
FUNET (Finnish university network) 7

g

G-REUNA (Gigabit-Red Universitaria National) project 211
GARR (Gruppo Armonizzazione Reti della Ricerca) 77, 189, 202
gateway 172, 295
Gbps circuits 235, 245
GÉANT (gigabit European academic network technology) service 26, 31, 112ff., 128ff., 151, 180ff., 193ff., 207, 235ff.
– configuration 241
GÉANT+ 247f.
GÉANT2 231, 242
– complex procurement 243
– configuration 246
– exchange 231
– gestation period 242
– Joint Research Activity (JRA) 243
– network 58ff., 113ff., 128ff., 188, 200
– networking activity 243
– NOC 247
– service activity (SA) 243
GÉANT3 130
GIGA (gigabits networking research) 212
GIX (global Internet exchange) 92
GLIF (global lambda integrated facility) 125f., 187f., 229ff.
– open lightpath exchange (GOLE) 229
global connectivity 249ff.
GlobalTeleSystemsGroup, Inc. (GTS) 93
GLORIAD (global ring network for advanced applications development) project 197, 217, 231
GMD (Gesellschaft für Mathematik und Datenverarbeitung) 91
GOPHER 121, 295
GOSIP profile 107
Green Report 43
grid 175, 231, 295
– community 59
GRIP (guidelines and recommendations for incident processing) 169
GRNET (Greek research and technology network) 143, 199f.

h

HD (high definition) distribution   197
HEAnet (Higher Education Authority network)   7, 47, 146
HEP (high energy physics)   5
– community   175
HEPnet (high-energy physics network)   22, 73ff.
– planned configuration   75
HKOEP (Hong Kong open exchange portal)   229
home area network (HAN)   298
host   295
HPIIS (high performance international Internet services)   184
– program   227
HTML (hypertext markup language)   295
HTML/HTTP   173
HTTP (hypertext transfer protocol)   295
hub   296
HUNGARNET (Hungarian academic and research networking association)   193ff.
hypertext   296

i

IBDNS (international backbone data network service)   103ff.
IBERPAC (servicio IBERico de conmutacion por PACkets)   8
ICEAGE (international collaboration to extend and advance grid education)   176
ICM program   184
ICT task   189
IDWG (Intrusion Detection Working Group)   169
IEEAF (Internet Educational Equal Access Foundation)   228
IEEE (Institute of Electrical and Electronics Engineers)   294
IETF (Internet Engineering Task Force)   41, 173, 255ff.
IETF WG X.400-operations   173
ILAN   201f.
IN2P3 (Institut National de Physique Nucléaire et de Physique des Particules)   249
incident response team support   167
INCS   106
INFN (Istituto Nazionale di Fisica Nucleare)   8, 143, 189
INFNet (INFN network)   171
INNOVA|RED   212
INRIA (Institut National de Recherche en Informatique et Automatique)   223
interconnection of national hosts   137
intercontinental connectivity   150
international hybrid network   242
Internet   258, 296
internet background noise   165
Internet2   130, 184ff., 296
– network   231
internetwork packet exchange (IPX)   298
interoperability   158
IP (Internet protocol)   22, 179ff.
– multicast   245
– network   142
– QoS   245
– service   245
IPsphere Forum (IPSF)   157
IPv4   240
IPv6   186
– network   197, 240
IRIS (interconexión de los recursos informáticoS)   8
IRNC (international research network connections) program   230
ISDN (integrated services digital network)   71
ISO   255
ISO FTAM   74
ISO/ITU discussion   108
ISO-OSI protocols   120
ISP (Internet service provider)   69, 133, 223ff.
IST (Information Society Technologies)   12
– project   214
ITN (international transit network) service   150
ITU (International Telecommunication Union)   255ff.
ITU-T (ITU-telecommunication standardization sector)   294
IUCC   228
IXI (International X.25 infrastructure)   21, 65, 126ff., 182
IXI (international X.25 interconnect) network   120
IXI/EMPB network   99

j

JAMES (joint ATM experiment on European services)   138f.
JANET (joint academic network)   5, 95, 159, 185, 195, 229
– coloured book protocol   74
– operations team   6
JANET-CERT   166
JANET-SINET link   195
JINR (Joint Institute of Nuclear Research)   218
JISC (Joint Information Systems Committee)   229

Subject Index

JIVE (Joint Institute for Very-long-baseline Interferometry in Europe) 122
JNT (joint network team) 6
JUNET (JapanUNIXnetwork) 195

k

KISDI (Korea Information Society Development Institute) 196
KOREN (Korea advanced research network) 196
KPN (Koninklijke PTT Nederland) 22
KPN/Qwest 85ff., 128, 239, 152
KRLight 229
KTH (Kungliga Tekniska Högskolan) 81

l

L3 link 224
lambda 188, 296
lambda grids 187
lambda networking 187, 229
LambdaGrid fabric 231
LAN (local area networks) 294
– technology 155
largescale international IPv6 pilot network (6NET Project) 186, 240
– consortium 197
LDAP (lightweight directory access protocol) 110
leased line connection 195
LEP (large electron positron collider) 73
LHC (Large Hadron Collider) 106, 175
– network 122ff.
– OPN (optical private network) 125
lightpath 297
LISTSERV 121
LSP (label switched paths) 245

m

MAC (media access control) 294
mailer 297
MAN (metropolitan area networks) 155, 298
MAN LAN (MANhattan LANding) 229ff.
management and policy and control layer 156
MBGP (multicast border gateway protocol) 151
MBONE (multicast backbone) 219
MBS (managed bandwidth service) 144
MCC (Metro Core Connect) 245
MDNS (managed data network service) 21
MECCANO (multimedia education and conferencing collaboration over ATM network and others) project 146
MEDA (Mediterranean economic development area) program 203

MHS (message handling service) 40
migration 245
MIME (multipurpose Internet mail extensions) 173
mosaic 297
MoscowLight 229
MPBS (multi-protocol backbone service) 86ff.
MSDP (multicast source discovery protocol) 151
MSUNet (Moscow State University Network) 218
MTA (message transfer agent) 173
multicast 297

n

NACSIS (National Centre for Science Information Systems) 150
NASA (National Aeronautics and Space Administration) 40, 131
national host 137, 297
national infrastructure 191
NATO (North Atlantic Treaty Organization) 190
NCP (network control programme) 4
NetherLight 229ff.
network development 197
Network News software 80
networkshop resolution 10
NEUCC (Northern Europe University Computing Centre) 6
NGI (next generation Internet) 184
NGIX-East (Next Generation Internet Exchange-East) 229
NICE (national host interconnection experiments) 138
NIKHEF (Nationaal Instituut voor Kernfysica en Hoge Energie Fysica) 39
NIST (National Institute of Science and Technology) 4
NJE 52
NLR (National LambdaRail) network 231
NLUUG (NL UNIX Users Group) 80
NMC (Network Management Committee) 47
NOC (network operation centre) 141
NorduGrid 186
NORDUnet (Nordic university network) 14, 47, 84ff., 164, 179ff., 223ff.
NORDUnet2 program 186
NORDUnet3 186
NorthernLight 229
NREN (National research and education networks) 299

Subject Index | 313

– service   120ff., 132
NSF (National Science Foundation)   4, 183, 224ff.
NSF HPIIS program   230
NSF IRNC program   230f.
NSFnet (National Science Foundation network)   4, 84, 183, 195
NTT (Nippon Telegraph and Telephone)   197

o

OC-3 (optical carrier level 3)   150
off-fiber research networks   247
OMII (Open Middleware Infrastructure Institute)   176
on-fiber research networks   247
ONP (open network provision)   138
OPN (optical private network)   125
organized cooperation   39ff.
OSI (open systems interconnection)   3, 107ff., 128, 172, 181
– implementations   172
– model   298
– networking model   294
– reference model   298
OSI protocols   119, 133f.
OTE (Hellenic Telecommunication Organization)   123, 298
OTEGlobe   200
OU   42ff., 87
– acceptable use policy (AUP)   90
– management and staff   50f.
OUSC (operational unit steering committee)   44ff., 90

p

Pacific Wave   229
packet   298
PAD (packet assembler-disassembler)   9
Pan-European connectivity
– CEEC   192
partnership period   228
PASCAL   298
PCR (peak cell rate)   196
PDH (plesiochronous digital hierarchy)   294
PEM (privacy enhanced mail)-enabled email client   164
PGP (pretty good privacy)   164
PHARE (Poland and Hungary: assistance for restructuring their economies) program   96ff., 190f.
PIM-SM (protocol independent multicast-sparse-mode)   151
PMDF (PASCAL-based memo distribution facility) e-mail package   195

PNO (Public Network Operator)   24, 96ff., 135ff., 160
PNWGP (Pacific NorthWest gigabit point of presence)   231
point of presence (PoP)   70, 144
– housing   153
POL-34   146
porting   79
POS (packet over SONET)   149
Premium IP service   240
protocol war   106ff.
PSNC (Poznań Supercomputing and Networking Center)   213
PSPDN (packet-switched public data network)   24
PTO (public telecoms operators)   24
PTT (post, telephone, and telegraph operating entities)   2ff.
PTT Telecom   95
PVC (permanent virtual circuit)   136

q

Q-MED   146, 202
QoS (quality of service)   137ff.
QUANTUM   143ff., 193ff., 236
– test program (QTP)   151f.
Qwest   85

r

RAG (requirements action group)   235
RARE (Réseaux Associés pour la Recherche Européenne)   11, 27ff., 52ff., 95, 109, 181ff.
– activities   39
– CERT Task Force   165
– constitution   16
– MHS experimental project   172f.
– OU   87f.
– Security Working Group   164
– WG   172ff.
RAS (Russian Academy of Sciences)   215
RASNet (Russian Academy of Sciences Network)   218
RBNet (Russian backbone network)   217ff.
RBNet PoPs   217
RBS (regional boundary systems)   87
RCCN (Rede da Comunidade Científica Nacional)   146
RCnet   149
RDIG (Russian data intensive grid)   219
REACCIUN (Red Académica de Centros de Investigación y Universidades Nacionales)   207
RECAU (det Regionale Edb-center ved Århus Universitet)   6

Subject Index

RECKU (det Regionale Edb-center ved Københavns Universitet)   7
RedCLARA   204ff.
– network   207ff.
– PoP   208
– topology map   209
RedIRIS (Red de Interconexión de Recursos Informáticos)   143ff.
regional identity   165
RELARN-IP (Russian electronic academic and research network-IP)   218
Relcom (Reliable Communications)   216
RENATER (Réseau National de Télécommunications pour la Technologie, l'Enseignement et la Recherche)   48, 93, 143, 166, 196, 228
research and development (R&D)   152ff.
research and education (R&E)   152ff.
– networks   154
research networking
– impact   250ff.
RESTENA (Réseau Téléinformatique de l'Education Nationale et de la Recherche)   46
RETINA (Red Teleinformática Académica)   207
REUNA (Red Universitaria National)   207
RFC 1405   175
RIPE (Réseaux IP Européens)   39, 68f.
– IRT object   169f.
– NCC (network coordination centre)   42, 68f.
RIPN (Russian Institute of Public Networks)   217
RIR (Regional Internet Registry)   69
RISC (reduced instruction set computer)   109
RN1   235
RN2   235
RNP (Rede National de ensino e Pesquisa)   207ff.
ROC (Russian Operation Centre)   219
RoEduNet   200
roll-out   245
router   298
RSCS   74
RSCS/NJE protocol suite   119
RSSI (Russian space science Internet) project   216
RSSI NOC   216
RTP (real time protocol) video conferencing   219
RUHEP/Radio-MSU (Russian HEP/ Radio-Moscow State University)   216
RUNNet (Russian university network)   216ff.

S
SARA (Stichting Academisch Rekencentrum Amsterdam)   223
SCR (sustained cell rate)   196
SDH (synchronous digital hierarchy) network   127
SDN (system development network)   195
security   163
SEEREN (South-East European research and education networking)   199f.
– configuration   201
SEEREN2   200
seismo   84
– server   81
SERC (Science and Engineering Research Council)   6
SERENATE (Study into European Research and Education Networking As Targeted by eEurope)   58
server   298
service and business layer   156
SGML (standardised generic markup language)   110
SHARE Europe   159
SIIT&T (State Institute of Information Technologies and Telecommunications) Informika   217
SINET (science information network)   195, 249
SINTEF (Selskapet for INdustriell og TEknisk Forskning ved Norges Tekniske Hoegskole)   40
SMTP (simple mail transfer protocol)   174
SNA (systems network architecture)   77, 128, 172
SNA/OSI   107
SNMP (Simple network management protocol) data definitions   110
SOA (service oriented architecture)   157
SOAR (Southern astrophysical research) telescope   213
SoftEng (software engineering)   8
solicitation   227
SONET (synchronous optical network)   149
SouthernLight   229
SPAN (space physics analysis network)   163
StarLight   187f., 219, 231
STARTAP (science, technology, and research transit access point)   150, 184, 219
STM-1   200
STM-4   217
STM-16   217
STM-64   217
SUNET (Swedish university network)   8

Subject Index

SURFnet 87ff., 118ff., 132, 185, 228ff.
– CERT 165
– B.V. (Besloten Vennootschap) 132
SUSIE 149
SVC (switched virtual connection) 136
SWITCH 48, 143, 298
– CERT 166
Switched Point-to-Point (p2p) Connection 245

t

T-carrier 298
T-LEX (Tokyo Lambda Exchange) 229
TaiwanLight 229
TCP (transmission control protocol) 108
TCP/IP 4, 35, 40, 107ff., 121ff., 133f., 172f., 181, 224
TDM (time-division multiplexing) 86
– equipment 224
TEIN 196f.
TEIN2 249
– configuration 198
TEIN3 249
Telebit (Denmark) 143
Telecom Operators 152
telecommunication 299
Telemanagement forum (TMF) 157
Telematics 299
TEN-34 (trans-European network at 34 Mbps) 36, 77, 106, 113, 128, 135ff., 185, 193
– management committee 159
– topology 142
TEN-155 (trans-European network at 155 Mbps) 113f., 128f., 142ff., 185, 193f., 235ff.
– configuration 145
TEN-34/155 202
TERENA (Trans-European Research and Education Networking Association) 28ff., 39, 53ff., 117ff., 128, 165ff., 182ff.
– technical task forces 211
– CERTs in Europe task force 166
Tier-1 299
– network 129
Tier-2 299
– center 129
Tier-3 299
– center 129
TIFR (Tata Institute of Fundamental Research) 196
TF-OU (task force operational unit) 43
TF-TANT (task force testing of advanced networking technologies) 151
trans-eurasia information network 196

transatlantic connection 221ff.
transatlantic link 224
TransLight/Pacific Wave 231
TransLight/StarLight 230
TransPac2 231
TRIXI 89
Trusted Introducer service 169

u

UBN (unisource business networks) 102
UbuntuNet Alliance 299
UDP (user datagram protocol) 108
UERJ (Universidade do Estado do Rio de Janeiro) 213
UIC (University of Illinois at Chicago) 227ff.
UKERNA (United Kingdom Education and Research Networking Association) 135ff., 159, 188
UKLight 188, 229
UKUUG (UK UNIX Users Group) 80
UMOS (South Moscow backbone network) 218
UNI·C 299
UNICOM-B (universal integrated communication-Bulgaria) 199
UNINETT 8, 299
United Kingdom Coloured Books 172
UNIX (UNICS, uniplexed information and computing system) 4, 16, 180
UNIX operating system 79
UNIX to UNIX copy protocol (UUCP) 79, 194
USENET 81
USENIX 80
UUCP 206
UUCPnet (UNIX to UNIX copy protocol network) 80, 223
UUG (UNIX Users Group) 80

v

VAX/VMS (virtual address extension/virtual memory system) 77, 125
vBNS (very high speed backbone network service) 150, 227
VBR (variable bit rate) services 136
virtual circuit network 108
VLANs (Virtual LANs) 245
VM (virtual machine) 16
VMS (virtual memory system) 16
VPN (virtual private networks) 129
VRVS (virtual room videoconferencing system) 219
VusTelecomCentre (Universities Telecommunication Centre) 216

W

WAIS (wide area information server)   121
WAN (wide area networks)   297
WCW (Wetenschappelijk Centrum Watergraafsmeer)   39
WDM (wavelength division multiplexing)   296
web   300
– application   300
– browser   300
– page   300
– protocol   300
– server   300
– traffic   300
welcome guest period   221
WG1   172f.
WHOIS   300
WHREN (Western hemisphere research and education networks)   231
WHREN/LILA (links interconnecting Latin America)   210
WIDE (widely integrated distributed environment) project   197
WIN (Wissenschaftsnetz)   95
WorldCom   252
WWW (World Wide Web)   84, 176, 296

X

X.25   2ff., 111ff., 182, 300
X.29   300
X.400   173, 300
– e-mail address   172
X.500   301
– set of OSI protocols   164
X.509   301
X.EARN project   180
Xbox   124
XML (extensible markup language)   110

Picture Credits

Figure 1.5(a): Rob Greer Photographer
Figure 3.1: Jan van der Woning, Audio Visual Design & Fotographie
Figure 3.2(c): Maaike Neggers
Figure 3.7(a): Michael Manni Photographic
Figure 3.7(b): Michael Manni Photographic
Figure 3.9(a): Chris van Houts Fotografie
Figure 4.2(a): Jeroen Strack/SURFnet
Figure 4.2(b): GTS
Figure 4.5(a): Rob Greer Photographer
Figure 4.5(e): Lars Marelius

Though the editors have undertaken every effort, unfortunately not all of the photographers of pictures printed in this book could be identified.